MEDICAL ASSESSMENT OF FITNESS TO DIVE

BIOMEDICAL SEMINARS

MEDICAL ASSESSMENT OF FITNESS TO DIVE

**Proceedings of an International Conference at the
Edinburgh Conference Centre
8th - 11th March 1994**

Edited by
David H. Elliott, O.B.E.

Published by
Biomedical Seminars

Published by

BIOMEDICAL SEMINARS
*7 Lyncroft Gardens,
Ewell,
Surrey KT17 1UR, England
Fax. 44 (0)181 786 7036*

Copyright D.H. Elliott on behalf of individual contributors, 1995

*Printed and bound by BIDDLES LIMITED
in Guildford and King's Lynn, England*

*Distributed in North America by
BEST PUBLISHING COMPANY
P.O. Box 30100, Flagstaff, AZ, U.S.A. 86003-0100
Tel. 1 (602) 527 1055*

All rights reserved; no part of this publication may be reproduced, stored in a retrieval system, or transmitted in any form or by any means, electronic, mechanical, photocopying, recording, or otherwise without the prior written permission of the Publisher, Biomedical Seminars.

First published 1995

ISBN: 0-9525162-0-9

PREFACE

The assessment of medical fitness for an individual intending to dive, whether for work or recreation, is rarely easy. The available guidance from authorities such as the navy, sports diving agencies and government bodies contain a number of pass/fail criteria and recommendations. These may provide useful advice for some but for many individuals the deciding factors are not obvious and a decision will depend on the training, experience and judgement of the examining doctor.

Historically, the navies of the world were the first to lay down medical standards for their divers. Many of these are based on what are predominantly theoretical considerations. A navy can afford to select only "perfect specimens" for training and later also to remove from diving those who acquire some medical or other condition which might impair their underwater safety or effectiveness. In achieving a good record in the avoidance of medical complications during diving, the navies have set standards which may have been unnecessarily high. Probably they also eliminated many who could have dived in safety. In contrast, recreational divers, who can choose when and where to dive, have not been subject to strict regulation and some, by insisting on their rights of personal freedom, have demonstrated that, in some circumstances at least, safe diving is compatible with medical conditions which would certainly exclude them from military diving.

Between these extremes of regulation and liberality are the non-military working divers. Their fitness is assessed against published standards which were based upon those used for naval divers and which, since then, have developed much further. In the United Kingdom, the Health and Safety Executive (HSE) issued guidance on the medical examination of divers which has been used successfully for many years and similar standards now exist in many other countries.

This volume contains the proceedings of a 4-day conference which was held at Heriot-Watt University, Edinburgh, 8-11 March 1994. The meeting was planned as a workshop aiming towards consensus on the assessment of fitness that is essential for the health and safety of the diver. Each medical condition which could affect in-water safety can affect any category of diver and experience from recreational divers proved to be the foundation of much of the discussion although the emphasis in Edinburgh was upon the working diver. The category of working diver refers to all those who dive for reward. Professional instructors of amateur divers, recreational dive guides, diving scientists, fish farmers, police divers, inland, coastal and offshore divers are among those included. The medical fitness of compressed air workers, such as tunnellers, was not specifically addressed at this meeting but consideration was given to those who never dive in the water but who, for instance as medical attendants, enter raised environmental pressure in dry compression chambers.

The structure of the clinical sessions was based upon the wording of the U.K. Health & Safety Executive's guidance "MA1. The medical examination of divers" and the relevant extracts are reproduced in the text. Each section, together with a number of prepared questions, was reviewed first by an appropriate consultant and then was opened to discussion by the attendees. More than 200 persons from some 20 nations were present, the majority of them being diving medical examiners.

Some conclusions and recommendations arose from this conference and also from a meeting of the European Diving Technology Committee which was held in Luxembourg one month later under the sponsorship of the European Union. This meeting was dedicated to a much broader objective, the Harmonisation of Diving Standards in Europe. Concurrent sessions were held on:

- Diver training and competencies
- Design and certification of equipment
- Operational safety, and
- Medical standards of fitness

The workshop organised by the European Diving Technology Committee was attended by a number of the speakers and delegates from the Edinburgh meeting but importantly there was a similar number of newcomers. The Luxembourg meeting, for which no detailed proceedings are to be published, largely confirmed and consolidated what had gone before, but it also took a number of the considerations further forward. For this reason an additional feature of this volume is the inclusion of several editorial commentaries and a Conclusion in an attempt to summarise the outcome of the two related meetings. These conclusions and recommendations should, however, be regarded as no more than a personal view and interpretation by the Editor. They are intended to reflect the consensus view of a large international group of experienced diving doctors but they must not be construed as representing the views of the sponsors or of individual participants. Nevertheless they are views that need to be considered by any doctor who tells someone whether or not they are fit to dive.

David H. Elliott
January 1995

ACKNOWLEDGEMENTS

To plan an international conference, but to have no guarantee of funding at the date of the deadline for booking the venue, seems unwise and then to promise to publish its proceedings from the verbatim recordings made at the time seems, from past experience, even more rash. But it worked, and it worked primarily because of the enthusiasm and practical contributions of all who took part. It is therefore a pleasure to acknowledge all who made it possible, especially those who came to the Edinburgh Conference Centre to participate in the wide-ranging discussions or to just listen.

In particular all the help given by many persons in the U.K. Health & Safety Executive is acknowledged with gratitude. Within weeks of the initial proposal the HSE had promised funding support for this workshop and provided a wealth of questions for the workshop to address. The HSE then provided the Keynote Speaker and other speakers for the sessions. The pharmaceutical company, ASTRA, are to be thanked for their supplementary funding specifically of the pulmonary session. The HSE funding was sufficient to support attendance by invited clinical consultants whose task it was to advise on standards in appropriate specialities and to curb some of the clinical speculations of the diving doctors.

The experience of the world of recreational diving is invaluable and, in particular, Dr. Alessandro Marroni, on behalf of DAN-Europe, is to be thanked for arranging contributions from each of the principal European sports diving authorities.

There were many helpful contributions in Edinburgh from members of the European Diving Technology Committee. This group met in Luxembourg a few weeks later and the summary notes and conclusions published within these Edinburgh proceedings draw heavily on the debate which continued at the EDTC meeting.

Dr. Nick McIver and Dr. Eric Botheroyd shared with Professor David Elliott the responsibilities of the Programme Committee. With Dr. Harry Rycroft, Dr. McIver also secured for the general practitioners at the meeting approval for Post Graduate Education Allowance. Dr. McIver appreciates the help given to his first contribution by an international group of colleagues. Indeed all the speakers are thanked for giving up their time to prepare their presentations and later to review their transcripts. The work involved is appreciated.

Matthew Curtis designed the cover: he was given many ideas but used his own.

The final and perhaps the largest debt of thanks is to Karen Reeves who, behind the scenes and largely unpaid, quietly did all the administration for this meeting. She has since listened to all the tapes, parts of them for many times, to produce these proceedings.

This was a team effort.

CONTENTS

PREFACE	v
ACKNOWLEDGEMENTS	vii
CONTENTS	ix
LIST OF CONTRIBUTORS	xiii
KEYNOTE ADDRESS R. Mavin - Chief Inspector of Diving, Health & Safety Executive	1
THE BASIS FOR MEDICAL EXAMINATION OF THE DIVER Chairman : D.H. Elliott	3

D.H. Elliott:	*Chairman's Introduction*	3
W. Maas:	*Why have fitness examinations?*	5
B. Minsaas:	*What is the relevance of an in-date fitness examination to the individual's in-water safety?*	7
R.I. McCallum:	*What is the relevance of an in-date fitness examination to the long-term health of the diver?*	9
S.J. Watt:	*What is the effect of ageing upon the diver?* Discussion	12
R. Ramaswami:	*Who should be examined? Should the standards be the same for all categories?*	16
N.K.I. McIver:	*What regulations exist? Who for, and in which countries?*	18
H. Örnhagen:	*What are the international differences of potential significance?*	24
D.H. Elliott:	*Is harmonisation appropriate? Would international recognition of national standards be sufficient?* Discussion & Commentary	32

RECREATIONAL DIVING Chairmen : A. Marroni and N.K.I. McIver	39

N.K.I. McIver:	*Introduction*	39
A. Marroni:	*Recreational diving safety*	40
R. Cali-Corleo:	*Special medical problems in recreational divers:*	
	- *Diabetes*	44
	- *The diver over the age of 40*	45

Y.G. Mebane:	*Recreational diving medical standards: DAN in the United States*	50
C.J. Edge, J. Douglas & P.J. Bryson	*Recreational diving medical standards: in the United Kingdom*	57
J. Seyer:	*Recreational diving legislation and medical standards in France*	62
W. Welslau:	*Recreational diving medical standards in German-speaking Europe*	66
J. Wendling:	*Recreational diving medical standards in Switzerland*	68
F. Wattel:	*The role of the European Committee for Hyperbaric Medicine for the safety of the recreational diver*	69
	Discussion	

CARDIOLOGY AND PHYSICAL FITNESS 75
Chairman : T. Nome

M.R. Cross:	*Cardiovascular problems commonly found in divers*	77
P.T. Wilmshurst:	*Cardiological investigation and assessment*	84
	Discussion	
J. Madsen:	*Exercise tolerance tests for divers*	93
	Discussion	
P.T. Wilmshurst:	*Intracardiac shunts*	98
	Discussion & Commentary	

PULMONARY 109
Chairman : T.J.R. Francis

T.J.R. Francis:	*Pulmonary fitness - an introduction*	111
D. Denison:	*Mechanics of pulmonary barotrauma*	112
S.J. Watt:	*Current criteria of pulmonary fitness to dive*	114
	Discussion	
P.J. Benton:	*Vitalography as a predictor for pulmonary barotrauma*	118
D. Denison:	*Lung function testing of divers*	123
J.W. Reed:	*Lung function changes associated with diving*	134
E. Thorsen:	*Changes in pulmonary function: Norwegian experience*	139
	Discussion	

E.N.T., VISION AND ENDOCRINOLOGY 155
Chairman : H. Örnhagen

W.D. McNicoll:	*Otorhinolaryngology*	156
P.J. Benton:	*Are divers deaf?*	159
	Discussion & Commentary	

CONTENTS (cont'd)

M.R. Cross:	*Vision*	168
	Discussion	
J. Seckl:	*Endocrine Disorders*	172
	Discussion	

MUSCULO-SKELETAL AND HAEMATOLOGY 177
Chairman : I.M. Calder

E. Macdonald:	*Musculo-skeletal*	179
	Discussion	
R.I. McCallum:	*Bone necrosis*	185
	Discussion & Commentary	
J. Risberg:	*Haematology*	190
	Discussion	

GASTRO-INTESTINAL, GENITO-URINARY SYSTEMS AND DERMATOLOGY 197
Chairman : I.M. Calder

N.K.I. McIver:	*Dental, gastro-intestinal & genito-urinary fitness*	199
	Discussion	
R. Aldridge:	*Dermatology*	205
N. Moe:	*Special considerations of "the diver's hand"*	212
	Discussion	

NEUROLOGY AND MENTAL FITNESS 213
Chairman : N.K.I. McIver

B. Lunn:	*Mental fitness to dive*	215
	Discussion	
D.J. Dick:	*Neurological assessment*	224
I.M. Calder:	*Accident investigation and neuropathology*	230
M. Grønning:	*Prospective epidemiological investigation of possible effects of diving on divers' health*	232
	Discussion	

RETURN TO DIVING AFTER UNFITNESS 243
Chairman : T. Nome

D.H. Elliott:	*Return to diving after surgery or accidental injury*	244
S.J. Watt:	*Return to diving after accidental injury*	245
	Discussion	
P.B. James:	*Return to diving after in-water loss of consciousness*	247
	Discussion	
M.R. O'Connell:	*Post-traumatic stress disorder*	250
	Discussion	

CONTENTS (cont'd)

F.W. Smith:	*Imaging techniques*	253
D.J. Dick:	*Evoked potentials*	256
B. Lunn:	*Cognitive function testing following a dive injury*	258
	Discussion	
I.M. Calder:	*Problems in diving pathology*	261
T.J.R. Francis:	*Criteria for return after decompression illness*	262
	Discussion & Commentary	

THE FUTURE HEALTH OF DIVERS 267
Chairman : H. Örnhagen

B. Minsaas:	*Training doctors to examine for fitness of divers*	267
	Discussion	
M. Kromberg:	*Proposal for a diver health service in Norway*	273
	Discussion	
D.H. Elliott:	*The need for specialist centres*	275
	Discussion	
E.M. Botheroyd:	*Appeals*	280
	Discussion	
D.H. Elliott:	*Recording the occupational exposures*	285
	Discussion	
R.I. McCallum:	*Long-term health surveillance: national/central registries for occupational exposure histories*	289
	Discussion & Commentary	

CONCLUSIONS 295
D.H. Elliott

EDINBURGH PARTICIPANTS 301

CONTRIBUTORS

Roger D. Aldridge
    Consultant Dermatologist, Royal Infirmary, Edinburgh, U.K.

Peter J. Benton
    Senior Medical Officer, Undersea Medicine, Institute of Naval Medicine, Gosport, U.K.

Eric M. Botheroyd
    Senior Employment Medical Adviser, Health & Safety Executive, Aberdeen, U.K.

Ian M. Calder
    Wellcome Laboratory for Comparative Neurology, University of Cambridge, U.K.

Ramiro Cali-Corleo
    Hyperbaric and Undersea Physician, Hyperbaric Unit, St. Luke's Hospital, Malta

Maurice R. Cross
    Director, Diving Diseases Research Centre, Fort Bovisand, Plymouth, U.K.

David M. Denison
    Emeritus Professor of Clinical Physiology, Royal Brompton National Heart & Lung Hospital, London, U.K.

Jordi Desola
    CRIS - Unitat de Terapèutica Hiperbàrica, Barcelona, Spain

David J. Dick
    Consultant Neurologist, Norfolk & Norwich Hospital, Norwich, U.K.

Jim Douglas
    Medical Adviser Scottish Sub Aqua Club, Fort William, Invernesshire, U.K.

Chris J. Edge
    Chairman, Medical Committee, British Sub Aqua Club, Ellesmere Port, Cheshire, U.K.

David H. Elliott
    Occupational Health Unit, Robens Institute of Health & Safety, University of Surrey, U.K.

James T.R. Francis
    Head of Undersea Medicine, Institute of Naval Medicine, Gosport, U.K.

Marit Grønning
    Department of Occupational Medicine, Haukeland Hospital, Bergen, Norway

Philip B. James
: Senior Lecturer, Wolfson Hyperbaric Medicine Unit, University of Dundee, U.K.

Marit Kromberg
: Deputy Director General, Norwegian Board of Health, Oslo, Norway

Brian Lunn
: Lecturer in Neuro-Psychiatry, School of Neurosciences, University of Newcastle upon Tyne, U.K.

Walter Maas
: State Supervision of Mines, Rijswijk, The Netherlands

Ewan B. Macdonald
: Senior Lecturer in Occupational Health, Department of Public Health, University of Glasgow, U.K.

Joop Madsen
: Associate Professor in Physiology, Medicinsk Fysiologisk Institut, Copenhagen University, Denmark

Alessandro Marroni
: President, DAN Europe, Roseto Abruzzi, Italy

Ralph Mavin
: Chief Inspector of Diving, Health & Safety Executive, London, U.K.

R. Ian McCallum
: Professor of Occupational Medicine, Institute of Occupational Medicine, Edinburgh, U.K.

Nick K.I. McIver
: Director, North Sea Medical Centre Limited, Great Yarmouth, U.K.

William D. McNicoll
: Consultant Otolaryngologist, King's Mill Hospital, Mansfield, Nottinghamshire, U.K.

Yancey G. Mebane
: Divers Alert Network, Durham NC, U.S.A.

Børge Minsaas
: Deputy Director General, Norwegian Board of Health, Oslo, Norway

Nils Moe
: Anestesi-Service A/S, Haugesund, Norway

Tor Nome
: Medical Director, Phillips Petroleum Co., Norway

Morgan R. O'Connell
: Consultant Psychiatrist, Royal Naval Hospital, Haslar, U.K.

Hans Örnhagen
: Research Director, National Defence Research Establishment, Naval Medicine, Sweden

Ravi A. Ramaswami
　　Employment Medical Adviser, Health & Safety Executive, Aberdeen, U.K.

Jim W. Reed
　　Respiration Laboratory, Department of Physiological Sciences, University of Newcastle, U.K.

Jan Risberg
　　Diving Physician, NUTEC, Bergen, Norway

Jonathan R. Seckl
　　Wellcome Senior Fellow and Honorary Consultant, Molecular Endocrinology Laboratory, Department of Medicine, The University of Edinburgh, U.K.

Jerome Seyer
　　President of the Medical Committee of the FFESSM, University of Rouen, France

Frank W. Smith
　　Consultant in Nuclear Medicine and MRI, MRI Centre, Aberdeen Royal Infirmary, U.K.

Einar Thorsen
　　Diving Research Division, NUTEC, Bergen, Norway

Stephen J. Watt
　　Senior Lecturer, Department of Environmental and Occupational Medicine, University of Aberdeen, U.K.

Francis Wattel
　　Professor of Intensive Care and Hyperbaric Medicine, Calmette Hospital, Lille, France

Wilhelm Welslau
　　Westfälisches Institut für Sauerstoff-Therapie, Hamm, Germany

Jürg Wendling
　　Safety Committee, Swiss Society of Underwater & Hyperbaric Medicine, Biel-Bienne, Switzerland

Peter T. Wilmshurst
　　Consultant Cardiologist, Royal Infirmary, Huddersfield, U.K.

KEYNOTE ADDRESS

R. Mavin : Chief Inspector of Diving, United Kingdom

Ladies and Gentlemen, on behalf of the HSE, the sponsors, it gives me great pleasure to welcome you to this meeting to discuss the fitness standards that are essential for the health and safety of the working diver.

The present Diving Operations at Work Regulations 1981 were entered on the statute books in 1981 - some thirteen years ago. Since then technology has advanced and this has been reflected in the work practices. During this time there has been greater involvement with Europe particularly in the latter years. On the home front there has been a significant move towards deregulation and with a greater emphasis on a more goal-setting approach to new regulations rather than the prescriptive approach.

With reference to the UK Diving Regulations preliminary work has already started on a rewrite of these regulations. It is planned for a consultative document to be with the public in the third quarter of this year. The present plan is for there to be a set of goal-setting regulations common to all forms of diving supported by approved codes of practice for the various diving sub groups e.g. offshore, inshore, scientists etc.

From Europe there is talk of a Directive on diving but there are no firm indications on the timescale. All one can say is that if it does happen we need to be ready for it and be in a position to make firm, positive inputs.

The consolidated outputs resulting from the papers and discussions of this meeting will ensure HSE are well prepared for such a directive should it happen.

Over the last thirteen years the offshore diving industry in particular has made great improvements in the standard of equipment and diving procedures related to their diving operations.

These improvements have been prompted by the feedback from field operations. Shortcomings have been identified over time and the divers, supervisors and managers have made suggestionS for modification of plant and equipment inventories to ensure the improved efficiency and safety of the diving operations. These efforts have ensured the equipment is fit for purpose.

It is obvious that nothing will be achieved without the diver having the appropriate skills and knowledge to follow these improved procedures and to use the equipment safely. The appropriate skill level will be achieved by training which produces safe, competent divers. Since 1981 there has been some evolution on this front but HSE recognise that it is time to look at diver training afresh to ensure the skills provided satisfy the needs of the various client-markets. The present action is to progress the training along the lines of a National Vocational Qualification. Some problems have been identified but the methodology is sound and the project to identify the needs should be starting in the next month or so. This approach will ensure the diver has the appropriate skills to do the jobs required by the clients and is hence fit for purpose.

Which brings me to the subject of this week's meeting - the purpose of which is to review the essential fitness standards required of the diver to ensure that he is fit for purpose. The task is not easy as the result has to be valid for a very wide spectrum of the population working in a variety of environmental conditions and carrying out an infinite number of tasks: the scenarios vary between a one-off shallow familiarisation dive to a 300 m or deeper saturation dive on a physically demanding engineering task. To complicate matters further the diver may also be required to deal with an emergency at any stage during these dives.

Because recent market forces encourage the retention of the experienced and hence older divers rather than risk delays to a project by using younger less experienced men, the average age of the commercial air diver from a recent survey is ageing by some 6 months per year. I have no reason to suppose that this is not the case with the saturation divers who are an older group anyway. Could this ageing population produce safety problems for the divers? Maybe there is a need for a more detailed examination in certain medical areas for divers above a certain age.

My main concern is for the diver. The objective of the meeting makes reference to the "fitness standards that are essential for the health and safety of the working diver" - and I stress the word "essential".

Whatever standards HSE decide upon they will need to be well defined: divers are very good at detecting anomalies in the system which they can use to their advantage. The examination should be relevant to the risks the diver will undertake - the majority are self-employed and they require value for money.

It is essential that the fitness standard is defined in enough detail to ensure consistent implementation - anything else will only bring the system into disrepute.

Of less immediate concern, but still relevant to the fitness of the diver, are the long term health effects of diving. Can we be sure that the health of a diver, who has not been involved in any form of diving accident has not been affected by the years of working in the industry. There is a great deal of experience from the years of carrying out routine divers medicals but the indications are that to look for these more subtle changes in the diver's physiology or psychology requires more specialised techniques. Is there a need for a more specialised medical early in a diver's career to act as a base line for any post incident evaluation at a later date?

As I said earlier, not an easy task, but we have a wealth of experience in this meeting to help provide solutions. The expertise is not just here with the undoubted subject experts but also out there with the approved doctors amongst you. For it is the approved doctors who have much of the practical expertise of dealing with the divers on a day to day basis. Many of the approved doctors see the same diver from year to year. Is this not a source of information which could be used to flag cases which need further investigation? It is from you, the approved doctors, that I on behalf of the divers am expecting an injection of practical realism into the proceedings should it be seen to stray into the more esoteric medical areas. I should add that I do recognise that many of the experts here are also 'hands on' approved doctors.

Finally, can I on behalf of the HSE and you thank the programme committee - Professor David Elliott, Dr. Eric Botheroyd and Dr. Nick McIver, for putting together such an excellent programme.

And to you the delegates once again welcome. I look forward to the presentations and subsequent discussions with interest and in particular, the final outputs which will be used to assist the HSE in formulating their fitness to dive policy.

Thank you Ladies and Gentlemen.

THE BASIS FOR MEDICAL EXAMINATION OF THE DIVER

Chairman : Professor D.H. Elliott

CHAIRMAN'S INTRODUCTION

For the purposes of providing a structured basis for this meeting, the original agenda included a number of sections in italics and these will be found also in these proceedings. Each represents an extract from "The Medical Examination of Divers", a guidance published by the Health & Safety Executive (HSE), or from "Health Notes" which have been issued subsequently.

My contribution at this stage is merely to outline the objectives and structure of the meeting and its published proceedings.

The first question is "why is fitness needed for diving?" There seems to be four reasons. First of all is the personal in-water safety of the diver and then, second but equally important, there is the safety of the other divers who might have to look after him or her. The exacerbation of existing disease is a third reason and this can be related to safety. The fourth is a possibility of long term sequelae and this will also be covered in the scope of this week.

In Norway there has been a tendency in "Health & Safety" to split "Health" from "Safety" and to say that safety is the area that government is rightfully involved with, but that the health of the diver is a matter between the diver and his employer. That is not so in the U.K. Thus this makes an important point for debate but we must remember, particularly with the possibility of Norway and others coming into the European Union, that we need to have similar standards throughout Europe.

In the review of medical standards a secondary objective of this meeting is to look towards the harmonisation of diving medical standards across Europe. We must debate the fitness standards, not only from a UK standpoint but also, for those of you who are Approved Doctors from overseas, we should also relate them to the medical standards for diving in your own country.

At the end of the week, having considered the medical assessment of each of the organ systems, we will review the associated issues : such as training standards, audits, organisation and epidemiology.

So the scope of this meeting is very broad. It is broad in terms of the types of diver, it is broad in terms of organ systems and it is broad in covering not only the basic policy of fitness to dive but also in considering the administration of diver fitness medicals, the documentation of records and epidemiology.

We have much to achieve. The Chairmen will need to be ruthless with the clock which is why we have introduced forms for the submission of written questions and comments that can be supplementary to a busy session. Every person present thus has an opportunity to contribute to the debate. These written questions and comments will be identified in the proceedings by ** after the name of each person making a written submission.

We must keep to time and therefore I am immediately going to ask Dr. Walter Maas to begin.

WHY HAVE FITNESS EXAMINATIONS?
Dr. W. Maas

It is rather ironic that I stand here before you telling you why you should perform a diving medical while, in my own country, the Netherlands, the Minister of Social Affairs in his latest diving regulations has decided that we don't need one. Luckily, he is not my Minister and I can say, on behalf of the State Supervision of Mines which looks after diving in the oil and gas industry, that we differ in opinion on this matter and that we, at least for the diving on oil and gas installations, still and will in the future, ask for a medical.

Why should we perform fitness examinations? Going through the textbooks on diving medicine I noticed that every one of them start with "a medical shall consist of ....", followed by all those things one should do, but no one actually asks why are we doing the medical? The easy way out is to say that the regulations require it, but then you successfully by-pass at least two dilemmas that are part of the question.

First, there is the moral dilemma. Everybody in this room will agree with me that one cannot let a severe asthmatic dive. You will probably also agree with me when I say that no man or woman shall be medically examined against his or her will. Nevertheless, to be able to answer the question of fitness in the case of a diver, those of you who are government-approved doctors (which by the way narrows the diver's constitutional free choice of a doctor to a very select group), must perform the medical examination to get the information, even though the diver does not like it and losing his job may be his penalty when he refuses. In the example of the severe asthmatic, because it is rather obvious, the diver will be a danger not only to himself when he dives, but also to other members of the team if he has to be rescued. He will also create financial loss to the diving company due to non-productive time, or even material loss. In other words, one may have to put the common interest above that of the individual which is something that they didn't teach at medical school!

Second, there is the practical dilemma. What do we mean when we are talking about a medical examination. Ask 20 of your colleagues and you will get 20 different answers, but they will all have in common:

- that, whenever possible, only non-invasive diagnostic techniques should be used;
- that because these techniques have not been initiated because of a specific medical complaint, there is no real focus;
- that the doctor has to take into account several non-medical issues, such as diving hazards and the work of the diving team.

The use of relatively simple diagnostic techniques must lead to a very crude diagnosis by exclusion ("we cannot find anything serious, so he must be fit to dive"). This is on an individual whom we see, at most, only once a year.

To put these points together: how can I, as a government regulator, justify the diver medical examination and, if so, what is the bare minimum I think that the doctor should look at? Diving is not a dangerous profession if you look at the number of dives against the number of accidents. It is, however, a profession with a high risk of serious and possibly permanent damage if something does go wrong. Decompression illness is just one of the hazards involved and it is not always possible to prevent it. Diving accidents are an ever-present hazard and the only thing we can do is try to control the external factors i.e. with "good" decompression tables, procedures and certified equipment. At the same time we must identify and minimise the risk factors involved and, when something does happen, make sure that the diver and all others involved, are in the best possible situation, that they will survive without residual damage. One of the major risk factors is and will always be "man" himself. Therefore if we can make sure that he is in a healthy condition, we do reduce the risk of permanent damage for him and therefore also reduce the hazards for others. Here lies my justification for the medical, it is not only for the protection of the individual against himself, but also for the benefit of all the other members of the team.

A healthy mind in a healthy body, and all our problems are solved. We will skip the mind of the diver and concentrate on the body. Traditionally we look for the absence of serious abnormalities on certain key fields known to our medical profession. To be safe we will, in the near future, be checking everything there is to check and we will do it because we will be afraid to miss even the smallest abnormality. We will become haunted by the thought that even after a very detailed 3-day medical the diver still develops a diving medical problem, meaning we had missed something. This is not what I, as a regulator, have in mind. A good, well-performed medical examination "yes", but not at any price. Where to draw the line on how much must be put into legislation, be it national or European, is a very difficult question to answer. How much and what kind of diagnostic ammunition we are going to use on the poor diver is something we must try to solve in these next 4 days.

WHAT IS THE RELEVANCE OF AN IN-DATE FITNESS EXAMINATION TO THE INDIVIDUAL'S IN-WATER SAFETY?
Dr. B. Minsaas

The title of my lecture is a question which has no answer. This is because nobody has ever subjected the problem to a proper and reproducible scientific study. We simply assume that a diver will be better off being examined at periodical intervals than not being subjected to any medical examination at all. When accepting such a concept : what can be achieved by a periodical medical examination?

The medical conditions which, so far, are quoted as barring divers from diving are often the result of bits and pieces of medical investigations done over many years. They are very rarely the result of hard scientific knowledge like that available for aseptic bone necrosis.

Even with the condition commonly called acute decompression sickness we are confused. The new term "decompression illness" is an admission both of the inadequacy of our overall knowledge as well as our increasing understanding of some detail of what is taking place. To quote the opening lines made by Jim Vorosmarti of the U.S. Navy in my first course on diving medicine in 1980: "I have been asked to talk about decompression sickness. What can I say? In a person who just dived, any medical sign or symptom can be that of decompression sickness: it is just a great mimicker." There is no disagreement that medical symptoms and signs do arise from time to time as a result of a fall in ambient pressure. So, even with the most well-known medical condition of diving, we are surprisingly confused and unknowing.

Modern technology cannot replace such basic confusion in medicine. Regulations cannot solve the problems either. It is basically the problem we are faced with all the time as medical practitioners: how do we made a good qualitative judgement in the absence of hard and absolute facts? We move in a land of shadows where reality hovers at the edge of our knowledge and senses.

What is needed is perhaps a critical look at what good medical practice is all about. The answer is not in governmental regulations: the regulations serve another purpose.

I was first faced with the problem a long time ago when I saw a man who wanted to be a diver and who stated he was healthy. I found his abdomen was criss-crossed with surgical scars. He had had a kidney transplant and was on six different drugs but the surgeons had told him that he was now "as good as new" which, to him, meant he was "healthy". An extreme case, but not uncommon. The term unhealthy or fit is a concept that has no single and clearcut meaning, neither in the population nor in medical society. This is the reality we are facing. What are we to base our judgement on when we accept that it is better to have a periodical medical examination than none at all?

The United Kingdom is going through profound changes in their handling of offshore matters and the term "de-regulation" is employed. This is similar to the Norwegian concept of "functional requirements" in our offshore regulations. The concept behind these regulations is very close to the U.K. concept of the "safety case".

I am often asked for our new regulations in Norway for divers. It must be emphasised that there are regulations for divers: they are those which apply to anybody going offshore. These regulations contain several references to the divers as a population. The basis for these regulations are based on a safety concept: for the diver it would be the in-water safety concept. The purpose of these regulations, dated 12th November 1990, are outlined in their Chapter 1 with the relevant guidelines:

"To ensure that persons engaged in the petroleum activities are medically fit for this from a safety point of view based on whether they may constitute a risk to themselves or others as a result of their condition of health."

Unless the regulation is considered as a whole this does not make a basis for medical practice. Certain concepts can, however, be grasped. The basis for anyone being offshore (including divers) is their safety. There is no referral to their work ability: that is part of the contract between the employer and the employee. The judgement of the fitness of the diver has to be a qualitative judgement, as indicated from the word "may". This is the task of the medical practitioner and we will return to what this means for his training later in this conference.

Section 12 of the regulations elaborates on the reasons for the medical evaluation to be performed and Section 13 lists certain basic medical requirements. These apply to everybody expected to stay on an installation offshore. The diver has first to meet these requirements and then he has to meet the requirements imposed by the fact that he is entering an extreme hostile environment imposing particular hazards to the health. What is the risk to the diver? His greatest risk is the loss of his protective systems against the hostile environment. Can his health help him survive such a situation or will it be a serious impediment to his health?

The word risk, like the word safety, is confusing. If the risk is, for example 1 in 10,000 man-hours underwater, then safety will be maintained for 9,999 of 10,000 hours. If you double the risk it will be 2 in 10,000 man-hours and the safety will be maintained in 9,998 of 10,000 hours. How can one evaluate the risk of any medical condition with the real scarcity of medical problems? What is statistical variation and what is significant? The answer for the medical community has been to base its evaluation of what is seemingly an absurd term: the probability of risk. Based on what the medical practitioner knows about the diver and his environment, he makes an evaluation of a probability of risk. Medical practitioners will disagree with this approach but that is what they do for so many medical conditions under normal environmental conditions. Uncertainty then can only be removed by referrals, second and third opinions, as is done in ordinary medical practice. We will return to this in the session on training doctors for diving medicine, later.

Finally, I propose a simple matrix in which each organ system and special investigation can be listed against five columns representing the principal medical examinations for diving:-

- Initial examination
- Annual for safety
- Annual for fitness
- Long-term effects
- Return to diving

If we can complete all the boxes in such a matrix we may be on the road to a sensible structure for the examination of the health of divers.

Elliott (Chairman): That raises one of the fundamental questions which we will need to discuss. To what extent can one be prescriptive and to what extent can one set targets? And, if one sets targets, how is one going to audit the performance and effectiveness of those examinations? But, to begin with, we must review the scope and benefits of the annual fitness examination.

WHAT IS THE RELEVANCE OF AN IN-DATE FITNESS EXAMINATION TO THE LONG-TERM HEALTH OF THE DIVER?
Professor R.I. McCallum

The main purpose of a statutory medical examination is to satisfy legislators as to the fitness of people to dive. In the past it has been difficult to get beyond that. The old diving regulations in the UK dating from 1960, now superseded of course, required an annual medical examination which included what was rather quaintly described as "a chest examination by radiography" and sometime in the 1960's the Decompression Sickness Panel said to the representatives from the Ministry of Labour, "what are the results of these examinations"? The answer was they didn't know and it was extremely difficult to find out. There was no central recording of results of those examinations and no means of saying whether or not the chest radiography was performing any useful function. I have no doubt that it had a function, maybe in those days to detect tuberculosis, and maybe it had other functions as well.

But, at a statutory medical examination, there is the possibility of establishing data which can be used for comparative purposes, checked at subsequent examinations and which can be used for epidemiological studies. There is no reason why the examination should not fulfil both functions and this was accepted in principle in the late 1970's when the CIRIA examination form, sponsored by the U.K. Construction Industry Research and Information Association, was introduced (Fig. 1). These were filled in by examining doctors and collected in the Registry at Newcastle over a period of some years. There was also a form for the diver to set down what he had done in diving during the previous year and which could be matched with this medical form.

This examination procedure was the result of considerable discussion amongst doctors concerned with diving and with quite conflicting views on everything, from the desirability or not of measuring chest expansion to whether an EEG should be used routinely. From the start it was thought that baseline information was necessary, not only for the diver personally and particularly early in his career, but for the diving profession as a whole. The medical form was concerned with a number of things which were thought to be relatively simple to deal with. We introduced skinfold measurements of fatness on the grounds that fat and decompression sickness were related. We included audiometry in the examination of ear, nose and throat, and simple ventilatory testing in the examination of the respiratory system. Data on the cardiovascular system and on the CNS were gathered by ordinary clinical means and we later introduced more detailed blood testing, particularly for sickling.

All of these areas are still relevant to the long-term health of divers but there are problems relating to the way in which data are collected and the specificity and repeatability of the tests which are used. There is also some doubt, certainly in my mind, about the adequacy of what has been collected on the basis of this detailed medical examination.

Bone necrosis was perhaps our greatest interest in the 1970's and 1980's and, in fact, the natural history of bone damage in divers has been well explored. Even the limitations of conventional radiography are adequate in dealing with this problem at the moment. The CNS is much more difficult and the problem here is that conventional clinical examination is probably inadequate. It is arguable therefore, that this kind of assessment, if it is to be done properly, should not be part of an annual medical but should be carried out on a special occasion in a special place. The same applies to psychological testing, if that is to be done, because it is not really suitable for routine and annual occasions. Similarly, the apparently simple procedure of recording lung volumes (FEV_1 & FVC) may not be worthwhile or adequate. If more complex tests are indicated then one wants specialist help and so these should be taken out of the annual medical and done on an entirely different basis. There are questions about other body functions which have not been considered, certainly in this scheme, which may lead to the inclusion of further tests. Again I feel that these may be more appropriate done at longer intervals and in the proper specialist background.

My answer to the question of whether the annual examination is appropriate for a survey for long term occupational illness is yes and no, there are certain things which are useful and I hope at a later stage in the proceedings to refer to some epidemiological investigations which have been quite valuable on the basis of information from this type of examination. It is quite time consuming and quite expensive, but I think it is possible to justify it.

CIRIA UNDERWATER ENGINEERING GROUP **Medical examination of commercial divers**

Book No.

Section 2 To be completed by the doctor   Cross out YES or NO whichever is incorrect

Surname 8   Forenames 6   7   16
DOB
SEX: Male/Female   23
22   Height ☐☐ Metres   Weight ☐☐☐.☐ kg
Computer No. 1 (Office Use) 26

EAM normal? R. Yes / No L. Yes / No Any sinus abnormality? R. Yes / No L. Yes / No Audiometry normal? R. Yes / No		ENT normal? 49 Yes / No
Ear drums normal? R. Yes / No L. Yes / No URT Infection R. Yes / No L. Yes / No R. Yes / No		
Eustachian tubes patent? R. Yes / No L. Yes / No Nasal airways normal? R. Yes / No L. Yes / No L. Yes / No		

Are teeth and gums in good condition? Yes / No Any dentures? Yes / No FEV₁ ____ FVC ____		Respiratory system normal? 50 Yes / No
Lungs normal? Yes / No Current CXR normal? Yes / No FEV₁/FVC % 30 ☐☐		

Apex beat in normal position? Yes / No   32 syst 35 diast   37
Heart sounds normal? Yes / No   Blood pressure ☐☐☐   Heart rate (beats per minute) ☐☐
Heart murmurs? Yes / No   39
Peripheral circulation normal? Yes / No   Sickle cell trait? Yes / No   PCV? ☐☐
Varicose veins? Yes / No   ECG Normal? Yes / No

Cardiovascular system normal? 51 Yes / No

Is abdominal palpation normal? Yes / No   Hernia? Yes / No   Skinfold 41   43
Skin rashes, infections or infestations? Yes / No   L.Biceps ☐   L.Triceps ☐
Lymphatic glands normal? Yes / No   45   47
External piles? Yes / No   L.Subscapular ☐   L.Sacro-Iliac ☐
Genito urinary system normal? Yes / No

Alimentary system normal? 52 Yes / No
Skin normal? 53 Yes / No

Limbs normal? Yes / No   Spine normal? Yes / No   Current joint x-rays normal? Yes / No

Limbs & bones normal? 54 Yes / No

Are the cranial nerves normal:
 I Yes / No   V Yes / No   IX Yes / No
 II Yes / No   VI Yes / No   X Yes / No
 III Yes / No   VII Yes / No   XI Yes / No
 IV Yes / No   VIII Yes / No   XII Yes / No

Are reflexes normal:
 Rt. Tri. Yes / No AJ Yes / No   Lt. Tri. Yes / No AJ Yes / No
 Bi. Yes / No Abdo Yes / No   Bi. Yes / No Abdo Yes / No
 Sup. Yes / No Plantar Yes / No   Sup. Yes / No Plantar Yes / No
 KJ Yes / No   KJ Yes / No

Nervous system normal? 55 Yes / No

Power and tone of limbs normal and equal? Yes / No   Proprioception normal? Yes / No   Cerebellar function normal? Yes / No
Normal sensation to: Pinprick? Yes / No   Light touch? Yes / No   Temperature? Yes / No
Vestibular function normal? Yes / No   Rombergism? Yes / No

Vision without glasses: R. 6/   L. 6/   Vision with glasses: R. 6/   L. 6/
Visual fields normal? R. Yes / No L. Yes / No   Colour vision normal? Yes / No   Fundi normal? R. Yes / No L. Yes / No

Eyes normal? 56 Yes / No

Normal exercise tolerance test? Yes / No   General appearance

ETT normal? 57 Yes / No

Urine: Identifying features, scars, tatoos, etc.
Albumin? Yes / No   Sugar? Yes / No
Blood? Yes / No   Ketones? Yes / No

Urine normal? 58 Yes / No

Comments on any abnormalities mentioned above:

Fit? 59 Yes / No

Fig. 1. : Part of the CIRIA form
(by permission of the Construction Industry Research and Information Association)

WHAT IS THE EFFECT OF AGEING UPON THE DIVER?
Dr. S.J. Watt

The first question is "What is the relevance of ageing to the diver?" It is very difficult to separate biological effects from the importance of ageing to the diver's career. It is important to understand the structure of industry, the way in which it works and the influence it will have upon the diver's career when an assessment has to be made of someone's fitness to work.

The first career logistic which is important relates to minimum age. The regulations suggest that it is unlikely that divers will wish to have a medical examination before the age of 18. Realistically that is correct, especially as other career entry factors will be of importance. It's unlikely that anyone will get into a police diving team, for example, and it's unlikely that anyone will have the necessary qualifications to be a scientific diver, below that age. The current regulations, I think, deal with this probably quite adequately. It is likely that most people at the age of 16 to 18 have the physical makeup and ability to undertake most diving activities but it is probably questionable whether all people of that age have the necessary emotional maturity. We also need to consider in the next few days, whether young divers might be at greater risk from the biological effects of diving. Within oilfield diving there is an ageing population of divers. What is happening is that client companies are producing a specification for the competency of the divers whom they wish to undertake their work. This specification is becoming increasingly more complex and he may well require to have spent up to 10 years in the industry to achieve the necessary qualifications. So undoubtedly, we have an ageing population.

The next point is that there is a marked difference between chronological and biological age and that that difference is most pronounced at each end of the working age spectrum.

At the other end of the spectrum, should there be an upper age limit? Based on the precedent of persons in their 70's and 80's who continue to dive (no longer working perhaps) it seems unreasonable to define any statutory upper age limit. I know that medical certificates are issued to working divers in their 60's, and I don't see any reason why people who meet the necessary physical standards, should not be passed fit to dive. The question that arises of course, is "what are the physical standards and how to take age into account in arriving at a physical standard?"

If one looks at physical fitness, it may suggest the approach which would be appropriate in assessing a diver's physical fitness and the impact of age. In most of the present medical assessments we compare the diver with an index which has been reached from a study of the general population. That seems to be a very appropriate way of doing it. We know that the physical fitness of the general population diminishes with increasing age and one can measure it in terms of maximum oxygen uptake, heart rate response and so forth. The ability to undertake physical work declines quite markedly between the ages of 18 and 65. So how do we take that into account? One can continue to compare divers with the general population but, because of the physical nature of the work activity, the standard relative to the general population has to go up as divers age. Age, in itself, does not become an obstacle to diving, but maintaining the necessary physical fitness clearly becomes more difficult. If, for example, the average level of fitness at age 25 was consistent with being able to undertake the diving job, then I would suggest that that percentile would need to go up as the diver ages.

Another example in which we need to consider the effects of ageing in more detail, is in lung function testing. Unlike physical fitness, which we know declines steadily in the general population from the age of 18, lung function does not. Although we use prediction equations which suggest there is a slow and progressive decline in lung function, there is good evidence which suggests that lungs actually continue to grow in terms of size until late 20's or even early 30's. So, during the period in which divers are likely to be active, their lung volumes may normally be growing before they then start to decline, and we may need to take that into account in their assessment.

Of the other effects of age, blood pressure goes up and we take that into account routinely when we do medical examinations. We know also that hearing deteriorates with age and take that into account in assessment of audiograms. So in the discussions which follow, clearly age will be a major consideration.

We need to consider the frequency with which we conduct medical examinations and the implications of age. A recent audit of a 1,000 offshore workers, who attended for periodic examinations, was studied by age group. It gave an indication that the percentage of people presenting for examination who are not fully fit goes up fairly steadily with age. There is a substantial increase in the number of abnormalities found as the population ages and the audit is strongly supportive of the practice in many other areas of increasing the frequency of examination as the population ages.

We need also to review some aspects of the examination which we conduct on an annual basis. Is the frequency with which we carry out certain examinations justified? It is, for example, unlikely that in other industrial situations one would consider annual audiometry in a population who's noise exposure is similar to divers. Certainly there are some groups of divers, for example scientists, for whom noise exposure appears to be minimal.

What are we actually achieving in the annual medical examination? Can we actually justify conducting large numbers of tests on this body of people, and make them pay for it, when the yield rate from some of these investigations is remarkably small? We know that the population of divers do have some diving-related health effects. We know from discussions that we have had already that the tests we routinely perform during the annual medical examination are not particularly sensitive to such changes. So, the obvious question that arises is "what are we actually achieving by doing these examinations so frequently?" Perhaps we could achieve a satisfactory standard by reducing the frequency of the examinations, particularly in the younger age group.

DISCUSSION

Elliott (Chairman): Our speakers have highlighted very well the basic problems that we are facing in this field. When we open this up for discussion, we are likely to disagree with the Social Affairs Department in the Netherlands and agree unanimously that some degree of medical examination is appropriate. We have been challenged by Norway: should this be goal-setting? Should we define the functional tasks the person has to do and train the doctor to assess the diver? Or should standards be prescriptive? If they are, then as Professor McCallum suggests, are they specific, are they reproducible and how often do they need to be done?

These questions, should be reviewed in detail later as we go through each of the organ systems.

We now have a few moments for discussion of fundamental principles. Why do we need examinations? What are we trying to achieve? If we are to decide we will include only the items that are really essential, what would they be?

Risberg: I was impressed by the arguments of Stephen Watt when he proposed the personal limits for the ageing diver. It was a smart idea. On the other hand it is not wise to change with age the physical or medical standards. We do need to use functional goals, the diver has to achieve some standard of physical fitness to do his physical tasks. That is why I do not think we can compare him to the age-matched group of the general population.

Elliott: In 1981 we did put a target into the original guidance (MA1) "providing all the medical standards can be met there is no upper age limit." For example if the standard for physical fitness is now set at a particular value, something like 13 METS or 47 ml oxygen/kg/min, then that is not chronologically-linked.

Watt: What you have suggested is perhaps the ideal way of going about it but could you please tell me what the metabolic requirements for doing the task are? The problem is that we do not actually know, and until we do know exactly what it is, it's not reasonable to set a standard based on anything other than, I think, the general population.

I am reminded of the calculations that the physiologists made about ascending Everest without oxygen. They worked out in great detail that in order to undertake this they would have to have the most enormous ability to utilise oxygen and then they looked at climbers who had actually made the ascent and found that their ability to use oxygen was well below what had been calculated. So we need to know in considerable detail what is actually required if we were going to use that approach to set a standard. Another point which relates to ageing is that younger divers may be physically fitter but in practice they are often less effective. Older divers have experience which enables them to undertake tasks more rapidly and more efficiently. That is a very difficult factor to assess in a medical examination.

Elliott: In the field of psychological fitness, I once tried to define, as a standard, that the successful candidate would be somebody to whom you would entrust your own life. With physical fitness surely one is again looking at the extreme physical requirements, for example, whether the diver, experienced or not, can rescue a buddy from a life-threatening situation. The physical standard to be met is that of extreme physical hard work and therefore, as saving a buddy's life is part of the safety requirement, then to set a <u>maximal</u> sustainable limit for every diver, should meet the requirement?

Watt: I don't have problems with that approach. In fact it may work out to be exactly the same thing, when compared with the normal declining fitness in the general population. However, if we are to make a decision about a diver's fitness which may effectively terminate a career, we need to do that on fairly firm evidence. If we are saying that the standard is one which you must achieve to rescue a buddy, we need to know what is actually required to undertake that task. I think that we are short of that information at the moment.

Bennett: This comment is in relation to recreational diving. There seems to be less of a problem in commercial diving today, in the broad sense that there are very few accidents. If you look at the USA we have 800 recreational diving accidents a year and 90 deaths on average. Of those deaths over the age of 40 who are examined by coroners, 75% have cardiovascular pathology. So we are seeing an ageing population too and we are seeing more evidence of disease causing death. You may not see it so much in the commercial diver, perhaps because he is not diving to the ages that recreational divers do.

Rogerson: I would like to throw a new subject into the discussion, and I think it is important. It is the necessity of keeping very tight control on notes and repeated tests, in case of litigation. Last year solicitors actually subpoenaed all my medical records for one diver for the last 10 years. If we do not repeat all the tests every year then we are lost when we have to stand up in court and give chronological detail.

LeDez: At this meeting we need to address in detail the ethical issues involved. Who are we working for in doing these medicals? I think that we have to give that a great deal of thought, are we working for the divers or the employers? That is a critical issue.

Nome**: The examining doctor, in Norway, "approves" the fitness of the diver for his employer. (The doctor in this context is not the "patient's friend and protector"!)

WHO SHOULD BE EXAMINED?
SHOULD THE STANDARDS BE THE SAME FOR ALL CATEGORIES?
Dr. R. Ramaswami

The aim of this presentation is to review briefly the range of diving activities that are covered in the United Kingdom by the Diving Operations at Work Regulations, to mention some of the hazards associated with particular types of diving and to stimulate discussion on the question of variability of standards. What are we trying to achieve by having medical standards of diving? Is it appropriate to have the same standard for a saturation diver and a dry diver? Should there be an age variability and is an annual examination appropriate for all?

The Diving Operations at Work Regulations require that all divers must have an annual medical to be conducted by a doctor approved under the regulations, to a standard laid out in the Guidance Note MA1 and to be recorded on a form MS80. Just about all divers who are diving for remuneration are subject to the Diving Operations at Work Regulations. Form MS80 on completion is returned to the Employment Medical Advisory Service (EMAS) in Aberdeen, but from this form we cannot tell what type of diving is being done by any particular diver.

Approved doctors carry out medical examinations under the Regulations and each is approved in response to a perceived HSE requirement for examinations to be conducted in a particular location. They should have a knowledge of diving medicine, and have access to suitable facilities to conduct the examinations. Approval may be withdrawn at any time and this is usually in response to a failure to conduct a sufficient number of examinations. There were 205 Approved Doctors in the U.K. in June 1993, and another 92 located overseas. Since then about 3 more have been approved making around 300 in all. About 4,750 examinations are carried out per year and are theoretically to the same standard.

However it is up to the individual doctor to use his or her judgement as to the interpretation of the standard. Examination in accordance with the Guidance Note is based on a clinical examination followed by certain basic investigations:

- radiography
- haematology
- spirometry
- electrocardiography
- exercise testing

and is designed to be a relatively low cost procedure.

Divers covered by the Diving Operations at Work Regulations include offshore saturation divers, offshore air divers and inshore and inland divers. The inshore and inland divers work in civil engineering, fish farming, harbours, for search and rescue, police duties, for scientific and research purposes and there are also the remunerated instructors of amateurs. Then there are dry divers, such as doctors, who are not covered by the regulations but are often examined in spite of that.

The effects of medical conditions on fitness to dive are primarily directed towards the in-water safety aspects. The condition must not expose the diver to unacceptable risk and not expose his diving companions to risk. It is generally found that the criteria are interpreted rather more stringently at the initial examination as the loss of career is not relevant at the initial exam. Long term health considerations should also be taken into account.

Approximately 1% of medicals result in failure. About 50% of the primary causes of unfitness to dive are cardiovascular or respiratory. It is likely that the number of cardiovascular failures may increase with the increase in the age of the diving population.

AGEING DIVERS

At the moment the youngest diver covered by the Diving Operations at Work Regulations is 17 and there are two divers at 68 who have medicals. We do not know what these people actually do but only that they have current medical certificates. The average age of North Sea divers in 1984 was 29.9 and in 1990 it was 33.4 years.

I should remind you that some of the particular hazards encountered by saturation divers are: exposure to high pressure; use of mixed gases; long periods of inactivity; relatively high oxygen concentrations; exposure to pathogens and exposure to noise hazards. Noise hazard is also a factor for some divers working in harbours along with poor visibility, underwater debris, often quite demanding manual handling tasks, and cold from the waters of the harbours.

Civil engineering divers suffer similar considerations but in addition may be in remote locations, a long way from any form of medical help.

A group which are often forgotten are the police divers who operate in shallow waters, usually less than 10m with poor visibility. Discarded sharps are a frequent hazard, they have a requirement to handle corpses and quite often they are required to dive in sewage. Police divers are exposed to rather different hazards than the offshore divers and perhaps there is justification for asking for a different medical standard.

The dry divers have no in-water hazards but may have delicate tasks to perform. Their dives may be of long duration and may involve manual handling. The standards for them should not be the same as for saturation divers.

WHAT REGULATIONS EXIST?
WHO FOR, AND IN WHICH COUNTRIES?
Dr. N.K.I. McIver

"M. Paul Bert has recently drawn the attention of the Academy of Sciences, through M. Claude Bernard, to the great danger of sudden transition from compressed air to the outer atmosphere ...... Before men are detailed for diving they should be examined as to their fitness by a Medical Officer".   Siebe (1873)

Physical fitness for work forms part of the expanding legislation covering Occupational Health and Safety. At entry level to any occupation there may be simple "Pass/Fail" criteria and the candidate should be examined by a doctor with experience of that occupation. The employee and his employer both have a duty towards health surveillance and detection of long term health hazards. The medical examination of a commercial diver is the first stage in this process.

There is a great variety of legislation and guidelines internationally. A brief review of legislation and regulations in 11 Countries was made by Mebane & McIver (1993) but much has taken place since then.

EUROPEAN COUNTRIES

Belgium

Dr. Herman van Bogaert, 1994 : There are no statutory regulations or medical guidelines for commercial diving operations. The Ministry of Labour is drafting regulations which should be ready in a few months. No examinations are required but most of the physicians use the British or Dutch standards. Much responsibility is vested in the supervising occupational physician, as already occurs for caisson workers. The number of commercial divers in Belgium is small and most work is for foreign companies.

Denmark

Prof. J. Madsen, 1994 : There are regulations governing medical examination of professional diving candidates and professional divers (1981). There are guidelines concerning examination of commercial divers (1985) and a Diving Act of 1988.

There is a requirement for initial examination before entry to a commercial diving school. British divers working in Danish waters are required by the Maritime Authority to satisfy British statutory requirements. Under the Diving Act 1988 all professional divers between the ages of 18 and 39 years must have a medical examination every five years, every two years between the ages of 40 and 59 years and thereafter annually. For offshore and mixed gas divers there is an annual examination.

There is also an requirement for periodic examination after more than 20 days sickness absence from work, after hospital admission, pregnancy, "the use of optical or mechanical aids", regular medical treatment, or where there is any doubt about the diver's health. There is no fitness requirement for hyperbaric medical staff and attendants.

France

M. Jean-Claude Le Péchon, 1994 : There are regulations under the Hyperbaric Work - Health and Safety Act (28th March 1990) and guidelines dated 28th March 1991. These are extremely detailed and have been offered as a basis for international adoption. They cover training standards and fitness standards for all varying classes of hyperbaric exposure. There is an initial medical followed by annual periodic review until the age of 40 years, and an annual medical with a 6 monthly clinical review above the age of 40 years. The lower limit is 18 years and there is no upper limit (medical discretion). No diving candidates are accepted above the age of 40 years.

A Certificate d'Aptitude à l'Hyperbarie (CAH) is issued by the Institut Nationale de la Plongée Professionale on behalf of the French Ministry of Labour. The decree of 1990 already covered all those exposed to raised ambient pressure, breathing gases, equipment and procedures. Medical fitness was covered by the Arrêté of 1991. This also covered safety, training and certification according to exposure. The Arrêté of 1992 covered working conditions, decompression tables and therapy. In future, equipment, including all chambers and locks, will be covered by a "Code du Travail".

Medical examination on return after illness or injury is left to the doctor's discretion.

Hyperbaric medical staff require a Certificate of Training and a medical examination. Age limits are 18 to 55 years for new personnel, with no upper age limit for active personnel.

Germany

Prof. J. Holthaus, 1992 : Commercial air diving to 50 metres and the treatment of decompression illness has been covered by legislation since 1985. Special dispensation and advice is required for diving beyond this. Some companies have dispensation for breathing mixtures such as Nitrox. Research diving is covered by guidelines that are almost identical and fitness to dive deeper than 50 metres is also subject to special permission.

Dr. J. Wendling, 1994 : There are detailed guidelines for medical examination of sports divers in Germany under the auspices of the German Diving & Hyperbaric medical Society.

Greece

Dr. B. Zachariades, 1994 : The Greek Navy follows NATO diving medical standards. For civilian divers there are existing standards requiring an annual medical, investigations including: chest x-ray, urinalysis, ECG and blood test which may be performed by any physician at any hospital and by a doctor who is not required to have any diving medical knowledge. Medicals are performed in response to demand of the divers and their companies rather than any requirement by legislation and all look to the EDTC to set standards which should be formally adopted.

Italy

Dr. A. Marroni, 1994 : There are regulations covering compressed air diving, harbour underwater activities and professional underwater fishing. For offshore and oilfield diving there are guidelines recommending adoption of North Sea regulations. There is an initial medical, periodic review annually (age limits 18 to 60 years). The Unions are pressing for the adoption of updated EDTC Guidelines in the absence of commercial diving regulations.

The Netherlands

Dr. W. Maas, 1994 : For commercial divers, working under the "Mining Regulations", legislation has been in force since 1988 with guidelines on medical fitness to dive. All doctors must be appointed by the Minister of Economic Affairs and use this guide when examining commercial divers.

Surgeon Commander R.A. van Hulst, 1994 : For the Royal Netherlands Navy there are additional respiratory function tests and oxygen tolerance test requirements, with annual review to the age of 45 years. There is no regulatory requirement for medical examination after illness or injury for commercial divers, but naval divers are assessed at one week after limb pain decompression illness and after one month for neurological decompression illness and arterial gas embolism. Other assessments are left to the discretion of the diving doctor. There is no additional requirement for hyperbaric medical staff attendants.

Norway

Dr. B. Minsaas, 1994 : Under the existing regulations concerning manned underwater operations (Norwegian Petroleum Directorate 1990), there is a mandatory certificate of fitness required for offshore divers based on an evaluation of whether the medical condition represents a danger to him/herself or others.

The medical practitioner must have approval from the Director of Public Health and examinations must be carried out in accordance with the guidelines. The emphasis is placed on safety and all advice and fitness decisions are based on the effect of safety on diving. Long term effects do not affect safety and so are the responsibility not of government but of the employer.

Earlier today, Dr. Minsaas has described the new guidelines (Section 1) which have the purpose of ascertaining medical fitness from a safety point of view. Section 12 ascertains fitness first to be on an offshore installation, and thereafter to take part in manned underwater operations. This involves assessment of risk and safety factors. The diver must be able to detect alarms, to be psychologically able to handle an evacuation and must be carefully assessed if taking any medication. The guidelines contain a short list of disqualifying conditions (any perceived risk may lead to disqualification). The medical examination must be performed by an Approved Doctor who must have knowledge of divers.

Spain

Dr. J. Desola, 1994 : Regulations for professional divers are issued by the Secretary General of the Ministry of Fishing and Agriculture. These include a detailed pre-employment examination which must be performed by an approved doctor with a diploma in underwater medicine (but is rarely followed). There is no age limit but annual review is advised. There is no specification for examination after illness or injury, no regulation of hyperbaric medical staff. There is legislation covering compressed air workers.

There are therefore detailed regulations differing from the EDTC and HSE (U.K.) Guidelines, but these are not necessarily followed. Divers and companies may conform voluntarily. At the Hospital de la Creu Roja in Barcelona the EDTC and HSE (U.K.) Guidelines are followed, but they feel that they are in a minority in doing so.

Sweden

Prof. H. Örnhagen, 1991 : The employer is responsible for a register of employed divers who are certified medically fit. Pregnant divers may not dive professionally

Prof. H. Örnhagen, 1994 : There are new regulations (1994) which govern the fitness to dive examination but the performance is covered by guidelines. The guidelines recommend detailed lists of investigations although a certificate of fitness may be issued without these. Frequency of examination is 5 yearly up to the age of 40 and every 2 years beyond that age. After illness or injury a new medical examination must be conducted if fitness to dive could have been affected. Hyperbaric medical staff and attendants are covered by the guidelines.

Switzerland

Dr. J. Wendling, 1994 : Switzerland authorises the State insurance "SUVA" to analyse accidents and causes of occupational ill health. The SUVA doctors may also issue instructions for preventative medical examinations and technical modifications of the worksite. The regulations of SUVA are obligatory for employees, but not for independent professionals such as a self-employed commercial diver for whom there are no obligatory health standards. The law demanding SUVA to control commercial divers and other professionals with special risks is VUV 78 ("Verordnung uber die Verhutung von Unfällen und Berufs-Krautheiten") ratified by Swiss Parliament, Bern 1983.

Turkey

Prof. M. Çimsit, 1994 : There have been regulations covering professional divers (Regulations for Professional Frogmen and Divers, T.C. Ministry of Transport 1966). For the last two years commercial diving medical examinations have been conducted according to guidelines and there is a proposal that these be accepted as regulation.

There is an initial pre-employment medical including extremely detailed investigations: blood counts, biochemistry, urinalysis, ECG, cardiovascular performance testing, chest x-ray, paranasal sinus x-rays, pulmonary function tests, bleeding and clotting time, audio-vestibular tests, vision tests, skinfold measurements, oxygen tolerance test, 110 ft. pressure test, dysbaric osteonecrosis screening and a detailed physical examination. There is a periodic review every two years, when all the tests are repeated. The lower age limit is 20 years, upper age limit for beginners is 30 years and above the age of 40 years periodic review is required annually.

An examination is conducted before return to diving after decompression illness: three weeks after limb pain DCI, six months after neurological DCI if there are no residua. The hyperbaric medical staff and attendants follow the same medical examination and periodically at two year intervals. There is a dysbaric osteonecrosis investigation after acute DCI and four months following therapy. Psychomotor tests are being prepared.

There is a requirement for any diving operation using deck decompression or surface decompression on oxygen for depths deeper than 30 metres to have a medical officer on site. All mixed gas diving operations require a medical officer on site.

United Kingdom

As already described under the Diving Operations at Work Regulations 1981 as amended by the Diving Operations at Work (Amendment) Regulations 1990, the diver must be in possession of an in-date Certificate of Medical Fitness issued after an examination carried out by a doctor approved by the Health and Safety Executive (1987). This regulation imposes a duty on persons who have any responsibility for or control over the diving operations to ensure that diving is safe so far as is reasonably practicable. The diver has a responsibility to declare fitness to dive on any diving operation. These regulations cover all commercial divers in the U.K. including anyone exposed to pressures exceeding 300 millibars above atmospheric (1.3 atmospheres absolute, 131 kPa). This covers all divers at work including professional scuba diving instructors.

COUNTRIES OUTSIDE EUROPE

Australia

Dr. J. Williamson, 1994 : The Australian Medical Association has reviewed the Australian standards (AS 2299-1992) and given a draft code of practice for occupational diving. This covers inshore air diving to 50 metres depth. Offshore deeper than 50 metres and mixed gas diving requires compliance with the U.K. regulations. There is an initial pre-employment medical and periodic review from the ages of 18 years to 40 years, annually. After return from illness or injury there is no specific regulation, but each case is decided by an appropriate experienced diving doctor using his discretion.

There is a requirement for an experienced hyperbaric registered nurse as inside chamber attendant, and for a suitably trained hyperbaric doctor, technicians and nursing staff outside the chamber.

While medical fitness to dive is reasonably well regulated, the manning of commercial (inshore) chambers for on site recompressions is not. There are differing opinions about lay off time after successful treatment of acute decompression illness between the centres.

There is a move to apply the new standards from 1994 onwards. The South Pacific Underwater Medicine Society has been in debate with the AMA over the preparation of this uniform document.

Canada

Dr. M. Lepawsky, 1994 : The Canadian Association of Diving Contractors has issued guidelines and codes of conduct in conjunction with the Defence and Civil Institute of Environmental Medicine (DCIEM). These cover initial and periodic diving medical examinations.

Malta

Dr. R. Cali-Corleo, 1992 : There is legislation covering diver training schools and guidelines are in preparation for commercial diving activities. Under the joint Police and Health Authority Diving Regulations 1979 (with minor amendments since then pending total revision in 1995), there is a requirement for a pre-employment medical, periodic review between the ages of 18 to 50 years annually (air diving only).

There is no specific requirement after illness or injury, this being left to the medical officer's discretion. There is no requirement for recompression facility at the dive site as the distances to the hyperbaric unit on call are small. The hyperbaric unit staff undergo an annual examination to recreational diving standards. The regulations apply only to employed divers and only air diving is carried out in Malta.

U.S.A.

Dr. Y. Mebane, 1994 : The initial OSHA standards have been abandoned in favour of the adoption of new standards by the Association of Diving Contractors. Member companies agree to abide by these standards when they become ADC members. The small time salvage operations and commercial fishing are unregulated at present.

The guidelines recommend a pre-employment examination, periodic examination every two years until the age of 35 years and annually thereafter. There is a minimum age of 18 years and no upper age limit. This requirement applies to anyone who may enter the hyperbaric environment in the course of employment. After injury or illness requiring hospital treatment of more than three days, or any decompression illness, a physical examination is required before return to work. Some companies require physical examination if the length of disability exceeds 30 days. There is no uniform requirement of medical standards for hyperbaric medical staff, each centre using its own.

The consensus standards for commercial diving operations adopted by the Association of Diving Contractors were last revised in 1994.

REFERENCE

Mebane, Y.G. & McIver, N.K.I. *The Physiology and medicine of Diving, 4th Edition.* Eds. P.B. Bennett & D.H. Elliott. Saunders: London 1993. Pp 53-76.

WHAT ARE THE INTERNATIONAL DIFFERENCES OF POTENTIAL SIGNIFICANCE?
Professor Hans Örnhagen

As a preparation for the harmonisation of diving regulations and medical standards for diving in Europe, the European Diving Technology Committee (EDTC) decided in 1993 to identify the current situation in the member countries. A questionnaire was sent to the doctors or, in countries with no EDTC medical representative, to the responsible person, usually the government representative, in the 16-member countries. Eleven questionnaires were returned. The answers were categorised and tabulated in 17 tables. The bottom line in each table gives the EDTC recommendations from the 1986 Guidance Notes for Safe Diving.

Although it was pointed out that it was the official opinion, as expressed in the national regulations, that was being asked for in my questionnaires, it was obvious that in some cases the opinions given were the opinions of the of the organisation to who the questionnaire had been sent or the personal opinions of the doctor delegated for reply. As long as the doctor is using a higher standard or is doing more than required it is acceptable but this focuses on an important question viz "can doctors do what they think is best even if it does not meet the minimum standards?" My impression is that generally, doctors want to do more than the regulations require.

As seen in Table 1, only 7 of the 11 responding countries have a registration or license for doctors who examine divers. Four of the 11 countries have a central registry of names of medically-approved divers or of the diving medicals, while 4 countries have issued a specific form for the fitness to dive examination to guide the doctor. From this information an impression of the degree of authority control can be estimated. Using these criteria Sweden is a country with the lowest level of official control since all questions were answered "no", while Spain has a high level of control since all answers were "yes". Surprisingly, in many of the questionnaires, no answer was given regarding the special forms for examination results.

TABLE 1 - DEGREE OF CONTROL BY AUTHORITY

N = No; Y = Yes; - = no answer

	Central registry for diver medicals	Special license for doctors	Special form for examination results
Belgium	Y	N	Y
Denmark	Y	N	Y
Finland	N	N	-
France	N	Y	-
Germany	N	Y	-
Iceland	Y	Y	-
Italy	N	Y	-
Netherlands	N	Y	-
Spain	Y	Y	Y
Sweden	N	N	N
United Kingdom	N	Y	Y
EDTC-86	Y	Y	Y

Table 2 indicates that most countries only have one level of requirement which is valid for all kinds of diving, while some countries have special examinations for saturation divers. It is my interpretation that shallow air and nitrox diving is the most commonly used and hence this type of diving deserves harmonisation first. The specialised forms of diving such as heliox and/or saturation diving should be easier to address if the minimum requirements for air/nitrox diving have been agreed. Military diving is specific for each country and harmonisation of medical standards may not be needed for this type of diving.

TABLE 2 - HEALTH CERTIFICATE VALID FOR:

All types of military diving (none for civilian	Belgium
All types of diving	Denmark
All types of except saturation	Finland
All types of diving	France
Only air diving (none for mixed gas?)	Germany
Only air diving (none for mixed gas?)	Iceland
All types of diving	Italy
All but SCUBA (Mining Regulations)	The Netherlands
All but sat. (Military Regulations)	
Other diving: no requirements	
All types of diving	Spain
All types of diving	Sweden
All types of diving	United Kingdom
All types of diving	EDTC-86

TABLE 3 - THE INTERVAL BETWEEN MEDICALS

Belgium	1
Denmark	age <40, every 5 y
	age 40-60, every 2 y
	age >60, annually
Finland	1 - 3 y
France	1
Germany	1
Iceland	1
Italy	1
The Netherlands	1
Spain	1
Sweden	age <40, every 5 y
	age >40, every 2 y
United Kingdom	1
EDTC-86	- (annual was intended)

Intervals between medicals vary in European countries according to Table 3 from "annual" in most countries to "every 5 years" in Denmark and Sweden for divers younger than 40. The rationale for the relatively long interval in Sweden for young divers is that only very rarely something was found during repeated medicals in fit divers. At an age above 40, the cardiovascular problems start to occur and hence there are good reasons to undertake more frequent medicals.

In this context I would like to stress the value of the contact between a diver and his doctor, not only when it is time for the medical examination that is compulsory, but also when the diver has experienced something that could affect his or her fitness to dive, such as a severe cold, a trauma or a gastro-intestinal problem. Each diver should have a "company doctor" and the name and telephone number of this doctor should be noted in the diver's logbook.

Coupled with the question about "company doctors" is of course the competence of these doctors. How are they educated? How do they maintain and/or increase their competence? If the doctors have a high level of competence, the need for specific instructions on how to perform the fit-to-dive medical is less than if with no specific training in diving physiology and medicine a doctor is allowed to perform the examination. Most countries have, as a help and guidance to the doctors, a list of medical conditions that are not considered compatible with professional diving while only few have a list of drugs that disqualify for diving if used (Table 4).

TABLE 4 - LIST OF LIMITATIONS

	Medical Contraindications	Drugs not compatible with diving
Belgium	N	N
Denmark	Y	N
Finland	Y	N
France	Y	N
Germany	-	N
Iceland	N	N
Italy	Y	Y
The Netherlands	Y	Y
Spain	Y	N
Sweden	Y	N
United Kingdom	Y	N
EDTC-86	Y	N

Although cardiovascular and physical fitness problems probably pose a more severe threat to the health and survival of the working diver than do respiratory problems, there is and has always been a heavy focus on pulmonary x-ray and spirometry in the medical examination. Table 5 shows that all responding countries have a requirement for spirometry in the fitness to dive examination and all but one have specified limits on minimum performance at such tests.

TABLE 5 - SPIROMETRY : MINIMUM REQUIREMENTS

	Compulsory	Vital Capacity (VC)	FEV 1.0	FEV %
Belgium	N	-	-	-
Denmark	Y	-	-	>70%
Finland	Y	>80% of standard	>80% of standard	>90% of standard
France	Y	>80% of standard	>80% of standard	>70%
Germany	Y	>70% of standard	>60% of standard	-
Iceland	Y	-1 SD of standard	-1 SD of standard	>75%
Italy	Y	Special table	-	>75%(>70%)
The Netherlands	Y	-	>65% of standard	-
Spain	Y	>80% of standard	>80% of standard	>80% of standard
Sweden	Y	<-0.5 l of standard	>80% of standard	-
United Kingdom	Y	-1 SD of standard	-1 SD of standard	-2 SD of standard
EDTC-86	Y	-	-	-

Table 5 also summarises the minimum performance requirements and there is a good deal of agreement in these limits between different countries. Important in this context is that the equipment used is well calibrated and that common sense and good knowledge is practised when an individual diver performance is compared to these limits, so that fit divers are not excluded from diving. An example of this is the relatively low percentage forced expiratory volume (FEV%) seen in persons with larger than normal lungs. This limit is known to have disqualified fit divers although a lower than normal FEV% in persons with larger than normal total lung capacity (TLC) by specialists is not seen as an increased risk in diving.

The x-ray is mandatory in all countries, but the intervals vary from annual to every 5 years. In certain countries such as the Netherlands and the United Kingdom, the doctor decides if and when an x-ray is needed.

TABLE 6 - THE INTERVAL BETWEEN PULMONARY X-RAYS

Belgium	<40 every 3y, >40 annually
Denmark	Annually
Finland	Every 2 - 5 years
France	Every 4 years
Germany	Every 3 years
Iceland	Annually
Italy	Annually (sat. divers only)
The Netherlands	Doctor's decision
Spain	Every 3 years
Sweden	<40 every 5y, >40 every 2y
United Kingdom	Doctor's decision
EDTC-86	-

Additional respiratory tests such as Forced Expiratory Flow at 25 and 75% volume (FEF 25-75), Peak Expiratory Flow (PEF), Flow Volume (F-V) loops, Closing Volume (CV) and Residual Volume (RV) measurements are seldom requested (see Table 7) although most modern spirometers give some of these parameters as an automatic bonus.

TABLE 7 - ADDITIONAL PULMONARY TESTS

	FEF$_{25-75}$	CV	Other
Belgium	Y	N	PEF
Denmark	N	N	N
Finland	Y	N	PEF
France	N	N	N
Germany	N	N	N
Iceland	N	N	N
Italy	N	N	N
The Netherlands	N	N	N
Spain	N	N	N
Sweden	N	N	N
United Kingdom	N	N	N
EDTC-86	N	N	N

The electrocardiogram (ECG) is probably one of the most widely used special examinations in the investigation of fitness to dive. Some countries require an ECG annually while others require ECG's less often (Table 8). The fact is that there are some divers who have died because of coronary sclerosis shortly after an ECG that showed no abnormality. The true value of an ECG is when it is performed during an exercise test. This makes it more complicated and expensive, but this should not be an argument when discussing the medical examination of professional divers. The need for work-tests with ECG's calls for additional education of the doctors who examine divers.

TABLE 8 - RESTING ECG's

Belgium	Annually
Denmark	1 examination then only on medical indication
Finland	Every 2 years <40, then annually
France	Annually
Germany	Y
Iceland	Every 2 years <30, then annually
Italy	Y
The Netherlands	Y
Spain	Only on medical indication
Sweden	Every 5 years <40, then every 2 years
United Kingdom	Annually
EDTC-86	Y

The physical fitness of a diver can be investigated in many ways. The most standardised and widely spread in Europe is probably the bicycle ergometer test (Table 9). To get the most out of this test it should be combined with the ECG. For those doctors who do not have this already as a standard, it will require additional investment but there is no doubt that this is worthwhile when divers over 40 are examined.

TABLE 9 - TEST OF PHYSICAL FITNESS

	Test	Minimum limit for approval
Belgium	Bicycle ergometer	Heart rate <170 at 10 MET
Denmark	Step test	Resting heart rate 45 sec after 15 sec of chair climbing
Finland	Only on medical indication	
France	Bicycle ergometer	∇O_2 max >40 ml x min-1 x kg-1
Germany	Bicycle ergometer	5 min at 120 W
Iceland	Bicycle ergometer	∇O_2 max >50 ml x min-1 x kg-1 (new divers)
Italy	Y	-
The Netherlands	Y	-
Spain	Rufier-Dickson	<9
Sweden	Bicycle ergometer	<40 yrs; >6 min at 200W, then >6 min at 150 W
United Kingdom	Army Physical Fitness Test	Sum of pulse counts <190
EDTC-86	Y	

When something is easy to measure and the normal variation is small, it is likely that this parameter ends up in a fitness examination. Blood pressure is such a parameter. The diastolic should not, in general, be over 95 and the systolic over 160 to be approved for diving (Table 10). The U.K. limits are so low 80/140 that this must cause a problem for many divers and doctors. On the other hand, the German limit 100 diastolic seems to be a little too high because such a person should be treated for his high blood pressure even if he is not a diver.

TABLE 10 - BLOOD PRESSURE (maximum allowed)

	Diastolic	Systolic
Belgium	90 - 95	140 - 150
Denmark	90	150
Finland	90 - 100	140 - 160
France	95	165
Germany	100	100 + age in years
Iceland	90	160
Italy	90	150
The Netherlands	95	N (doctor's decision)
Spain	90	150
Sweden	N	N (doctor's decision)
United Kingdom	80	140
EDTC-86	90	140

Hearing and vision are senses of great importance for operational reasons. From a medical standpoint it is good to have a base-line value so that any deleterious effects of diving on the individual's hearing or vision can be observed. The capacity is easy to measure and hence there are a lot of numbers indicating limits for approval (Tables 11 and 12). Whether or not these are set at an appropriate level depends on the type of work which is done by the diver. There are many places where the diver could be blind or deaf and still do a good job but there are so many other things to consider. The diver must for example be able to read his instruments and hear communications. When limits are discussed it is of the utmost importance that it is clearly understood by the doctors and the divers that, in this case, there are no absolute values and hence some flexibility is available.

TABLE 11 - VISION

Belgium	9/10 with both eyes, difference <2/10, perfect colour vision
Denmark	6/12 with both eyes
Finland	N
France	N
Germany	0.5 without correction
Iceland	6/9 with both eyes, normal visual fields (Donder) N5 at 30-40 cm
Italy	6/10 with both eyes, normal retina, normal tonometry
The Netherlands	Diver should find his way without glasses, normal visual fields
Spain	N
Sweden	N
United Kingdom	6/9 with both eyes, N5 at 25-40 cm, normal visual fields and fundi
EDTC-86	6/36 worst eye and 6/24 both eyes; J16 (N24) worst eye and J15 (N18) both and no defects in visual fields

TABLE 12 - HEARING

Belgium	<4000 Hz 10dB, >4000 Hz 20dB
Denmark	Speech shall be understood by each ear at 2.5 m
Finland	250 - 3000 Hz 40dB best ear, one ear may have 80dB
France	Frequency weighted hearing loss must be <25dB
Germany	Conversational speech must be understood at 5 m
Iceland	Normal conversation understood
Italy	<3000Hz 20dB, >3000Hz 35dB (dip to 50dB at 4000 Hz accepted)
The Netherlands	<60dBat worst ear
Spain	N
Sweden	Understand normal conversation
United Kingdom	Understand normal conversation
EDTC-86	<4000Hz 30dB, >4000Hz 60dB

Extensive laboratory tests of blood and urine are difficult to justify and in some countries there are no requirements for such testing at all. Haemoglobin in blood and glucose and protein in urine seem to be a commonly agreed minimum (Table 13). In some regions of Europe HbS may be screened for.

TABLE 13 - LABORATORY TESTS

	Blood	Urine
Belgium	Sedimentation Rate (SR), cells, creatinine, glucose, uric acid, transaminase, lipids	Protein, blood, cylinders, amorphous phosphates
Denmark	Hb, Packed Cell Volume (PCV), cells, HbS	Protein, glucose, blood
Finland	N	Protein, glucose
France	Cells, glucose, uric acid, cholesterol, lipids	Protein, glucose, ketonic bodies
Germany	Hb, SR	Stick screening
Iceland	Hb, SR, PCV, cells	Protein, glucose, pH, acetone, blood
Italy	Cells, SR, gluc, creat, transam, coagulation time	Y
The Netherlands	Routine blood	Protein, glucose
Spain	N	Labstix
Sweden	Hb	Protein, glucose
United Kingdom	Hb, PCV, HbS	Protein, glucose, blood
EDTC-86	Hb, PCV, (HbS)	Protein, glucose, blood, pH

The musculo-skeletal system and the body as a whole are covered by bone x-rays, a maximum body weight, and requirements on mobility (Table 14). It is agreed that bone x-ray (Table 15) is less important in divers performing shallow air dives of relatively short duration. This means that a large number of the divers do not need to have bone x-rays. Examples of such professional divers are rescue divers and instructors in recreational diving.

TABLE 14 - OTHER SOMATIC REQUIREMENTS

	Muscle Strength	Age	Body
Belgium	N		BMI<27 and body fat <25%
Denmark	N	-	N
Finland	N	-	N
France	N	-	N
Germany	-	-	<30% over weight
Iceland	N; unimpeded mobility & dexterity	-	N
Italy	N	-	N
The Netherlands	N	-	N
Spain	N	-	N
Sweden	N	>18	<20% over weight
United Kingdom	N; unimpeded mobility & dexterity. Must be robust	>18	N
EDTC-86	N	>18	<20% over weight

TABLE 15 - HOW OFTEN IS BONE X-RAY PERFORMED?

Belgium	Every 3 years (will be changed to a bone scintigraphy every 5 years)
Denmark	Not specified (only performed on sat divers and tunnel workers)
Finland	Only at start of profession
France	Every 4 years
Germany	Never
Iceland	Never
Italy	Every 3 years (sat divers only)
The Netherlands	Doctors decision
Spain	Only recommendation every 3 years
Sweden	Every 3-6 years in personnel working >20h/week at pressure
United Kingdom	Doctors decision
EDTC-86	Deep dive (>50m) and after DCI annually; <30m or <4h, no x-ray

Table 16 was compiled to find out how the doctors of EDTC judged and weighed the importance of different organ systems when investigating fitness to dive. The ranking is difficult because the approval for diving depends on all systems in interaction but, generally speaking, a low sum means that the organ system is more important. There was no surprise in the result: focus was on the pulmonary, the cardiovascular and the central nervous system.

TABLE 16 - IMPORTANT ORGAN SYSTEMS

	Pulm	Cardio	Neuro	ENT	Soma	Endocr	G-Int	Blood	Skin	Uro-G
Belgium	4	3	4	1	5	6	7	7	7	7
Denmark	3	2	3	4	7	5	6	7	7	7
Finland	3	2	3	7	4	7	7	7	5	7
France	1	2	4	3	6	7	7	5	7	7
Germany	7	2	7	3	4	7	5	7	7	6
Iceland	3	4	3	2	5	7	7	6	7	7
Italy	2	1	4	3	5	7	7	7	7	7
The Netherlands	1	3	2	4	5	7	7	7	7	7
Spain	2	5	1	4	7	3	7	7	7	7
Sweden	2	3	2	5	6	4	7	7	7	7
United Kingdom	2	3	2	5	7	4	7	7	7	7
Sum	14	30	36	41	61	64	74	74	75	76
Rank	1	2	3	4	5	6	6	6	9	10

CONCLUSION

Within the two extremes, no medical requirements at all for commercial diving (other than offshore) as in regulations recently issued in the Netherlands and, on the other hand, annual examinations including exercise tests with ECG and other specialist examinations, as in some other countries, there are no major differences in the details of fitness for diving medicals in Europe. The interval between medicals and the minimum performance requirement in specific tests could of course be discussed, but the main issue will always be the competence of the doctor who is responsible for the examination.

If the requirements on education and experience of these doctors are the same all over Europe the fitness to dive examinations will be harmonised automatically.

DISCUSSION

Elliott (Chairman): The actual question was "do the differences between diving medical standards have any justifiable basis?" and the answer to that appears to be "No, they are just different". Have you come across anything where you would say that there is a valid difference between different countries?

Örnhagen: Of course the statement that "no medical is necessary" is a difference that is of significance, but then when their blood pressure is 140 or 120 systolic, it doesn't really matter.

Elliott: Is there a justifiable difference, for instance, in testing for haemoglobinopathies between different countries?

Örnhagen: I do not know if the difference is justifiable but only the U.K. and Denmark mention HbS. Something that is not covered here is, maybe, a more important question "is there anything between the sexes that could be of interest, is there anything that has to be covered in the medical for the female diver that is not covered?" That is probably more important than the possible differences between medicals from Greece, Italy, Norway and Sweden.

IS HARMONISATION APPROPRIATE?
WOULD INTERNATIONAL RECOGNITION OF NATIONAL STANDARDS BE SUFFICIENT?
D.H. Elliott

As Chairman it is my task to highlight what the speakers have brought out so well. "Is harmonisation appropriate?" and there can only be one answer to that, "yes". Harmonisation is appropriate. It is also essential for divers who wish to dive in different countries. "Would international recognition of different national standards be sufficient?" and my answer to that, even as a temporary expedient, is "no".

With that very lengthy presentation against my name I will now open this up for discussion because many important principles have been raised and we are aiming for consensus.

DISCUSSION

Anderson-Upcott: I wondered if I could put forward a plea, not only for the standardisation which we are aiming at, but also for simplicity in the form of the examination. Proposed so far, we may have:

- varying examinations for different categories of persons who may dive in the wet or dry;
- varying examination frequencies with age;
- different categories of diving doctor.

If we become too complicated we risk the practicability of carrying out the regulations and perhaps compliance by the divers themselves who have to pay, often out of their own money being self-employed, for these already quite expensive examinations. My plea is, can we have a thought for the end product, that form that we have to fill in?

Örnhagen: The important principle could be to consider that, from the very beginning, all persons who are interested in diving are healthy. We should then specify which diseases could later jeopardise his/her performance or could put the diver into danger. When we have defined which diseases these are, we then have to define the means of how we can assess them, even if the diver is not telling us the truth. If we can keep this simple, we can eliminate a lot of fancy and expensive examinations for the normal diver.

In Sweden we have taken the decision that one only needs a good medical examination when one starts diving. If the candidate is young then, over the next coming 5 years, there is no real reason to suspect that anything should seriously affect his or her health unless there is some specific disease, like pneumonia, in which case there should be another medical. There is no real reason, as I see it, to have annual medicals for young, fit healthy men or women.

Elliott (Chairman): Indeed, that is an important approach for discussion. The point you began from is perhaps the basic point I put forward originally: that diving should be open to "perfect specimens only". However, we must be careful because, in this modern world, one must not restrict the freedom of people to enter the employment of their choice. One must have good evidence, if a person is not a "perfect specimen", that the particular imperfection is relevant to safety in the water. So we should focus first on the standards of initial entry into diving.

Would we have consensus that the initial standard for diving safety should be the same for all categories of diving and should be the same internationally? *(Pause)*

Having agreed the initial examination then, as Hans has just suggested, instead of doing frequent examinations to measure this and to measure that, we should be considering whether this diver, who has embarked upon his career at great expense, has now acquired something which makes it imperative that he or she be stopped? We should be looking for those indications which, during his career, make us stop a person from diving. That is quite a different approach to fitness to dive from the traditional concept of pass/fail criteria which we have been using in the past. I would welcome debate and discussion.

Örnhagen: My approach does not cover the surveillance for long-term health effects; that has to be a separate issue.

Griffin: As far as I understand what you are saying to suggest that the standards ought to be the same for all kinds of diving, do you mean that someone who wants to go out and teach diving at the weekend should have the same basic requirements as someone who's going to be isolated in a saturation chamber for a month?

Elliott: For the safety of working divers that would be the implication. You obviously have a problem with this, would you like to be more specific?

Griffin: That does seem to eliminate a lot of people, who could be very effective instructors, for conditions that really are not going to impinge on their employability as instructors of diving.

Elliott: Well, that is UK law at the moment. Anybody who dives for reward is a "diver at work" and that applies to the saturation diver and it also applies to the professional instructor of scuba divers. The Chairman of the BSAC Medical Committee is at this meeting and may like to comment. The phrase "for reward", I understand, includes getting travel expenses which means that an amateur diver teaching others in return for travel expenses is a working diver. Donald Lamont (HSE) said quite firmly at last year's meeting of the Society of Underwater Technology that, for this category of diver (the HSE part IV diver), concessions may be made as to how they dive and in the procedures they use, but there are no concessions nor dispensations from the medical standards.

Griffin: I work as a dive instructor in Canada having got the qualification in the United States, and there is no requirement to be examined by a physician.

Elliott: Well, that demonstrates a basic difference between Europe and North America.

Griffin: What I'm saying is that half of the instructors would be unfit.

Elliott: Can I ask you a question? Do you not think then, when one is considering a professional instructor of recreational divers, who is a person who has a safety responsibility for his or her pupils in the water, that he or she needs to be as fit as any other diver?

Griffin: In order to be able to become insured as an instructor in Canada there are medical forms that have to be filled out with the questionnaire that the diver himself fills out, and a lot of times they misinterpret what the questionnaire means. The point is that, if somebody has been teaching scuba diving for fifteen years and has not had any problem, and I was to say to them "you are medically unfit", they are going to say to me that "well I have got fifteen years of proof that I am fit for what I do". I just offer this to you, because the people in North America would be aghast at this whole concept.

Botheroyd: Could I just say that it is open to Approved Doctors, when making their decision on fitness and what sort of certificate they are going to issue, to make a limitation on the type of diving which the diver will be permitted to do. If he feels that the diver is only fit to undertake say pool diving or pool instruction, or whatever, he can impose that sort of restriction on the certificates. So there is scope there for some variation. Similarly, when the HSE conducts a review on appeal for a diver found unfit, it is open to us also to issue a restricted certificate which would limit the type of diving to which the diver was permitted to work.

Elliott: I see that restriction as something which is applied to an individual who may have lost a foot, or one eye, and therefore would not comply with specific MA1 requirements. The HSE dispensation does not apply to a whole sector of the diving fraternity, such as the diving scientists, the police divers or the sports diving instructors. Those categories of divers in general must attain the standards recommended. Is that correct?

Botheroyd: That's correct. The generality of those groups are subject to the identical requirements.

Elliott: The response therefore to Dr. Griffin who has just raised that important issue, is that the medical standard applies within the UK to all categories of working diver. I think that that is also the way that Europe will go but there is, certainly in the UK, scope for individual dispensation on a one-off basis.

Mebane: Just a comment on the requirements for physical examination for amateur instructors in the United States. There is an organisation called the RSTC which is a consortium of the training agencies and others and they do set standards. I will read: "For instructors, minimum medical examination: the individual shall have a current medical examination and approval for diving by a licensed physician as required by the certified training organisation prior to engaging in scuba water skills". So from dive-master up in the United States, a physical medical examination is required.

Elliott: An examination is required, that is good, but to what standard? I can quote a doctor, who used to be in the HSE, who said "I have my office on the first floor and providing the diver can climb the stairs, he must be fit". To what extent are these examinations detailed?

Mebane: I have the form and if necessary we can review it later *(see page 50)*.

Le-Dez: I recently examined a diver in Canada who wanted to become a professional diving instructor, and he was an experienced sports diver. I found his pulmonary function test came in at somewhere between 20 and 30% of normal and that alarmed me a great deal. The fact is that, in Canada and the United States, divers just taking up sports diving are not required to meet any medical standard. In contrast to my Canadian colleague I would say that I think they ought to be. Many who become sports divers then go into professional sports diving instruction. I think that there are many sports divers, when examined later, who would certainly come in that range that should be excluded.

Could I also ask a question relating to scientific divers, because there's a lot of diving sponsored by University institutions where they are diving not strictly for reward, but in pursuit of their research projects. My own University and other academic institutions are facing this question of what standards should be required in these people? How do you see that fitting in?

Elliott: They are required to fit in to the same medical requirements.

Musgrave: I would like to emphasise the filthy environment that some of our divers have to work in, particularly police divers. Would there be time in this conference to look at the question of immunisation status for divers or is it perhaps something for the HSE to consider at a later time?

Galway: With reference to the frequency of diving medicals, I think that some divers can be lazy. If it is at anything other than annual, I suspect that a lot of divers will put off the effort of remaining physically fit until they have to come up for the next medical, by which time they cannot easily get fit again.

Zachariedes: We all agree that the main difference must be between the commercial diver and the amateur. The difference between the Northern and Southern countries of Europe is due to only one element - oil. You have all these regulations in Britain, Norway and Sweden, because 80% of your diving activity is commercial diving activity. In the Mediterranean countries 90% of the diving activity is for pleasure. Our problem, and I think all my colleagues from the Mediterranean countries will agree, is not what to examine for someone to be a diver, our problem is how we persuade our governments to have any rules for someone to become a diver. For example that means to have some guidelines so that before you enter the diving school, you must, for the first time, get a proper medical examination. I think that this is simple, we don't have to dispute about the blood pressure or the ECG or the spirometry and all those other things. We must agree that there must be regulations from the government to require divers to go to the doctor. It is not the examination *per se*.

Örnhagen: The data that I presented here was regarding professional divers. The sports divers usually have their own regulations and there are many such organisations. It would be difficult to persuade the different governments to interfere with this when it is just a sports activity.

Glanvill: I agree with John Galway's comments about the frequency of medical examinations as many divers seem to get very casual about their physical fitness throughout the rest of the year.

I also wish to comment that it seems a paradox that we do a fairly extensive medical every year and the results of this medical are kept in our own record files. There is no adequate way that the records can follow the divers around. I am sure that there are many divers of marginal health who shop around and, with the anticipated increase of movement of individuals across national boundaries, this will become an increasing problem. It's all very well having standards, but you need to have some way of making sure that they are not being abused.

Ramaswami: I thought that I should quote from the regulations about who is actually covered by the Diving at Work Regulations. It is all employed or self-employed divers except those:

(a) who use submersible chambers or craft or pressure-resisting diving suits in which they are not exposed to a pressure exceeding 300 millibars above atmospheric pressure during normal operations;

(b) those who use no underwater breathing apparatus and members of the armed forces employed on military diving operations.

All others are covered.

Elliott: That is likely to be standard within Europe.

Minsaas: Dr. Watt mentioned the rarity of finding anything on the annual medical examination, and that is good news. Finding conformance with regulations, finding that people are normal, is a very important reason for doing preventive examinations. Sports diving, is the most complicated issue and that is where people die. We have a requirement in Norway that, if you dive for money, then you are covered by the regulations, but if you dive entirely in your free time and are not paid for it, we have no way of making any requirement.

Elliott: The sports diver will be the focus of Dr. Marroni's session later.

COMMENTARY

The meeting in Edinburgh was a milestone in the review and potential harmonisation of medical standards for diving in Europe. As mentioned in the Preface, this meeting did not occur in isolation and it is possible to draw some conclusions at the end of each major section which can also take into account some of the discussions at the subsequent EDTC workshop in Luxembourg. Given that the Edinburgh proceedings have been transcribed verbatim from video and audio recordings and sent to the speakers for checking, this selective summary and additional commentary by the Editor does not affect the integrity of the Edinburgh conclusions but may serve to amplify them. The following should, however, be regarded as a personal interpretation. It is intended to reflect the consensus view but should not necessarily be construed as representing the views of the sponsors or the participants.

The need for medical examinations

There was consensus that the medical examinations of divers are essential because they can reveal conditions which are incompatible with safety in the water. Not only are these and other conditions hazardous to the individual diver but, when an incident occurs, the circumstances could well put companion divers at risk. Once in-water safety has been satisfied then the effects of diving on health can be considered.

The selection of fitness criteria

The examination needs to focus upon the in-water safety of the diver and, unless requested, need not consider additional fitness standards that might relate to the vocational requirements of a particular occupation, such as the eyesight of divers also required to drive boats at night.

Some medical standards for in-water diver safety should also be related to activities in the bell and at the surface. These include, for example, the ability to tend another diver with a lifeline, and the ability to respond to aural and visual stimuli.

There is little scientific evidence to validate the fitness standards which are used to assess divers. The majority were originally derived from extensive military experience, guided by clinical judgement and anecdote. They do not rest upon documented data, largely because of the obvious ethical difficulty of any controlled experiment to test fitness criteria.

The view was expressed that some, but not all, of the current routine examination is of "low yield" and unlikely to demonstrate anything of relevance to diving safety, particularly in the younger age range of divers. This is reviewed in later sessions.

Using the qualitative criteria of the guidelines, an examining doctor must assess the fitness of an individual in relation to the hazards and demands of the job, but there is a lack of functional targets for what may be required from a diver in the water. For example, any diver may need to call upon all his reserves of effort in a life-threatening emergency. The required duration for that emergency effort is unpredictable and this makes it difficult to specify a required level of physical fitness. When functional goals can be defined, these should be independent of age and gender and yet allow for the fact that the experience of older divers may make them more effective functionally than fitter younger divers.

There was consensus that, in the provision of appropriate health and safety measures for the diver, there is also a need to monitor the effects of the occupation of diving upon the continuation of the individual's good health.

Different categories of diver

It was generally agreed that all candidates for diving training should meet identical standards of fitness.

For those components of the medical examination which relate to in-water safety, there is no justification in having different standards for different categories of diving.

In particular, the conclusion was reached that there could be no lesser standard of safety in the medical assessment of the instructors of recreational divers. Indeed, a view was expressed that, based upon their responsibilities for novice divers, there is an ethical requirement for the amateur instructors to attain the same medical safety standards as those demanded of the professional instructors.

For the criteria of fitness that relate only to health, it is reasonable to have, for saturation diving, a different standard from that for the other categories of diving. This is because there is a need to consider disorders which, though compatible with in-water safety, may require the person to have access to treatment at short notice. In saturation diving the patient can be isolated by the need for a decompression which extends over several days. If otherwise fit, such persons could be excluded from saturation but made fit for the other types of diving.

Effects of age

After the initial examination at entry, there are some components of the examination that need not be repeated regularly during the early years of a career. Indeed, in some European countries, no further medical examination is required until after several more years. On the other hand, as the years pass by, so some additional investigations may need to be introduced and possibly repeated at an increasing frequency.

There was no argument with the statement that, providing all the medical standards can be met, there is no upper age limit for divers.

RECREATIONAL DIVING

Chairmen : Dr. A. Marroni & Dr. N.K.I. McIver

INTRODUCTION
Dr. N.K.I. McIver

IS DIVING FOR YOU?

"There is an element of risk inherent in diving as in other adventure sports, but this is reduced to acceptable limits by the observation of basic safety disciplines ... and sound training".

So states the British Sub Aqua Club Diving Manual (1985) and it is the purpose of this evening to look at the medical aspects of that fundamental principle.

DAN Europe has assembled a notable group of international experts who will discuss, among other things:

- the novice diver
- the asthmatic diver
- the diabetic diver
- the physically handicapped diver
- the over 40 year old diver

RECREATIONAL DIVING SAFETY
Dr. A. Marroni

Our aim is to consider what is the real risk of recreational diving and secondly, using the figures derived from the DAN Europe network, to look at the possibility of common standards for the fitness of recreational divers. The recreational diver is a travelling diver which emphasises the need for this international approach.

The Divers Alert Network (DAN), a membership-supported non-profit organisation based at the Duke University Medical Center in Durham, North Carolina, was founded in 1980, under the guidance of Professor Peter B. Bennett. One year later, IDA - International Diving Assistance - also a membership supported non-profit organisation, was founded by me in Italy. In 1984 the Diver Emergency Service (DES) was started in Australia and New Zealand by Drs. Des Gorman and "Fred" Gilligan and in 1987 the Civil Alert Network (CAN) began assisting diving emergencies in Japan, under the guidance of Professor Yoshihiro Mano of the University of Tokyo Medical School.

Although independent and not yet collaborating, the four organisations were supporting diving safety by providing very similar 24-hour Diving Emergency Hotlines and non-emergency Diving Medicine Information Services. In case of a diving accident, qualified hyperbaric and diving medicine specialists would be available to assist the injured diver and to consult with local emergency medical personnel to co-ordinate medical evacuation and treatment and to provide the best care possible. Other important objectives were also pursued by the four organisations in very similar ways and with similar results, such as the regular collection of recreational diving accident data and the elaboration of periodical statistical reports on recreational diving accidents.

The need for an international organisation that would be available to all divers, wherever they dived around the world, became increasingly apparent and, during a meeting at DAN Headquarters in the U.S.A., in 1991, the process of forming an International DAN was started. DAN Europe, DES/DAN Australia and DAN Japan became parts of the INTERNATIONAL DAN (IDAN) organisation, together with DAN U.S.A.

Today the International DAN is a worldwide network of multi-lingual 24-hour diving emergency centres, over 300 hyperbaric facilities and many diving-hyperbaric specialists to treat diving emergencies and to accept diving medicine referrals. Every year the DAN "Hotlines" respond to more than 1000 diving emergency calls and to over 12,000 medical and safety questions. Over 100,000 DAN members around the world have access to the same unlimited emergency medical evacuation service and to insurance covered medical-hyperbaric treatment worldwide, as well as to diving safety information and diving medicine training programs.

Alert Diver, DAN's bi-monthly magazine in the U.S.A., and its regional versions in Europe and Japan, regularly convey essential diving safety information to the thousands of DAN members in the world. Recently, the introduction of the *"Oxygen First Aid in Dive Accidents"* training program, which is now taught by over 1,000 DAN Oxygen Instructors worldwide, further contributed to the improvement of effective first aid procedures for diving accidents. DAN promoted an international diving accident evaluation protocol and regularly publishes annual reports on recreational diving accidents. Finally DAN started a prospective dive profile/bubble production research project which will involve International DAN members, diving instructors, diving doctors and the diving equipment industry.

RECREATIONAL DIVING ACCIDENTS AND RECOMMENDED MANAGEMENT

Although not very common, decompression diving accidents do occur in recreational diving. The incidence of decompression illness (DCI) in the population of DAN Europe Members from 1989 until 1993 has been 1 case of DCI in every 6,604 dive exposures (0.015%) and of 1 bent diver out of 264 divers (0.38%); these data match well with the ones reported by the international literature (Refs. 1 - 9). Interestingly, if diving stress is reduced by diving to less than 30 metres and within the no-decompression limits, the incidence of DCI cases among the DAN Europe population from 1989 to 1993 has been of 1 case over 40,227 dive-exposures, thus corroborating the internationally shared opinion that the major and most recurrent DCI risk factors are deep and prolonged dives.

When a diving accident occurs, immediate treatment is essential to obtain a satisfactory clinical outcome without significant sequelae, but DAN's statistics show that the delay to call for assistance and, consequently, the delay to treatment, is rarely less than 4 hours and exceeds 12 hours in almost 50% of cases of recreational diving DCI (Refs. 3 - 11).

It has been demonstrated by Wolkiewiez *et al* (Ref. 12) that a protocol for medically assisted transportation of decompression accidents to the hyperbaric facility could improve the success of hyperbaric treatment and the overall clinical outcome by over 70% and the use of 100% oxygen and fluid therapy is now a widely recommended practice in the first aid of decompression accidents. DAN recommends that all divers know how to provide adequate oxygen first aid in a decompression accident and recently introduced the *Oxygen First Aid in Dive Accidents* program, to train divers to recognise decompression diving accidents and to provide 100% oxygen first aid, while activating the local emergency medical services or DAN (Refs. 11 - 13). Since the inception of the program in 1992, the use of oxygen in the first aid of dive accidents reported to DAN increased from less than 18% to more than 37%, with very satisfactory results. Anecdotally, twelve cases of DCI with neurological involvement, one of which was a case of gas embolism, were assisted by European DAN Oxygen Instructors in 1993; in 7 cases the response to oxygen first aid was so good that no further recompression treatment was considered necessary after transportation to the hyperbaric center. Immediate administration of oxygen and fluids is routinely recommended by the emergency operators of the DAN Hotlines, both to divers and to local EMS personnel, as one of the first actions to take in the management of a diving emergency.

DAN publications and guidelines for optimal management of diving emergencies are available and regularly circulated among the recreational diving and the diving medical communities. DAN operates through an international network of Diving Emergency Hotlines, staffed by specially trained emergency operators and backed-up by a network of Diving-Hyperbaric Specialists on call. Diving Accident management and data collection criteria are standardised and a list of over 300 hyperbaric centers and of many diving-hyperbaric medicine specialists is regularly controlled and updated by the International DAN organisations worldwide.

The four main DAN Hotlines are in Australia at the Royal Adelaide Hospital, in Europe at the REGA Foundation in Zurich (REGA is a corporate member of the International Red Cross), in Japan at the Tokyo University Medical School and in the U.S.A. at the Duke University Medical Center in Durham, North Carolina.

Due to the many languages and nationalities in Europe, a network of regional alarm centres is active in Germany, Italy, Malta, Spain and Switzerland with DAN Europe National Hotlines and in France, Holland and Scandinavia with specific alarm centres.

In the recreational diving world today, DAN is not only an important service for divers, but also for the medical community and for the emergency medical services personnel, who often refer to DAN for consultation about the management of a relatively infrequent and unusual kind of emergency.

When any of the DAN Hotlines is called concerning a diving accident, qualified Hyperbaric and Diving Medicine Specialists are immediately available to assist the injured diver, to consult with local emergency medical personnel, to co-ordinate medical evacuation and treatment and to provide the best care possible, wherever the diving accident occurred around the world.

In order to assure adequate and timely assistance, especially when emergencies occur in remote areas of the world, DAN co-operates with SOS Assistance/Assist America and with some of the leading insurance companies in the world, to provide every DAN member with a global assistance plan, including unlimited evacuation or repatriation and insured medical/hyperbaric treatment. By simply calling one of the international DAN Hotlines and Alarm Centres, any DAN member will access the DAN network being entitled to the same emergency assistance anywhere in the world.

DAN'S DIVING SAFETY RESEARCH PROGRAMS

From the very beginning, DAN's activity focused on research projects that would improve the safety of recreational diving.

With time the annual reports on diving accidents and the many papers published by DAN became the classic references for reliable statistical evaluation of the risk connected to recreational diving. Relatively new risk factors, such as multi-day repetitive diving, were demonstrated with statistically significant evidence, while more commonly known risk factors, such as deep diving, decompression diving, age, etc. were corroborated with statistically reliable data.

DAN Europe is now starting a new prospective double blind study on the safety of diving. The scope is to evaluate the safety of unrestricted normal recreational diving activity. Other goals are to compare the performance of different dive tables and dive computers with respect to real time/depth exposure and to the actual/estimated bubble production ratio. The study will involve standard recreational divers as well as professional scuba instructors and dive masters.

The dive profiles will be recorded with dive computer-recorders, provided by a major European dive computer company. The instrument will act as a diver's "black box" and be carried in a way that the diver will not be able to look at it (to avoid influencing the dive profile). The diver will be stimulated to follow a profile according to personal plans or preference, without any restriction. After the dives, the recorded data will be unloaded into a PC for subsequent analysis by a "blinded" team. At the end of the dive, as the only imposed procedure, the divers will be examined for clinical signs and symptoms and monitored with a precordial ultrasound Doppler probe, over a period of 40 minutes after surfacing. All clinical data and Doppler tapes will be saved for subsequent evaluation by a second "blinded" team.

Finally, the dive and clinical records will be examined and correlated, after recalling the dive profiles with the appropriate Doppler recordings and clinical files. The study will start in 1994 and will take place during a series of DAN-sponsored research trips and research weekends over an estimated period of three years.

REFERENCES

1. Marroni, A. Diving Habits and Diving Accidents in a Recreational Diving Population in Italy. *Proceedings of the XVIII Annual Meeting of the EUBS.* Basel 1992, page 197.

2. Cali-Corleo, R. Analysis of Diving and Diving Related Illness in Maltese Registered Divers during the period 1979-1991. *Proceedings of the XVIII Annual Meeting of the EUBS.* Basel 1992 page 45.

3. *DAN Report on 1987 Diving Accidents.* Divers Alert Network, Durham 1988.

4. *DAN Report on 1988 Diving Accidents.* Divers Alert Network, Durham 1989.

5. *DAN 1989 Report on Diving Accidents and Fatalities.* Divers Alert Network, Durham 1990.

6. *DAN 1990 Report on Diving Accidents and Fatalities.* Divers Alert Network, Durham 1991.

7. Bennett, P.B. DAN, Sports Diving Accidents and Deaths in the U.S.A. First DAN Europe Workshop. Proceedings of the III European Conference on Hyperbaric Medicine. *Acta Anesth. Italica,* suppl. 2/91, 1991; **42**: 119.

8. Marroni, A. Le emergenze subacquee trattate dal DAN Europe nel 1990. *Seminario DAN Europe sul primi intevento nella Malattia da Decompressione dell'immersione sportiva.* DAN Europe Publisher, 1991.

9. Marroni, A. Chiamate d'emergenza alla centrale DAN Europe nel 1991, valutazoni statistiche ed epidemiologiche. *DAN Europe News* 1992; **1**(1): 4.

10. Marroni, A., Catalucci, G. et al. Some observations on 551 cases of sport diving decompression sickness treated in Italy during the period 1978-1983. *Proceedings of the XII Annual Meeting of the EUBS.* Palermo 1987.

11. Marroni, A. Il protocollo DAN per la gestione sul campo delle emergenze da decompressione nell'immersione sportiva. In: *The Realm of Hyperbaric Therapy,* E.M. Camporesi, G. Vezzani and A. Pizzola (Eds). Dept. of Anesthesiology, SUNY Health Science Center at Syracuse, 1992.

12. Wolkiewiez, J. Bilan de 10 ans d'evacuation sous rèanimation mèdicale d'accidentès de plongèe. *CR Journèes Mèdicine de la Plongèe,* EASM-CERB Ed. Toulon Naval 1983: **38**.

13. *DAN Underwater Diving Accident Manual,* Divers Alert Network U.S.A. and Europe, 1991-1992.

SPECIAL MEDICAL PROBLEMS IN RECREATIONAL DIVERS : DIABETES
Dr. R. Cali-Corleo

It is the opinion of most diving physicians that diabetics on insulin or oral medication should not dive.

The present recommendation is that only diabetics who are well controlled on weight loss and dietary programmes should be permitted to dive.

The reasons for this recommendation are:

1. **Risk of hypo/hyperglycaemia:** Any alteration of the level of consciousness during a dive will put the diver at risk of drowning and also puts his buddy diver at risk.

2. **Insulin reaction:** This usually occurs in diabetics who have stopped and restarted their insulin or have changed brand. Sometimes production batch changes in the same proprietary preparation can be enough to provoke a reaction. Although this reaction is uncommon, the rapid onset and resulting impairment of judgement associated with such a reaction makes it a risk not to be ignored.

3. **Sudden death:** The earlier onset of atherosclerosis puts them at greater risk of sudden death due to an acute ischaemic episode or ventricular fibrillation during a dive than a non diabetic diver of the same age.

4. **Increased risk of decompression sickness:** The generalised small vessel disease found in diabetics alters peripheral perfusion and thus gas exchange, also the hyperviscosity and abnormal platelet aggregation (probably due to increased prostaglandin synthesis) found in diabetics will affect blood flow as well.

5. **Electrolytes:** Some diabetics also suffer hyperkalaemia due to the reduced renal secretion (from reduced aldosterone production caused by low plasma renin and hypoaldosteronism).

6. **Assessment of DCS:** Any diabetic neuropathy present, especially if undiagnosed before, may cause difficulty in assessing a suspected case of neurological decompression illness.

In most countries there are no laws or regulations prohibiting a sports diver continuing to dive against medical advice, however the examining doctor must fully document his findings and recommendations to protect himself against future legal problems.

In Malta sport diving is regulated and no diabetic on medication is permitted to dive. Any diabetic on diet and exercise only must be found free of glycosuria and with an acceptable blood sugar during the medical examination.

Diabetics may try to influence their doctor telling him that some world class athletes are diabetics and practice their sport successfully, however their doctor should try to convince them that any malaise happening while underwater may prove fatal.

SPECIAL MEDICAL PROBLEMS IN RECREATIONAL DIVERS :
THE DIVER OVER THE AGE OF 40
Dr. R. Cali-Corleo

There are no formal age limitations on the sport diver as there are on the commercial and military diver. Recent findings have indicated that divers over 40 years are more liable to serious medical problems when carrying out recreational diving. Research by Divers Alert Network has shown that there is a significantly higher morbidity and mortality in the "40 and over" diver age group than in the "under 40" group; in particular it has shown that there is a significantly higher incidence of decompression sickness (DCS) in the "40 and over" group.

In assessing a diver candidate it is important to determine the physiological age rather than the chronological age, however there are a number of conditions which although present in the older diver can be completely asymptomatic. These conditions include:

1. **Ischaemic heart disease:** Coronary artery stenosis starts at an early age but the stenosis will only become apparent when the peripheral coronary vascular bed can no longer compensate to ensure the normal coronary blood flow response to an increased work load. In fact the arterial resistance has been shown to remain nearly stable until the reduction in cross-sectional area reaches 75%.

   Rest studies may not demonstrate a significant lesion and the patient may be asymptomatic even on moderate exercise. With increased work there is usually only a small increase in oxygen extraction but there is a large increase in myocardial blood flow to match the increased oxygen needs of the myocardium. The imbalance between myocardial oxygen supply and demand when diving may cause myocardial infarction, ventricular fibrillation or a local/global reduction of contractile capability resulting in heart failure. The primary ventricular fibrillation in these asymptomatic individuals can result in sudden death. The vasotonic response to exercise and cold stress (catecholamine release causing coronary spasm) will worsen the ischaemia.

   Exercise stress testing with electrocardiographic and blood pressure monitoring in divers over 40 will help identify individuals at risk. However absolute certainty of the preventive and prognostic value of this type of testing is not possible and so a negative finding is not a guarantee of fitness to dive.

2. **Hypertension:** This is the most common illness in adults today and if untreated can cause coronary illness or strokes, treatment is for life. Hypertension causes a chronic overload on the heart which induces hypertrophy of the myocardium. This affects myocardial oxygen consumption, myocardial blood flow and blood flow distribution.

   All antihypertensive medication can cause physiological alterations and important variations in the individual's response to physical exercise and immersion. This inhibition of normal control mechanisms of cardiovascular function can result in reduced exercise tolerance, syncope and rapid onset of generalised weakness after exercise. The practice of stopping anti-hypertensive medication before a bout of diving is inadvisable because of "rebound".

In recreational diving any blood pressure more than 150/90 in a person on low dose diuretics should be considered a contraindication. Candidates should be encouraged to lose weight and improve physical condition as this often will result in a reduction in blood pressure sufficient to permit approval for diving.

3. **Increased airway resistance:** Diving increases the work of breathing due to the rise in gas density, the reduction in lung volume and airway diameter by the hydrostatic effect on the chest, and the resistance to breathing by the diving respirator used.

    Twenty per cent of smoking adults have some degree of chronic bronchitis and emphysema, often without recognised dysfunction. The increased airway resistance normal in diving when added to the bronchoconstriction and retention of sputum found in smokers with early chronic bronchitis may increase the risk of air trapping and gas embolism.

    Plain chest x-ray and basic lung function tests (e.g. spirometry) will assist in identifying individuals at risk although certain persons may have to be referred to a lung function laboratory for more specific tests. Again, even with these tests, it is not possible to be absolutely sure that there are no lung areas with raised ventilatory resistance in the young candidate and even more so in the "over 40". The ability of pulmonary function tests to identify minimal and very localised dysfunctions is doubtful. It is these minor dysfunctions which may have an important role in the higher incidence of decompression illness (DCI) in the "over 40" group.

4. **Physical condition:** The capacity to deal with exercise stress decreases with age, this is mainly because of lack of exercise. Regular exercise and training will help maintain good physical condition and there is no reason why a fit individual cannot carry on diving well into their 80's.

    One must take greater care when assessing a new diving candidate than an individual who has been diving regularly for many years.

    Peripheral vascular resistance increases with age due to reduced muscle mass and reduction of the microvascular channels in the peripheral muscular bed which potentially increases the chances of DCI. There is minimal reduction in myocardial contractile performance with age and in a fit individual maximal work capacity is only moderately decreased. Also, elderly divers show an increase in unventilated lung compartments even in the absence of chronic illness, and so they will suffer greater physical stress for the same task.

5. **Metabolic changes:** Changes include reduced thyroid activity with resulting increased sensitivity to cold and reduced response to stress which must be taken into consideration by the individual but should not affect diving as long as hypothermia is avoided. There is also an increased risk of glucose intolerance as one gets older and monitoring for this condition is recommended.

In Malta there are no upper age limits in the sports diving regulations and all that is required is that the diver is physically and mentally capable of coping with the stress involved in diving.

SPECIAL MEDICAL PROBLEMS IN RECREATIONAL DIVERS : THE NOVICE DIVER
Dr. J. Desola

In order to determine the medical fitness of a novice diver, careful medical assessment is needed. Some aspects are mandatory, others are needed in only some special situations, depending on the medical criteria. A third group of investigations are only recommendations and not mandatory.

MANDATORY

- history (anamnesis)
- complete physical examination
- chest x-ray
- spirometry
- ENT examination

OPTIONAL INVESTIGATIONS

They will be done only in selected cases as a result of the first mandatory part of the assessment :

- sinus x-ray
- electroencephalogram
- electrocardiogram

RECOMMENDED INVESTIGATIONS

These are not strictly necessary but it is good to do them as appropriate and if the diver agrees, in order to enhance information and, in some cases, to provide a baseline for future possible problems:

- audiometry
- impediometry
- exercise test
- blood analysis
- compression test
- oxygen tolerance test

As a result of these investigations, medical assessment for fitness may lead to temporary or permanent restrictions, or to absolute unfitness.

RELATIVE AND TEMPORARY RESTRICTIONS

The diver is unfit until any of the following disorders are resolved:

- ENT disorders
- acute airway disorders
- dental caries

RELATIVE RESTRICTIONS

There are physical alterations which are not by themselves a formal cause of unfitness, but which will need to be controlled because they can become a cause of unfitness:

- arterial hypertension
- pleural disorders
- asthma
- diabetes
- mild cardiac disorders

ABSOLUTE CAUSES OF UNFITNESS

The diver is, and will always be, unfit to dive due to:

- spontaneous pneumothorax
- epilepsy and other CNS diseases that can produce seizures or loss of consciousness

SPECIAL MEDICAL PROBLEMS IN RECREATIONAL DIVERS : THE PHYSICALLY HANDICAPPED
Dr. J. Desola

Witnessing a film of a paraplegic diver continuing to dive raises an important question : how do we allow a seriously bent diver to dive again and what is the real risk? Is there a recurrence rate that is statistically significant?

Diving should not be recommended for a newly handicapped person who was not previously a diver, but it can however be accepted in some cases. If the handicapped individual is a diver already, he or she will learn more easily a new technique for diving, and water sports can offer some benefits for the handicapped.

If the deficiency is in the upper limbs the diver will have good mobility underwater, but he will need special help to enter and leave the water, to enter the boat, and with equipment. A deficiency in the lower limbs will make underwater movement difficult but the diver probably will manage the equipment better, and to enter the boat on surfacing.

Considerations in such cases would be:

- no ENT, CNS or respiratory causes of unfitness

- good functional capacity of at least two limbs (both upper ones, both lower ones, or one upper plus one lower)

- good mouth control and ability to hold a regulator

- completion of specialised training

- diving to be allowed only in optimal sea and weather conditions

- only inland diving or when support boats are available

- presence of specially trained buddy is mandatory

We conclude that a trained diver who suffers a serious handicap can dive again after appropriate special training and, in these circumstances, diving may be very good for him or her. However, to teach diving to a handicapped person who has never dived before is also possible, but this is a more serious decision that must be taken carefully.

RECREATIONAL DIVING MEDICAL STANDARDS : DAN IN THE UNITED STATES
Dr. Y.G. Mebane

Divers Alert Network (DAN), a non-profit organisation, exists to provide expert information and advice for the benefit of the diving public. DAN's historical and primary function is to provide emergency medical advice and assistance for underwater diving accidents, to work to prevent accidents, and to promote diving safety.

Second, DAN promotes and supports underwater diving research and education particularly as it relates to the improvement of diving safety, medical treatment, and first aid.

Third, DAN strives to provide the most accurate, up-to-date and unbiased information on issues of common concern to the diving public, primarily but not exclusively, for diving safety.

DAN does not issue diving certifications of any kind nor does it attempt to establish standards of performance. DAN interprets and reports the diving medical literature to the diving public, avoiding bias and personal views to the greatest extent possible. The following position papers are presented on that basis and in our opinion represent the current consensus of diving medicine as practiced in the United States.

THE NOVICE DIVER

The definition of "novice diver" is somewhat elusive but might include student divers, divers making their first few dives after certification or those divers who complete less than 18-20 dives in two years following certification. Recently certified divers trained by a United States agency have met minimum requirements established by the Recreational Scuba Training Council (RSTC) plus additional requirements which may have been added by the agency.

The minimum RSTC standards for certification are the following:

1. **Age:**

    (a) 15 minimum
    (b) no upper limit

2. **Physical fitness and watermanship:**

    (a) continuous 200 yard surface distance swim
    (b) 10 minutes survival swim/float
    (c) without use of mask, fins, snorkel

3. **Medical history:**

    (a) "Out of ordinary medical history" (sic) *advised* to have licensed physician certification before scuba water skills portion of course.

4. **Knowledge-entry level:**

   (a) equipment
   (b) physics of diving
   (c) medical problems related to diving
   (d) pool/confined water scuba skills
   (e) use of diving tables
   (f) diving environment
   (g) general information
   (h) open-water training/scuba skills

The diver who completes this training is certified as an open water diver. A small amount of further training and experience may qualify the diver as an advanced diver. Although the terms are similar, the requirements vary considerably among the various agencies. The certification term, i.e. "advanced" may imply more skills than the diver actually possesses.

During 1992 there were 96 scuba deaths involving United States citizens reported to DAN. The certification levels of 74 of the deaths were known to DAN. Twenty-one of the 75 deaths (28%) occurred to divers at the novice level. The twenty-one deaths were distributed as follows. Five deaths occurred during training exercises, five deaths occurred in divers with less than five dives, and eleven deaths occurred in divers with 5-20 dives.

There was a similar distribution for decompression illness. DAN reported 465 DCI incidents in 1992 and 178 (38.3%) incidents involved student or inexperienced divers.

Certainly, thousands of new and inexperienced divers perform dives safely and well. However, the new diver does appear to be at increased risk for DCI or a fatal accident.

ASTHMA

At present the recreational scuba diver candidate with asthma is frequently denied training by United States training organisations. This denial results from the consensus of the majority of diving physicians who regard the presence of asthma as a contraindication to diving. The Recreational Scuba Diving Council lists asthma as a "relative contraindication" in their *Guidelines for Recreational Scuba Diver's Physical Examination (RSTC, 1986)*. The diver instructor usually refers a student candidate with a history of asthma to a physician for an opinion as to his medical fitness for diving. The physician is not required to have any knowledge concerning the physiology of diving, but receives a copy of the Guidelines which provides a list of disorders and a brief explanation. If the student, instructor and physician all agree that the student is fit, then the student will be accepted into the course.

Individuals with asthma quickly learn the method of evading restrictions on dive training and do become divers. It is not possible to estimate the number of asthmatic divers.

The physician charged with the evaluation of the asthmatic diver has difficulty because of the elusive nature of the diagnosis. Asthma is not a distinct entity. Asthma is a disorder characterised by increased responsiveness of the airways (hyper-reactivity) to various stimuli and by resultant smooth muscle contraction and obstruction. Asthma, manifested by cough, shortness of breath, wheezing, and exercise intolerance, results from acute airway hyper-reactivity and chronic inflammation. This response represents a spectrum from normal through mild and moderate to severe hyper-reactivity. The disease spectrum includes the individual with only episodic cough or wheeze; the individual with intermittent asthma with or without an identifiable cause; exercise-induced asthma; and persistent or chronic asthma. There are perhaps millions of people with mild asthma who require little or no treatment and frequently self-medicate themselves with inhaled epinephrine or similar agents. These individuals however do have asthma. At the other end of the disease spectrum are the persistent or chronic asthmatics who require chronic medical suppression to control their disease.

It may be possible to distinguish clinically between bronchial hyper-reactivity which is stable, and specific allergen mediated response which is labile. In a survey in the U.K. (Farrell & Glanvill, 1990) 12,000 dives had been performed by 104 respondents without sustaining pneumothorax or cerebral gas embolism. However, from Australasia it is reported that 9% of the deaths in recreational divers occurred in asthmatics and there are case reports of apparently mild or well-controlled asthmatics having life-threatening attacks while diving (Edmonds, 1991).

Exercise induced asthma is very common and probably occurs in every asthmatic patient with sufficient provocation (Strunk, 1991). The significant factors are the intensity of the exercise and mouth breathing of dry cold air.

Asthma in diving may precipitate an emergency if an attack occurs before the diver can reach the shore or the dive boat. A diver must have the ability to swim reasonably fast, to hold breath and cope with waves and spray at the surface. The evidence for difficulty in emptying the lungs as being the cause of death in asthmatics who dive is not convincing. A further problem may occur if an asthmatic diver needs to be recompressed therapeutically in a recompression chamber. Treatment of asthma under pressure may lead to compromise of the lung filter with subsequent decompression illness (Butler & Hills, 1979).

Asthma appears infrequently in DAN accident and fatality reports as a cause of, or contributor to either decompression illness or a fatal event.

> ***Case report.*** *A 38 year-old obese male was practising open water diving for the first time with his instructor. The dive was to 23 feet (7m) for 28 minutes and buddy breathing was practiced during ascent. At the surface the subject became unconscious floating on his back with head out. Resuscitation was not possible. After discovery of asthma medications in his dive bag, it was revealed that the diver had not reported a history of bronchial asthma. Autopsy was consistent with cerebral air embolism and chronic obstructive pulmonary disease (asthma).*

A survey of DAN members in late 1991/early 1992 received 306 asthmatic respondents. Eleven cases of decompression illness (DCI) were reported in eight individuals. The calculated risk of DCI in questionnaire respondents (1 in 5,100) significantly exceeded the estimated risk for unselected recreational divers (Wilmshurst, 1990) (Odds ratio = 4.16, p = 0.00001).

Previous retrospective studies of DAN data suggested an approximate two-fold increase in risk for AGE in asthmatics when comparing non-asthmatic accidents to asthmatic accidents. The data, however, do not reach significance (Corson et al, 1991).

Further investigation will be needed to quantify this risk according to the degree of severity of asthma. The restriction on asthmatics who wish to dive will not change in the near future. A change awaits the clear demonstration that diving is safe for certain asthmatics and a method to identify the individual at risk.

DIABETES MELLITUS

Physicians in diving medicine generally disapprove of individuals with insulin-dependent diabetes mellitus participating in underwater diving. The advice arises from knowledge of the pathophysiology of the disease and clinical experience.

The spectrum of disease with diabetes mellitus ranges from the person with end-organ disease and frequent episodes of hypo- or hyperglycaemia or keto-acidosis to the barely detectable abnormality of glucose metabolism. Just as the first individuals are clearly disqualified, the mild diabetic fully controlled by weight and diet management can be qualified for recreational diving. Lying between these two extremes are the patients who require insulin or oral medications in addition to diet to control their disease. The occurrence of a hypoglycaemic episode is totally unpredictable even in the most carefully controlled diabetic. A reaction underwater would be a very dangerous situation easily leading to drowning. At present most diving physicians advise against the medication dependent diabetic participating in diving because of the risk to the individual and companions and would bar anyone from commercial diving. There are two issues of concern.

The first issue concerns the adverse effects of insulin reactions in the diabetic patient which have constituted the principle basis for advising the insulin dependent diabetic not to dive. Hypoglycaemia is the most common complication of insulin treatment in patients with diabetes mellitus.

The risk of hypoglycaemia in insulin-treated patients with diabetes mellitus is determined in large part by the balance between the biologic actions of the administered insulin and those of counter-regulatory factors, particularly glucagon and epinephrine. This balance is shifted in favour of insulin action and the risk of hypoglycaemia is increased if insulin-dependent glucose utilisation is increased as it is during exercise. While diving can be a leisurely activity, the necessity for severe exercise is omnipresent. Glucose self-monitoring has made control of diabetes much better and reduced the risk for unrecognised hypoglycaemia. However, as the occurrence of hypoglycaemia remains unpredictable, the restriction that individuals with insulin dependent diabetes mellitus should not dive will persist for the time being.

The second issue concerns the major complication of vascular disease involving arterial, arteriolar and capillary vessels. Although the patient and physician maintain strict control, this problem may develop at an early age. This complication may have deleterious effects on inert gas transfer increasing the risk of decompression sickness and is a risk factor for the development of coronary artery disease.

Diabetes mellitus predisposes towards the development of atherosclerosis and heart attacks may occur as a result of this damage. The risk for this complication increases with the duration of the disease.

Diabetes mellitus is not a simple alteration in glucose metabolism, but a very complex combination of causes and effects on all organ systems. There are serious, life-threatening problems that can occur with diabetes and the diabetic diver must be prepared to address these problems at any time.

The insulin-dependent diabetic individual who chooses to become a diver must remember that diving is usually a social activity with others involved. Individuals who have an impairment of any kind are obligated to inform their diving companions. If they do not, the dive buddies have become responsible for their partner's problem without their knowledge or consent. The question remains an individual decision by the diver as each diver is unique in motivation, training, physical condition and control.

THE PHYSICALLY HANDICAPPED DIVER

Individuals with disabilities often wish to pursue scuba diving as a recreational activity. The response to these individuals varies, depending upon both the level of disability of the diver and the knowledge and ability of the instructor. There are several organisations in the United States devoted to the training of disabled divers.

In general, the focus of these organisations is on individuals with physical disabilities rather than medical disorders. Physical disabilities include individuals with post traumatic, surgical, or congenital spinal cord injuries, amputees, head injuries, hearing or vision limitations, cerebral palsy, and others. Quadriplegics at the C-4 level have performed pool work and C-5 quadriplegics have performed ocean dives.

Medical disorders such as insulin-dependent diabetes, seizures, or asthma are not generally addressed by these organisations. There is one program for young well controlled insulin-dependent diabetics in the U.S. Virgin Islands (Steven Prosterman, Director; Camp DAVI, University of USVI).

The two largest organisations in the U.S. for training individuals with physical disabilities are the Moray Wheels: Adaptive Scuba Association located in Boston, MA and Handicapped Scuba Association (HSA) in San Clemente, CA. There are several smaller groups throughout the country in the form of clubs, many of which are "spin-offs" from the above organisations.

The Moray Wheels originally started as a master's degree thesis in Occupational Therapy in 1981, and since has evolved into a self-sustaining club and non-profit corporation. The group runs several courses throughout the year held at Massachusetts Institute of Technology (MIT) in Cambridge, MA. MIT has donated the use of their aquatic training facility for this purpose. The skills taught to the handicapped diver are the same as those taught to the able-bodied diver. The handicapped diver learns to perform these skills to the best of his or her ability. If the diver is able to demonstrate proficiency and independence and meets the required standards, the diver is certified through a national training agency, such as the National Association of Underwater Instructors (NAUI) or the Professional Association of Dive Instructors (PADI). Club members, both disabled and able-bodied are encouraged to come to the pool sessions to practice and help with new students.

The Handicapped Scuba Association also began in the early 1980's, and offers training courses for instructors. The HSA issues their own certifications for both divers and instructors rather than using the national agencies.

Training standards are based on the national certifying agency standards (RSTC). Very few modifications are necessary for most individuals. There are a few obvious changes, however, such as a giant stride entry for individuals who are not able to stand. Instead, if the conditions allow, the diver learns to do a forward roll from a wheelchair. If the diver cannot perform proficiently to minimum standard levels required for safety (including rescue skills), the diver is either not certified and required to dive with one or two instructors, or in the case of HSA, given a modified "certification" which requires diving with two buddies.

There is no national standard for an Instructor Specialty in training the disabled. HSA offers their own Instructor Certification courses, but any instructor is allowed to train a disabled student. The Moray Wheels provide workshops, allow any instructor to monitor and assist with courses, or will assist with information over the phone or by mail.

Students should be medically cleared by a physician to ensure their safety. Courses are typically longer than the average course, and occasionally a student will take several courses in the pool before attempting an ocean dive. Some students are content to remain in the pool and use the time to exercise and socialise. Students pay for their own training at the same rate as an able-bodied student, although some groups may have access to funding for scholarships.

Restrictions vary with the level of ability of the diver. Some will require two or more instructors as buddies, and some will be certified as an independent diver. Everyone, both able-bodied and disabled, is taught to dive with a buddy, and to discuss with their buddy any special needs which may be necessary.

Certain dive sites will be more accessible to disabled divers than others. This is of course largely a concern in a diver with a walking disability. The diver may need assistance in getting into and out of the water. The pool training site will need to be accessible for wheelchairs if individuals with walking disabilities are to be trained. If any of the students have impaired temperature regulation, the pool should be warm and adequate wetsuit protection must be available. A few equipment modifications may be necessary, although it is best to minimise these. A diver who swims with arms only may prefer to use webbed gloves, as long as they provide adequate warmth and do not limit dexterity. Custom wetsuits are helpful, as temperature control is extremely important. Correct weighting is critical, as a slight imbalance will severely affect the diver's control. Other modifications are discussed at length in more detailed works (Robinson, 1991).

Disabled divers are integrated with able-bodied divers as much as possible. Typically divers with disabilities dive with people from the same club, but often they travel and dive with the general public. We are not aware of any problems developing from that arrangement.

THE DIVER OVER 40

The adult diver in the United States does not face any restrictions based on age alone. A candidate for dive training over the age of 45 may be asked to provide documentation as to physical fitness if there is a history of any one of the following:

1. tobacco smoking in any form
2. hypercholesterolaemia
3. family history of heart attack or stroke (RSTC, 1986)

Recreational scuba diving appeals to people of all ages from childhood to the senior years. Are there upper age limits for diving? Although the vast majority of divers are less than 40 years of age, there are many thousands of divers past 40. However, there are concerns for the diver who has entered or passed mid-life. Student divers past 40 and of either sex are part of many of today's scuba courses.

Near the age of 30, physical strength and exercise capacity begin a decline which continues throughout the remaining life span. The ability of the body to achieve maximum utilisation of oxygen in the production of energy reaches a peak in the late 20's and then begins to decline. This de-conditioning is the result of many causes. Some are fundamental changes in physiology with ageing. These changes may be accelerated if the individual follows an inactive life style. As they age, older individuals frequently reduce activities requiring muscular effort.

The reduction in physical fitness may be rapid or slow depending on the individual's physical condition and endurance training. The decline in physical endurance can be slowed by conditioning programs. There is increasing awareness that physical activity is a part of a healthy lifestyle for everyone. Recreational scuba diving requires good physical condition both for safety and to enhance the pleasure of the dive. The mid-life or older individual who enters a diving program will not be surprised to discover that a task is somewhat more stressful than it is for the younger diver. The differences in performance are due to more than reduced strength and endurance. Reaction time slows and muscle control is less precise with age. Muscle mass decreases, probably due to inactivity. New motor skills are harder to learn. The diving instructor needs to be aware of these changes and prepared to accommodate patiently the older student.

With ageing there is a reduced work capacity and decreased tolerance to heat and cold. It is uncertain that the risk of decompression sickness increases with age (Bove & Davis, 1990). As divers enter their middle and later years of life many chronic illnesses begin to appear. These may include diabetes, various lung disorders, arthritis and so on. However, the number one health problem of our society is heart and blood vessel disease. Is there increased risk for the diver with heart disease due to coronary atherosclerosis? We probably don't have an adequate answer to that question, but we do have some information. We have autopsy reports from the last four years on approximately 40 divers who died from heart attack while diving. We have another group of about 30 who drowned after having a heart attack while diving. In addition there are other fatalities which were probably due to heart disease, but no autopsy was done.

Obviously the diving did not cause the underlying heart disease in these individuals. However, the physical demands of the dive produced the acute episode resulting in the heart attack and a death while diving. Should we prevent these deaths by prohibiting individuals with heart disease from diving? Most of these deaths did occur in divers with known heart disease, but some of the deaths were the first symptom of the disease. We may not able to eliminate death from heart disease while diving, but we can reduce the numbers by establishing standards for qualification and educating divers and instructors in the risks.

REFERENCES

Bove, A.A. & Davis, J.C. *Diving Medicine* 1990; WB Saunders: Philadelphia

Butler, R.D. & Hills B.A. *J. Appl. Physiol* 1979; **47**: 537-543.

Corson, K.S., Dovenbarger, J.A., Moon, R.E. & Bennett, P.B. *Undersea Biom. Res. 1991;* **18** (Suppl): 16-17.

Edmonds, C. *SPUMS Journal* 1991; **21**: 70-74.

Farrell, P.J.S. & Glanvill, P. *Br. Med. J.* 1990; **300**: 166.

Robinson, J. *NOAA Diving Manual, Appendix A.* 1991; U.S. Dept. Comm: Washington.

RSTC 1986. *Revised instructional standards minimum course content for entry level scuba certification.* Recreational Scuba Training Council.

Strunk, R.C. *J. Resp. Diseases* 1991; **12**: 377-392.

Wilmshurst, P. *Progr. Underwater Sci.* 1990; **15**: 31-37.

RECREATIONAL DIVING MEDICAL STANDARDS : UNITED KINGDOM
Dr. C.J. Edge, Dr. J. Douglas and Dr. P.J. Bryson*

The medical standards of the British Sub-Aqua Club (BSAC), the Sub-Aqua Association (SAA) and the Scottish Sub-Aqua Club (SSAC) have evolved over the last twenty years. This evolution has taken place through the increased knowledge of the effects of pressure upon human physiology and a greater understanding of the pharmacological effects, both wanted and undesirable, of pharmaceutical agents that are increasingly prescribed for pathological conditions. The instruments through which this change has taken place have been the medical committees of the BSAC, SAA and the SSAC, together with input from diving medical experts, both military and civilian, within the United Kingdom and overseas. These medical standards are thus continually reviewed and updated as new knowledge and new ideas become available. The upholding of these standards is carried out in the United Kingdom and overseas by a team of medical referees. Qualification to be a medical referee can be obtained by attending the course run by the Royal Navy on diving medicine (or an equivalent course) and by holding an advanced qualification in diving skills from the BSAC, the SAA or the SSAC. The referee must be a practitioner of medicine and also a regular diver. The actual task of carrying out a medical upon any person seeking to join the BSAC, SAA or SSAC and learning to dive is most frequently performed by that person's local general practitioner, who will complete a medical form issued by the BSAC, SAA or SSAC. This medical form is updated regularly to conform to the standards issued by the medical committee and contains guidelines for the medical examiner to help him/her to decide whether the person is fit to dive. Should there be any doubt in the matter, the person is referred to his/her nearest medical referee for a further examination and decision. Such examinations are carried out by the medical referees *without charge*. Only in exceptional cases will the case be referred to the medical committee.

The BSAC, SAA and SSAC require that all new entrants **must** have a full medical before being allowed to dive in open water. A postero-anterior chest x-ray is mandatory at this first examination. The full medical must be repeated every five years for a person under 30 years of age, at three-yearly intervals for a person under 50 years of age and annually for persons over the age of 50. Further chest x-rays are not performed unless there is a clinical requirement for them.

The medical standards can be broken down into broad general areas, as with other diving organisations. The standards are stated briefly and **should not be taken as a definitive statement without consulting the appropriate medical body:**

General: A body mass index of greater than 30 is considered to bar the individual from diving. Any limb disease, amputation, deformity, arthritis or arthrodesis must be referred to a medical referee. If ability to rescue others is impaired, then the entrant will have to dive with two healthy experienced companions.

E.N.T.: Perforated eardrum or chronic vestibular disease in new entrants is a disqualifying factor. Factors that are allowed are perforated eardrum known to have been present during several years of diving, healed perforation, including "paper-thin scars", unilateral nasal block and sinusitis if not adversely affected by diving. Deafness may restrict the entrant to diving with a fit companion at the discretion of a medical referee.

---

* Dr. P.J. Bryson (Medical Adviser, Sub Aqua Association) *in absentia*.

Oral cavity: Dentures must be retained in place on fully opening the mouth and not be dislodged by placing jaws together in any position, or by movement of one denture against the other. They should extend to the muco-buccal fold. If dentures do not satisfy these requirements, they should not be worn while diving. A cleft palate is not acceptable without referee's opinion. Applicants should have regular dental checkups and be warned about bad teeth and fillings.

Respiratory system: Any suspicion of active tuberculosis, lung cysts or bullae is a disqualifying factor. Treatment of apical bullae by pleurodesis followed by a lung CT scan and a period of three years without a pneumothorax may be allowed. Traumatic lung injury, asthma, removal of lung tissue, chronic bronchitis or other serious lung disease must be referred to a medical referee.

Cardiovascular system: Clinical or ECG evidence of ischaemic heart disease, aortic valve disease, symptomatic or pathological arrhythmias, a systolic blood pressure greater than 160 mm Hg, a diastolic pressure of greater than 100 mm Hg in established divers or greater than 90 mm Hg in new divers, any evidence of hypertensive end-organ damage or other evidence of hypertensive disease will disqualify the entrant from diving. Intracardiac shunts or persons with well-controlled hypertension without evidence of end-organ damage may be permitted to dive. Persons with pacemakers should be referred to a medical referee.

Haematology: Haemophilia and thalassaemia may disqualify the entrant from diving depending upon the haematological parameters. Sickle cell disease and polycythemia will disqualify the entrant. Leukaemias and tumours must be referred to a medical referee. Sickle cell trait and mild anaemia may be allowable.

Abdomen/urogenital system: Significant proteinuria is a disqualifying factor until the cause has been established. Abdominal hernias should be repaired.

Neurological/ophthamological systems: Any history of epilepsy or post-traumatic fits must be referred to a referee, as must any serious head injury or disease of the central nervous system. Any current psychiatric or personality disorders must also be referred. Any episodes of decompression sickness must be referred.

Endocrine disorders: Any endocrine disorder must be referred to a medical referee. Diabetics allowed to dive by a medical referee must complete a set of forms and have a medical on an annual basis. No diabetic is allowed to dive with diabetic complications.

Pregnancy: Diving is not advised during pregnancy. However, in view of the fact that many women do dive whilst they are pregnant, the BSAC, SAA and SSAC recommend that should a pregnant woman choose to dive, she should subtract at least five minutes from any no-stop time. Diving to below 30 metres is strongly discouraged.

Drugs: Oral steroids, muscle relaxants, digoxin and psychotropic drugs are disqualifying factors. Abuse of alcohol, narcotics or drugs is also a disqualifying factor. If any psychotropic drugs have been used, complete cessation of therapy must have occurred for a minimum of 3 months before diving is allowed. Smoking is actively discouraged.

Medical standards, by their very nature, must always be an ever-changing compromise. In setting these standards, the medical committees of the three diving organisations have tried to open up diving to people who may not satisfy the most rigorous medical requirements. At the same time, divers' medical health and safety and the health and safety of those with whom they dive must not be compromised. Further, the medical committees are aware that if these standards are to be upheld, individual divers must play an important part in taking responsibility for the health and safety of themselves and their buddies.

- presented by Dr. C. Edge

THE ANALYSIS OF INCIDENT STATISTICS

Both the British Sub-Aqua Club and the Scottish Sub-Aqua Club have their own diving incident panels which examine incidents in great detail, and alter diving procedures accordingly. All this is done through dive clubs which are non-profit making associations, unlike dive shops and diver training associations. We also have a voluntary reporting system from the chambers that belong to the British Hyperbaric Association. The data are forwarded to the Royal Navy who maintain and analyse a database of all diving accidents.

ACCIDENT MANAGEMENT

Because of the National Health Service which treats the victims of diving incidents without charge and because we already have a diving emergency network based upon, for example, the Royal Navy at Portsmouth and the commercial diving medical centres, we have little need of DAN for diving within the U.K. There is also the communications network of HM Coastguard who co-ordinate the evacuation of diving casualties to a suitable treatment centre.

- presented by Dr. J. Douglas

Marroni (Chairman): DAN Europe would like to collaborate with the various diving accident databases around Europe and is currently discussing with the British Hyperbaric Association the retrieval of accident data.

DIABETIC DIVER ASSESSMENT

The British Sub-Aqua Club does allow certain diabetics to dive. I would like to tell you why we do that and tell you something about the various rules that we follow.

First there is no evidence to suggest that diabetics have a higher incidence of decompression illness. Up and until the mid-1970's the BSAC allowed diabetics to dive but, following one particular incident, a ban was placed by the Club on all diabetics. Reconsideration of that case led to the conclusion that the fact that the diver was a diabetic had no relevance to that person's death. So we then reviewed the case for diving diabetics. Stating the case very briefly we do not accept any diver who has any of the long-term complications of diabetes. These medical conditions will apply to both insulin-dependent and non-insulin-dependent diabetics. There are some references in the literature to the fact that non-insulin-dependent diabetics can exercise without fear of a deleterious metabolic effect. We have a form in which we ask some questions of the diabetic:

- has the diabetics medication regime altered within the past year?

- have any episodes of hypoglycaemia occurred within the past year and if so, under what circumstances did these occur?

The next few questions go on to ask about the control of diabetes:

- has the diabetic been hospitalised within the last year for any condition related to diabetes?

- has the diabetic's level of control been in any way unsatisfactory during the past year?
- is any microalbuminuria present (because this is one of the earliest signs of possible diabetic complications)?
- is any retinopathy, neuropathy or vascular disease present?

These questions should be answered by the consultant diabetologist who is looking after the individual. In addition the form asks the diabetologist to say whether in his/her opinion the diabetic is in any way mentally or physically unfit to undertake scuba diving, a recreation that includes degrees of stress and exertion. If the answer to any of these questions is yes, then the diabetic would not normally be allowed to dive. We usually make an exception if the diabetic has only a mild background retinopathy. In order to ensure that problems do not occur rapidly, we make the diver undergo a complete physical examination annually. This must be done by one of the medical referees within the clubs.

DIABETIC DIVING PROCEDURES

We advise diabetics to dive only once or twice each day and generally not to dive more than three days consecutively. We also feel that it is helpful both to the diabetic diver and to the club to which the diver belongs that the diabetic should give an annual lecture to the club on the problems of diabetes and diving. They must also give a demonstration of how they administer glucose to themselves and how they monitor their blood glucose. The general response to this is usually very good.

Pre-dive

The diving diabetic should be as fit and mentally prepared to dive as his/her non-diabetic buddy. They should preferably be wearing a bracelet to state that they are diabetic and also a diver, and that the possibility of decompression illness should also be considered. Adequate hydration of the diabetic is also very important and the dive marshal for the dive should be aware that the diver is diabetic and should be informed of the profile of the proposed dive. The diabetic diver's buddy should be his/her regular diving partner and familiar with the diabetic's individual problem. Alternatively, the buddy should be a trained medic or paramedic who understands diabetes. The buddy must not also be a diabetic. Additionally, most divers will take with them a small kit, containing either oral glucose tablets or preferably oral glucose paste. The other items of equipment include an emergency intramuscular injection of glucagon, also glucose testing sticks together with the necessary kit and instructions for the use of such testing kit. The normal diver safety equipment should be carried with one or more of the following items: surface marker buoy, flag, personal flares and/or an emergency beacon. Diabetics should plan to carry their glucose tablets or a tube of glucose paste with them in a small waterproof bag during the dive. The diving buddy must know the whereabouts of these and be able to administer these and if necessary, give the intramuscular injection of glucagon. Before diving, diabetics take extra glucose to ensure they have a higher blood level.

Dive phase

A diabetic diver should not dive deeper than 30 metres until a considerable experience of diving and its associated problems has been gathered by the BSAC Medical Committee. He/she should remain well within the tables and have more than two minutes no-stop time left on any dive computer. There are a few diabetic divers at National Instructor level who are diving deeper than 30 metres at this time. One of them has been diving for more than ten years and has encountered no problems.

Post-dive

On arrival back in the boat or onshore after a dive the diabetic should check his or her glucose level and correct it in the appropriate manner. We also say that any adverse symptoms or signs should be reported immediately to the diving buddy or dive marshal. Nothing should be passed off as "part of diving". The diving officer and all concerned with the diabetic diver are at pains to emphasise that the symptoms of low blood sugar may mimic those of neurological decompression illness. In this situation we emphasise that first aid therapy should be given as though both conditions are present i.e. 100% oxygen and treatment for low blood sugar. In the case of an unconscious diabetic diver the blood glucose level should be quickly measured if possible.

The scheme of allowing diabetics to dive has been going on for the last two and a half years and, as far as I am aware at the moment, there have been no adverse problems at all. There seems to be no reason why a well-controlled diabetic should not be allowed to dive.

- presented by Dr. C. Edge

Marroni (Chairman): That certainly raises some interesting questions but is the low number of diving incidents related to diabetes because they are now doing it safely or is it because there are so few diabetics for diving? We will have to wait and see.

RECREATIONAL DIVING LEGISLATION AND MEDICAL STANDARDS IN FRANCE
Dr. J. Seyer

In France the recognised practice of SCUBA diving is allowed : there is no "diving permit" but, none-the-less, a medical examination of persons practising this sport is required. This is especially so if it is either on a collective and/or a competitive basis. It is for this reason that the Fédération Français d'Etudes et de Sports Sous-Marins (F.F.E.S.S.M. French Federation of underwater studies and sports) was delegated the public service responsibility for training, diplomas and medical exams. The F.F.E.S.S.M. represents 150,000 divers throughout France. The medical commission is composed of 800 physicians who participate in diver training, surveillance and physical assessment.

In accordance with the 1984 Law 84-610, the sports physician has three tasks:

1. to determine if an individual is medically able to practice a given sport at a given competition level while it is probable that they will remain in good health.
2. in order to accomplish this task, the physician is asked to justify his clinical evaluation, based on established criteria. Specialised or technical advice can be obtained if necessary. The task is completed by issuing a medical certificate of "non-contraindications" (i.e. fitness).
3. to follow the athlete's state of health and to treat the athlete in case of injury.

The role of the F.F.E.S.S.M. includes the responsibility to develop, organise and encourage underwater activities both in France and in territories under French administration. The government endorses only one such Federation per discipline to supervise competition on an international, national, regional or local scale.

Underwater activities are understood as being:

1. those practiced while submerged;
2. those of mixed character: combining surface activity and submergence;
3. those which are exercised on the surface necessitating accessories (fins, mask, snorkel), or any accessories permitting respiration while airways are in a state of submergence;
4. and, on a broader basis, all underwater activities requiring a great degree of either skill or specific knowledge which permit man to exercise a sports activity underwater by means of aids, notably artificial means of respiration and propulsion.

ISSUING MEDICAL CERTIFICATES

Subject to legal provisions and regulations imposed on the Fédération, the issuing of medical certificates to licensed members of the F.F.E.S.S.M. is guided by the following dispositions. The means of establishing and issuing a medical certificate necessary to obtain a state diploma, is decided by ministerial decision.

A medical certificate specifying the absence of contraindications is required to obtain a *Fédération Diploma* in all disciplines, with the exception of an elementary SCUBA diving permit. This certificate must be issued by either a Fédération physician or a physician specialised in sports medicine.

The validation period of medical certificates required to pass Fédération diplomas is set at one year.

COMPETITIONS

In order to participate in any international, national or regional competition, a medical certificate issued by a qualified physician is required, specifying the absence of contraindications. The validity periods of a medical certificate issued to allow participation in French competitions are:

- 120 days in the case of the first issue of a competition licence;
- 180 days for renewals;

DIVING FOR PLEASURE

Non-competitive pleasure diving, breath-holding and swimming in open water with fins, do not require a medical certificate of fitness, unless stated by the concerned commission. However, taking the risks into account, a medical examination is strongly recommended.

Inaugural collective SCUBA diving in a pre-defined area does not require the possession of a medical certificate.

A medical certificate of fitness is required to practise SCUBA diving either individually or collectively. The medical certificate is valid for a maximum period of one year following its issue. A certificate expiring during a training period remains in effect during this training period.

The resumption of diving activities following a decompression or pulmonary over pressure accident associated with neurological signs, requires a medical certificate delivered by a Fédération physician and the agreement of the regional medical commission President.

Handicapped persons who wish to dive require a medical certificate delivered by a Fédération physician and the agreement of the regional medical commission President.

MEDICAL COMMISSION CONTRAINDICATIONS TO SCUBA DIVING

The following list of contraindications is relative. Certain problems have to be considered on a case by case basis, with an evaluation made by a specialist in relation to the technical level of the diver (beginner, experienced diver or instructor).

Cardiology - Definite contraindications

- advanced ischaemic heart disease
- heart failure
- obstructive cardiomyopathy
- valvular heart disease
- severe arterial hypertension
- congenital cardiomyopathy
- severe arteritis
- paroxysmal tachycardia
- syncopal heart condition
- second or third degree AV block
- treatment by antiarrhythmics, anticoagulants, beta-adrenergic antagonists

E.N.T. - Definite contraindications and temporary contraindications

- unilateral total deafness
- mastoidectomy
- tracheotomy

- infectious episode, acute or recent
- nasosinusal polyps
- obstruction of the Eustachian tube
- vertigo
- tympanic perforation, tympanoplasty
- significant audiometric deficit
- laryngocoele

Pulmonary - Definite contraindications and temporary contraindications

- chronic obstructive pulmonary disease
- interstitial lung disease
- asthma
- spontaneous pneumothorax

- infectious disease
- pleurisy
- sarcoidosis
- thoracic surgery

Ophthalmology - Definite contraindications and temporary contraindications

- vascular pathology of retina, choroid or papilla
- closed angle glaucoma
- hollow prosthesis or implant

- eye surgery
- curative or preventive treatment of retinal detachment
- keratoconus
- radial keratotomy

Neurology - Definite contraindications and temporary contraindication

- epilepsy
- deficits involving the extremities
- loss of consciousness
- intracranial surgery

- spasmophillia

Psychiatry - Definite contraindication and temporary contraindications

- severe psychiatric disease

- treatment by antidepressants, sedatives, neuroleptics

Traumatology - Temporary contraindications

- recent bone surgery
- severe head trauma

Gynaecology - Temporary contraindication

- pregnancy

Dentistry - Temporary contraindications

- unfixed dentures
- caries

Endocrinology - Definite contraindications

- diabetes, treated or not
- severe metabolic or endocrine disease

Dermatology

- various diseases can lead to temporary or definite contraindications according to their pulmonary, neurological or vascular involvement.

Gastroenterology - Temporary contraindication

- peptic ulcer

FUTURE PERSPECTIVE

In order to improve the present situation, we are studying the possibility of modifying the contents of the medical certificate of fitness for diving. Today, the physician can only answer "yes" or "no" on this certificate, without the possibility of modifying it. We plan to modify it according to two factors:

1. decompression susceptibility
2. decreased tolerance of exertion, cold, stress etc.

The answer to these two could be:

- fit
- fit, with restrictions
- temporarily unfit
- definitely unfit

A fit subject with a restriction on decompression would be limited to shallow water, a fit subject with restriction concerning exertion would be limited to effortless diving in warm water. These are now under study by the technical and medical commissions of the F.F.E.S.S.M. Thus we hope to have a better medical response to the real necessities of sub-aquatic activities without rendering the clubs mission too complicated.

RECREATIONAL DIVING MEDICAL STANDARDS IN GERMAN-SPEAKING EUROPE
Commander W. Welslau

Different to the situation in the U.K., we have in Germany 100,000 recreational divers, of whom 50,000 of them are organised in diving clubs. The vast majority dive only on holiday when in the Mediterranean or tropical waters after completing a basic course in a professional training school.

The "GTÜM" OR "Gesellschaft für Tauch- und Überdruckmedizin" is the German diving and hyperbaric medical society. The GTÜM was founded in 1983 and now has some 400 members. Of this number about 300 are physicians, the other 100 are diving instructors, technicians and nurses.

In 1992 a work group was begun by the GTÜM to create new guidelines for sport diver medical examinations and a suitable medical examination form. This was done with the idea of establishing a certain standard in a situation where every sport diving organisation has different or no medical standards, and where, as in other countries, there is no official regulation for sport divers health requirements. Here I would like to inform you about the development of the examination form rather than about the medical standards.

When developing the examination form our objectives were as follows:

- the form should not exceed four pages (including medical history, documentation of the examinations and certificate) to be easy to handle;
- we wanted to integrate as far as possible written responses the diver and examination comments for the physician;
- the certificate should be applicable internationally with texts in German, English and French;
- lastly, but not least, we wanted to replace as far as possible the often antiquated forms used by the different sport diving organisations in Germany.

The first 1½ pages of the form are to be filled in by the diver himself. Besides the personal data, the sport and especially the diving history are of interest. So we asked for previous diving accidents and minor diving incidents. After answering detailed questions regarding medical history the diver has to sign on the last line that the correct and complete answers have been given to all the questions above. This is very important for the examining physician (and for his civil liability insurance) because experienced divers have a quite good idea about the possible grounds for diving unfitness, and some think that they could handle problems arising by themselves. So they see no reason to point out a potential problem to the diving physician, and thus they avoid the risk of not being certified fit for diving.

Part A of the form relates to personal data, sport and medical history which I have mentioned above. Part B of the form starts with the physical examination and is to be completed by the physician. The fitness certificate is part of the last page and may be photocopied.

The diver's examination consists of:

- physical examination
- chest x-rays, which are obligatory for every first examination and should be repeated after severe lung disease

- pulmonary function test including vital capacity, forced vital capacity and forced expiratory volume in one second
- laboratory evaluation of blood count, ESR, fasting blood glucose, and urine analysis
- ergometry, preferably as a standardised bicycle ergometry combined with exercise ECG.

Because our aim was to replace the antiquated forms used by different sport diving organisations in Germany, we worked together with the diving doctors of some of these organisations. To promote the spreading of the GTÜM form we further encouraged the sport diving organisations to take our form and print it with their own letterhead. Now, two years after introduction, our form is distributed by most of the important organisations and the majority of German sport divers are examined according to our form and guidelines.

Most sport divers are interested in having an extensive medical examination but, because of the German health care system, many have problems in understanding that they will be charged for a service having to do with their health. In Germany an examination with chest x-rays will cost up to 400 German Marks which is equivalent to 160 U.K. Pounds Sterling or 230 U.S. Dollars. Follow-up examinations without x-rays will cost up to 270 German Marks equivalent to 110 U.K. Pounds Sterling or 160 U.S. Dollars. Unfortunately these figures are, for sport divers, the strongest argument against regular medical examinations as long as there is no official obligation to have a current fitness certificate.

RECREATIONAL DIVING MEDICAL STANDARDS IN SWITZERLAND
Dr. J. Wendling

In Switzerland we have no regulations which require recreational divers to have special medical examinations. Nevertheless most divers have a medical every few years conducted by general practitioners. The Swiss society for underwater and hyperbaric medicine has therefore produced guidelines on how this examination should be performed with checklists that doctors can go through.

We also have a manual which gives a list of the contraindications for diving but also gives more detailed information. The first part of the examination is the anamnesis (the history). This is taken by the doctor and not by completing a written checklist. We consider the direct contact between the doctor and the diver is very important.

The majority of limiting pathologies are not ones that can be measured but are the ones probably known by the family doctor. The clinical examination corresponds to the international standard but with no ECG or x-ray unless there is any suspicion of pathology. All the investigations that are necessary will then be performed as indicated clinically. This is in a manual which should be published towards the end of this year.

THE ROLE OF THE EUROPEAN COMMITTEE FOR HYPERBARIC MEDICINE FOR THE SAFETY OF THE RECREATIONAL DIVER
Professor F. Wattel

The European Committee for Hyperbaric Medicine is directly implicated in some aspects of recreational diving. On behalf of the committee I would like to tell you we have the opportunity to promote meetings and conferences with the goal to harmonise positions:

- with respect to standards elaborated by organisations (national federations, sub-aqua clubs, DAN etc);
- according to the regulations which exist in European countries.

The role of the committee is to make proposals. First to establish standards of treatment for decompression illness. Secondly, to organise a workshop on personal education and training procedures in diving and hyperbaric medicine and, for example, to answer the questions such as which treatment is appropriate for decompression sickness? Another workshop will deal with the appropriate training for those involved in hyperbaric medicine. The European Committee may also consider other topics such as those related to the prevention of diving accidents such as:

- medical contraindications to diving;
- diabetic diver;
- asthmatic diver;
- ischaemic cardiovascular disease;
- women in pregnancy.

A further proposal is to promote a debate about the correct and effective procedures for decompression and treatment following borderline diving and in relation to the inadequate use of the depth guage.

In conclusion I suggest that DAN Europe becomes part of the European Committee to be if possible more efficient than it is already.

DISCUSSION

Marroni (Chairman): The hottest spot is perhaps what Dr. Edge raised about the diabetic diver and he presented us with detailed procedures which were very interesting. Are there any questions therefore in relation first to the diabetic diver?

Örnhagen: I was most impressed by the programme presented about the diabetic diver but I wonder, is this a scientific test that has been put through ethical approval under the Helsinki declaration? This is against the recommendations existing in most countries and I would have to regard it as a test against scientific information.

Edge: Thank you for your kind words at the start of that. First, it is not a scientific test, it is no more a scientific test than diving organisations are allowing cigarette smokers to dive. Instead of being a group of people in the U.K. who are a disabling organisation, we are an organisation that is going to allow divers to dive unless there are specific contraindications. The evidence at the moment as far as one can find it in the literature, comes from the American Journal of Paediatrics, in which it says that "divers who are diabetic should not dive because of the risks of hypoglycaemia during the time they are underwater". There is no evidence for that statement and no evidence at all that diabetics who dive have any problems due to hypoglycaemia. They are probably more careful divers than the other members of the diving community. I therefore feel and my colleagues in this matter support me, that we should allow diabetics to dive within these very controlled guidelines. Who are we to turn round and say that they should not dive if they are well controlled?

Marroni: There is a significant difference between the two populations that are being discussed in this seminar. The commercial diver and the recreational diver, their freedoms and responsibilities are so very different. If the recreational diver is told he cannot dive with diabetes, he will dive anyway in all probability but without appropriate advice.

Saliba: If we allowed the diabetic diver, should we advise him to take the tablets on the day he is diving and another question, I recently had a request from a 42 year-old diver who had had a successful heart transplant in 1991. He now has a normal ECG, normal chest x-ray and he is on various drugs including lipid lowering agents as well as immuno suppressive agents, should we consider his application?

Desola: In Spain there is a heart transplanted diver who dives already.

Edge: The diabetic should carry on taking his normal insulin on the day of diving. In the U.K. we have certainly had one referral following a heart transplant. In that case we allowed him to dive but I need to check the records. Dr. Seyer knows another diver in France who is diving following a heart transplant.

Douglas: When we look at both diabetes and asthma we need to recognise that the monitoring and treatment of these conditions has made progress recently. There is a tendency for the responsibility for treatment and management of the illness to be handed back to the patient. Therefore we must find definite reasons if we are to stop anybody from diving.

Mebane: If we agree then we must accept morbidity and mortality. In the United States we have 5 or 6 diving diabetics who die each year, generally as a complication of coronary atherosclerosis but at least one teenager died last year of documented hypoglycaemia during training in a swimming pool. If one is willing to accept that, then there is no reason why diabetics should not dive.

Zachariedes: If we told sports divers they cannot dive, they would not come and ask us. Consider the diving paraplegic who presented Dr. Desola with the video of his continued diving. He said afterwards "look doctor, this is what I can do". In the Mediterranean countries diving is like a heroin addiction, once a person starts they can never stop it. The only time to intervene is before the person becomes trained as a diver, therefore at the first medical examination of a diver, the doctors have the responsibility to stop them. If somebody comes after 10 or 20 years experience of diving and with a medical problem, for example I know more than 10 Greek divers with cardiac bypass, our job is to help the diver to cope with his condition. In summary, let us do our best to stop persons with such potential problems joining the sports diving community, but once he is there let us do our best to make sure that he can continue safely.

Risberg: In Norway we have a single class of divers. Either you are a diver or you are not a diver. One must consider therefore the diver of being no hazard to himself or his companion. Will he be able to help his companion when he is perhaps a thousand metres from his boat or the shore? We do not have a handicapped diver association.

Edge: My first comment is, you talk about the diabetic as though he or she is a person who is different to everybody else. Admittedly he or she is diabetic but it is exactly the same situation as those people who have a smoking or a drinking problem. Are they able to tow their buddy a thousand metres to the shore?

Wendling: How to face the candidate for a fitness examination who has certain pathologies. In Switzerland we believe that the doctor must be the friend of the diver and help him but we must also understand the insurance companies who calculate the risk. The most important thing we have to do in doing the medical examination is to advise the diver about his individual risks. Maybe we should not give him approval but say "we will not give you the official approval, but if you dive anyhow then we will show you how to do it, how to avoid coming into hospital as a patient". If, however, it is an absolute contraindication then of course we will say "you must not dive" and that is quite different.

Marroni: It is too bad that the time has run out when we still have so many interesting questions to discuss but on behalf of the Executive Board of DAN Europe it is our intention to continue the work we have started. We must obtain a harmonisation for fitness standards within Europe.

Boonstra[**]**:** If insulin-dependent diabetics are allowed to dive, is it then not necessary to give rules as to the duration of the dive? This results from the observation that during hyperbaric treatment of clinical diabetes patients in the chamber, blood glucose levels drop rapidly and the amount of daily required insulin diminishes, while these patients are at perfect rest in the chamber! (Diving is in a similar hyperbaric environment).

Reply from Edge: I am interested that you refer to the hyperbaric treatment of clinical diabetic patients giving rise to hypoglycaemia whilst at rest in the chamber. Although you do not mention it in your question, I assume that these patients are being treated for diabetic ulcers or similar conditions with 100% O_2 at pressure? The insulin-dependent diabetics who scuba dive do not require rules as to the duration of their dive for the following reasons:

1. The dive takes place over a period of roughly 20-50 minutes, depending upon the depth, rather than the longer periods of time that are spent by the diabetic patients in the chamber. In addition, the dive is performed on air, rather than on pure oxygen, and my feeling is that oxygen may well play a role in the induction of hypoglycaemia. I therefore feel that the situation is really not comparable with the diabetic in the chamber.

2. The diabetic diver is always told to make him/herself slightly hyperglycaemic before the dive and to check that this is the case before going into the water by using a glucometer. Further, the diabetic diver carries glucose paste throughout the dive and dives with someone whom the diabetic knows well and is familiar with the signs and symptoms of hypoglycaemia.

3. As of 1st February 1994, the diabetic divers diving with the BSAC, the SAA or the SSAC here in the U.K. had logged over 750 man-dives in a 2.5 year period. During that time, to the best of my knowledge, there have been two occasions upon which the diabetic diver has felt slightly hypoglycaemic, and this has easily been rectified with the use of the oral glucose paste. The dives have been performed at depths of 0-40 metres and some of the dives have been decompression dives (although diving below 30 metres and doing decompression dives is not encouraged at present). The duration of the dives has been varied and obviously depends upon the depth to which the diabetic diver has been diving.

Lowsley-Williams (J.)**: I applaud DAN Europe's recommendation that each diver carry their own "Fitness for Diving" booklet with notes for the examining physician. This has become a proven successful way to keep medical records (patients look after their own notes better than the medical service). However, to make this system relevant and effective it needs:

- Europe-wide acceptance (is legislation by governments the way forward?)

- To take into account the different conditions in which European sports divers dive, i.e. Northern European and Mediterranean divers.

Reply from Marroni: Thank you for the kind comments on the action of DAN Europe and the usefulness of the Diver's Fitness Logbook. At the moment the logbook is the most widely accepted recreational diving fitness standard in Europe, as it was discussed, modified and eventually accepted by the members of the DAN Europe Scientific Board, in representation of practically all the European countries.

Matters like the differences in diving habits were also taken into consideration and the recommendations of the logbook reflect the minimal common denominator that the Board felt appropriate for recreational diving in general.

As for possible future European legislation, this may create limits rather than proving useful. Recreational diving is and should, remain a free individual activity and only general guidelines are appropriate and realistically applicable. Such guidelines should represent the view of the European diving medical community, and this is presently the object of DAN Europe's action, together with the European Underwater and Baromedical Society and the European Committee for Hyperbaric Medicine.

Wilmshurst**: In reply to Dr. Örnhagen's suggestion (*page 70 and in the discussion on asthma; see page 147*) that the decision of the British Sub-Aqua Club allows some diabetic divers to dive as members of the club is unethical: at the time that decision was made I was Chairman of the BSAC Medical Committee. Prior to that decision the BSAC had been requested by the British Diabetic Association to reconsider the issue, since the British Diabetic Association did not consider there was adequate scientific evidence to discriminate against diabetic divers. In particular we held meetings with Dr. Spathis, Secretary of the British Diabetic Association.

In 1975 the British Sub-Aqua Club introduced a ban on all newly diagnosed diabetics diving. At that time we allowed existing diabetic divers to continue diving with the club. Some of these had gone on to perform several thousand uneventful dives. We were also aware of other British diabetic divers outside the British Sub-Aqua Club. A survey of these individuals had been conducted by a British diabetic diver, who had submitted her findings to the Medical Committee for consideration. As a result of considering this information the Medical Committee decided that in the absence of cardiovascular and other complications resulting from diabetes, certain well controlled diabetics could be allowed to dive with the club.

However, before changing our advice I sought independent advice from Professor S.E. Smith, Professor of Clinical Pharmacology at St. Thomas' Hospital, London and Chairman of the Ethical Committee of that hospital. We asked Professor Smith to consider both whether there was evidence on which we could base a decision not to allow diabetics to dive and secondly the question of whether there were ethical problems with allowance of diabetics to resume diving. We asked Professor Smith to place the matter before the hospital Ethical Committee if he felt there were any problems with our plan of action. That plan involved our continued surveillance of diabetic divers to see if they had an unusually high incidence of complications which might cause us to reconsider our advice in the future.

Professor Smith felt that there was no good evidence on which to base refusal to allow well controlled uncomplicated diabetics to dive. He also felt that formal ethical approval was not required since no clinical trial was being undertaken, but merely audit of outcome. Rather than feeling that there was an ethical problem in allowing diabetics to dive, Professor Smith felt that there might be ethical problems in refusing individuals to dive unless one could clearly show good scientific evidence on which to base that refusal.

CARDIOLOGY AND PHYSICAL FITNESS

Chairman : Dr. T. Nome

The recommendations from the Guidance Notes on "The Medical Examination of Divers" are:

33. The examination of the cardiovascular system will consist of palpation of peripheral pulses and an assessment of the circulation; auscultation of the heart; recording of the blood pressure; the recording of an ECG before and after exercise. A resting ECG should be carried out at each annual examination. A recording of at least one lead should be made 1 and 5 minutes after the individual has exercised to a level sufficient to raise the heart beat to 180 per minute less his/her age. The following points should be particularly noted:

   (a) auscultation to the heart should be normal. Murmurs are acceptable only if deemed to be physiological: if the examiner cannot be certain, he should refer for a specialist cardiological opinion;
   (b) any organic heart disease is a cause for rejection;
   (c) coarctation of the aorta is a bar to diving;
   (d) disorders of rhythm, except for sinus arrhythmia and ventricular extrasystoles which disappear as the heart rate increases, should be referred for the opinion of a cardiologist. These should usually be a cause for rejection;
   (e) divers with ECG abnormalities should be referred for cardiological assessment. Such abnormalities will usually be a cause for rejection unless demonstrably benign such as isolated right bundle branch block;
   (f) any evidence of coronary insufficiency or myocardial ischaemia, clinical or electrocardiographic, is a cause for rejection. Coronary artery bypass surgery will not render a person fit for diving;
   (g) cardiomegaly should be fully assessed. It will usually be a cause for rejection except in those divers with 'athletic hearts', confirmed by a cardiologist;
   (h) the resting blood pressure at the **initial** examination should not exceed 140 systolic or 80 diastolic, using a sphygmo' and with the patient supine and taking the fifth phase as the indicator. Hypertension requiring therapy should be a cause for rejection;
   (i) the peripheral circulation should be adequate;
   (j) varicose veins, with evidence of eczematous change, are a cause for rejection. In other cases the decision will depend upon an assessment of the risk of potential complications.

Exercise testing

34. An exercise tolerance test should be carried out at each examination. Advice on appropriate tests, methods and interpretation of findings are given in an appendix This part of the examination can be usefully coordinated with ECG recordings as described in Paragraph 33.

Appendix to paragraph 34:

There are several means of testing the exercise response of an individual but the following methods are acceptable:

(a) **Army Physical Fitness Test** : The candidate is required to step at a rate of 30 times per minute, to a height of 43 cm, for 5 minutes. A standard of Sum of Pulse Counts, taken for 30 seconds, 1, 2 and 3 minutes post exercise, is made. The total should be less than 190.

(b) ***The Master Two-Step Test*** : *See details in Exercise testing and training of apparently healthy individuals. A Handbook for Physicians produced by the American Heart Association, 7320 Greenville Avenue, Dallas, Texas, USA 75231.*

(c) ***Bicycle Ergometer or Treadmill*** *systems where heart rate can be monitored against the exercise load. If the rate of oxygen uptake can also be monitored a very valuable assessment can be made.*

CARDIOVASCULAR PROBLEMS COMMONLY FOUND IN DIVERS
Dr. M.R. Cross

THE NORMAL HEART : ABNORMAL FINDINGS

If you examine the cardiovascular system of fit young men, then from time to time you will find abnormalities. Typically these may be in auscultation of the heart, on the chest X-ray or on examination of the electrocardiogram. It is worth our while getting out of the way at the start of this presentation a few "normal abnormals" which are found from time to time. These will be typically seen by those doctors who examine *ab initio* trainees who wish to become commercial divers. In the high-tech litigation-conscious world perhaps the philosophy might be that a cardiological referral is appropriate for each and every abnormality found but the competent clinician, possessed of few tools can do quite a good job in detecting true abnormality.

Typically, variations in normal which mimic the abnormal are found in:

1. the very fit
2. the very tall and skinny
3. those with pectus excavatum

All of the above groups are likely to have innocent murmurs. The very fit and those with flat backs have apparent cardiomegaly on radiography and the very fit have alterations in the electrocardiogram which reflect a very high level of vagal tone.

The innocent murmur

An innocent murmur is a cardiac murmur whose cause is not associated with any true cardiac pathology. Innocent murmurs which are almost invariably systolic in timing may be found in up to 60% of children of school age and most innocent murmurs fade with adolescence.

THE OLDER THE SUBJECT,
THE LESS LIKELY IT IS THAT THE MURMUR IS INNOCENT

In young adult subjects the most likely innocent murmurs are the pulmonary flow murmurs and the so-called "cardio-respiratory murmurs". These murmurs are uncommon in the third and fourth decades of life, after which time atherosclerotic murmurs arising from the aortic valve may replace them as the "innocent murmur of the elderly". In the age group of candidates for commercial diving medical certificates, innocent murmurs are extremely rare and any murmur heard should be presumed guilty until proven innocent.

Cardiac catheterisation was a daunting procedure and prior to the availability of the excellent non-invasive techniques there was pressure on physicians to regard a murmur as innocent till proven guilty in order to spare his patient a nasty invasive investigation. There is no excuse for this philosophy now that high-grade echocardiography with colour-flow imaging is available and the service should be used sooner rather than later. It is recognised however that some clinicians may not have ready and frequent access to this technique; some of those practising in far flung places, for example. For their benefit, some generalisations are possible.

Murmurs which are regarded as innocent usually arise from the right side of the heart. Their intensity fluctuates with respiration, being maximal towards the end of an inspiration. They are usually systolic and not associated with any other abnormal finding. They radiate poorly. The cardio-respiratory murmur is a highly positional systolic murmur heard in the thin-chested, typically at the heart-lung border. Its movement and change with position is the give-away. It may be confused with the systolic murmur of trivial mitral valve prolapse. In general, a systolic murmur arising from the base of the heart to the left of the sternum and transmitted to the neck is indicative of cardiac disease. This is particularly true if there is an ejection click.

In a typical published study, only one of twenty-one subjects with such a murmur was found to have no cardiac disease. Such murmurs in the age group which interests us are usually associated with the presence of a congenital bicuspid aortic valve. Such patients may be permitted to dive. However, they may be at increased risk of sudden death and also should have antibiotic prophylaxis for dental procedures. They should be reviewed by a cardiologist. This murmur may be falsely diagnosed when what is heard is an innocent supraclavicular bruit arising from the subclavian vessels.

Diastolic murmurs are almost inevitably pathological. However, innocent diastolic murmurs have been described in the literature but that's a distinction for a properly equipped cardiologist to make.

Innocent cardiomegaly on the x-ray

Athletes have big hearts. Their large ventricular volumes provide for the slow heart rate with the large stroke volume. Cardiomegaly is more often mis-diagnosed however in those with "The Straight Back Syndrome". These fit young men have a flattened antero-posterior diameter of the chest which displaces the heart downwards and leftwards giving the appearance of cardiomegaly on the chest x-ray. By the same mechanism, they have thrusting apical impulses which feel "meaty" and to finish off the picture, the proximity of the stethoscope to the heart (because of the chest wall) is a good source of innocent murmurs particularly of the cardiorespiratory type. Many endomorphic young men have been excused military service on this basis. The ECG will usually show high voltage complexes but should be normal in all other respects though T wave abnormalities may be found in this condition as in pectus excavatum.

Mitral valve prolapse

This is one of the two relatively common valvular conditions which may be found in normal individuals of professional diver age. It sits uncomfortably as being neither normal nor abnormal enough to warrant disqualifying the diver from his work. This condition was recognised early in the 60's and is very common. Its recognition was first based upon phonocardiographic criteria where it was recognised by its "click-murmur" nature. Since that time it has been renamed "floppy valve syndrome" and has finally settled in most cardiologists nomenclature as mitral valve prolapse.

What ever the name, the pathology is well understood. Most commonly seen in the second or third decades of life, the true incidence in the population may be between 1.4 and 17%; the condition is may be familial and probably occurs as an autosomal dominant trait. The predominant abnormality in this syndrome is the presence of excessive mitral valve leaflets and/or elongated chordae tendinae.

An abnormality of the valve is present in some patients and dilation of the mitral annulus may also be present. The condition is associated with a high frequency of skeletal abnormalities such as the Straight Back Syndrome.

Most patients with the condition are asymptomatic though a number have the features of the old-fashioned "neurocirculatory asthenia" which was said to be common in females. Patients may present with atypical chest pain, palpitations, dyspnoea and fatigue. The atypical pain has not been associated with ischaemia on perfusion studies however a small number of these patients have a congenital absence of the atrioventricular groove branch of the circumflex coronary artery and it has been postulated that associated with the prolapse they may have a minor degree of ischaemia of the basal portion of the left ventricle. Psychiatric manifestations are well described in association with mitral valve prolapse and specifically there appears to be an association with panic disorders. A common causation of all symptoms may be autonomic dysfunction.

On examination, there is a spectrum of abnormal findings with the stethoscope. Typically there is a mid-systolic click and a late short ejection type murmur. Sometimes the murmur which is maximal at the apex may have a whooping quality. The diagnosis is easily confirmed by echocardiography where the fluttering leaflet in time with the murmur is easily demonstrated.

In most cases of mitral valve prolapse, reassurance is all that is necessary. Some clinicians would advocate prophylactic antibiotics to prevent bacterial endocarditis. In patients with chest pain, a beta blocker may be administered and this is not incompatible with being a diver though the history of difficult-to-diagnose chest pain might make one think. Twelve-hour taping is highly desirable in cases of mitral valve prolapse who wish to be divers. Those with arrhythmias should not be considered as candidates.

The bicuspid aortic valve

The non-stenotic bicuspid aortic valve often remains undiagnosed early in childhood and rarely causes clinical sequelae. It is the commonest congenital heart lesion and affects about 1% of the population with a familial incidence. It is sometimes seen in association with Marfans syndrome, polycystic kidney and familial cardiomyopathies.

The valve leaflets are not of equal size, with one big and one small giving a characteristic appearance on echocardiography with the absence of the "Mercedes Sign". With age the relatively normal leaflets become thickened and an ejection click may be heard. Other echocardiographic evidence of its presence is the absence of ventricular dilatation and hypertrophy and often some dilatation of the aorta; eccentric opening of the leaflets may be seen on M MODE examination.

The condition is not benign though it may not have any haemodynamic implications. A significant number of patients (7% in one series) may develop endocarditis and just under one fifth may go on to develop a stenotic lesion requiring surgery. Trivial aortic regurgitation may develop in up to 10% but significant regurgitant lesions are seen in only 1% or less.

Bicuspid aortic valves may be associated with other cardiac conditions worthy of note by the diving doctor. These are a VSD, an aberrant origin of the left main coronary artery (MCA) and a dominance of the left MCA.

Divers with bicuspid aortic valves should have an exercise test and echocardiograms performed on a regular basis. Those who develop evidence of stenotic lesions or who have ischaemic changes on exercise studies should not be permitted to continue.

Electrocardiographic changes - normal and abnormal

It is in interpreting electrocardiographic changes that the doctor dealing with the young diver, particularly the trainee will have most difficulty. If a person becomes very fit through training, a number of events take place in their body. Most noticeably, there is an increase in size of the heart - biventricular hypertrophy - which is associated with the habitual increased cardiac work. Because of the considerable increase in cardiac reserve, there is usually a marked increase in vagal tone. This is manifest in the bradycardia of the fit, and the fast return of the pulse rate to basal levels after exercise. The high level of vagal tone also gives rise to a number of changes which are to be seen in the electrocardiogram and which are not pathological but which may mimic changes seen in other conditions. The term "Athletic heart syndrome" has been coined to describe the panoply of abnormal signs found in the very fit. Typically they have a systolic murmur, x-ray evidence of cardiomegaly and a sinus bradycardia.

Examination of the electrocardiogram in these fit individuals reveals a number of features:

a) the low sinus rate associated with the high vagal tone may also be associated with atrio-ventricular conduction defects such as A-V Block (typically of the Wenckebach variety) and the slow rate may permit a variety of escape rhythms such as sinus escape, atrial ectopics, nodal ectopics or occasional ventricular beats;

b) the cardiomegaly may be reflected in electrocardiographic evidence of ventricular hypertrophy and may be associated with right axis deviation. There may also be borderline ventricular conduction delays;

c) non-specific changes in repolarisation may be seen as T wave inversions or more rarely, ST segment alteration.

It is a useful general rule that many of the changes in the ST/T wave segment of athletes become more normal when the subject is exercised indicating their vagal origin and providing a useful means of distinguishing them from more pathological manifestations.

The athletic heart syndrome is seen in FIT YOUNG MEN and it is their very fitness which points up its origins. When they stop training the changes slowly reverse. The athletic heart syndrome must be distinguished from:

- mitral valve prolapse
- obstructive and non-obstructive cardiomyopathy

The best way to make the distinction, if doubt exists, is through echocardiography.

Electrocardiographic changes which suggest organic heart disease

The commonest form of heart disease to be diagnosed on the electrocardiogram is that of ischaemic or coronary heart disease. The cardinal features of the electrocardiogram which point to ischaemic heart disease are:

1. **Pathological Q waves**

    The Q wave is the hallmark of the transmural infarction. Abnormal waves are defined as being either as more than 0.04s in duration or more than 25% of the amplitude of the conjoined R wave. Q waves of pathological magnitude can be found in normal individuals if there is an abnormal QRS vector.

2. **ST segment elevation suggesting sub-epicardial change**

    Poorly applied chest electrodes particularly in coloured individuals probably accounts for most of the false ST segment elevations seen; a convex bowing of the ST segment reminiscent of pericarditis is typical of electrode misapplication. Pathological conditions and electrode misapplication apart, ST elevation has been described in hyperkalaemia and hypothermia as well as in carbon monoxide poisoning and cyanide poisoning. If there is no clinical evidence to support the abnormality then best check the electrodes!

3. **T wave inversion and ST depression suggesting chronic ischaemia**

   This is the most difficult to interpret. T wave inversion in lead V_1 is normal, sometimes it extends into V_2 particularly with sloppy electrode technique. An isolated T wave inversion in any V lead or in lead III is also normal and not evidence of ischaemic heart disease.

In dealing with ECG abnormalities in fit young divers, an open pragmatic approach is indicated. Remember that minor changes mimicking ischaemic heart disease are common and will always be grossly over-interpreted by computer driven interpretation systems. Ask yourself if the changes are reasonable and if other evidence supports a pathological diagnosis. If it does not then there probably is not one.

Arrhythmias

The response of ventricular ectopics probably causes more concern than almost any other finding in inexperienced clinicians.

Simple ventricular ectopic activity

The simple, unifocal ventricular ectopic beat is familiar to most clinicians possessing an electrocardiograph machine. Such beats express a simple uniform shape and occur beyond the T wave of the preceding complex. They are usually followed by a compensatory pause often perceived by the patient as a missed beat. Infrequent simple ventricular beats are seen in 35-50% of normal individuals during ambulatory monitoring. They occur at greater frequency after the age of 40. Complex multi-focal ventricular beats with varying morphology are better indicators of pathology.

The frequency of ventricular premature beats (VPB) is increased by stimulants such as caffeine and tobacco. Some would claim that suppression of VPBs by exercise is an indication of their innocent nature; by contrast an increase in frequency in the post-exercise phase points to a more pathological interpretation.

Atrial dysrhythmias

By contrast to the innocent ventricular premature beat, atrial ectopics frequently point to some underlying cardiac pathology, particularly in the older diver. The atrial beat is initiated by the sinu-atrial node and spreads through the atrial myocardium and is seen as the P wave of the electrocardiogram. The electrical front finally arrives at the atrio-ventricular node and after a programmed delay is conducted through to the ventricles. Atrial ectopic activity is part of a transition through atrial flutter to atrial fibrillation. Not infrequently, subjects with high levels of atrial ectopics will, on 24-hour taping, be found to have transient atrial flutter and fibrillation as well as nodal rhythm.

The presence of a high incidence of atrial ectopics and other atrial dysrhythmias may indicate a number of underlying conditions:

1. A sinu-atrial node with inadequate function - the "sick sinus syndrome" - in which periods of asystolic arrest or escape rhythm may occur. These individuals are considered likely candidates for insertion of a pacemaker.

   If atrial ectopics are frequent, look carefully at the P waves of the normal beats. If they are small, changing in morphology or have a varying P-R interval then refer the patient for specialist evaluation.

2. A high incidence of atrial ectopics may also point to atrial distension or overloading such as is associated with pulmonary hypertension or mitral or tricuspid insufficiency.

Problems of the atrioventricular node

Conduction through the atrioventricular node normally takes from 160 to 210 msec. This is measured as the P-R interval. Commonly in young divers, two abnormalities may be found. When conduction appears to be too slow and when it appears to be too fast.

Slowing of atrioventricular nodal conduction

When conduction through the atrioventricular node is slowed there is said to be atrioventricular nodal block. Complete block, when the atria and ventricles are beating completely independently, is quite rare but has been found even in normals. In the fit young diver, the common abnormality is the partial av block where the P-R interval gets progressively longer with each beat till one is "dropped" (it may not be) and then the process starts from the beginning. This is sometimes called Wenchebach Phenomena. This is a normal phenomenon. However, some workers believe that the sub-population showing Wenchebach Phenomena is a precursor to later cardiac pathology. If one considers that a normal ECG looks like this:

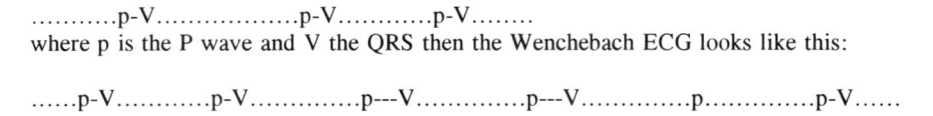

...........p-V....................p-V............p-V........
where p is the P wave and V the QRS then the Wenchebach ECG looks like this:

......p-V.............p-V..............p---V..............p---V..............p..............p-V......

This pattern is particularly seen during sleep recordings in the fit young subject. There is no reason to stop such individuals from diving.

Greater degrees of atrioventricular block and symptomatic atrioventricular block ("dizzy turns") require postponement of the certificate of fitness to dive and specialist investigation.

Accelerated atrioventricular conduction

Accelerated atrioventricular conduction is seen in a number of subjects. It appears to be associated with the presence of faster conducting bundles within the heart which bypass the slowing function of the atrioventricular node. Two manifestations of this syndrome are commonly seen and are termed: Wolf-Parkinson-White Syndrome (WPW).

In this syndrome there is an accessory bundle traditionally termed the Bundle of Kent which permits the rapid and uninterrupted conduction of the atrial impulse to the ventricles. The WPW electrocardiogram shows an altered shape P wave which almost slurs into the QRS with a delay in the QRS complex which is termed a delta wave.

A particular problem of WPW is the atrioventricular node which cannot protect the ventricle from being over-driven by an atrial tachycardia and thus atrial flutter-fibrillation can be conducted downwards with disastrous consequences. Studies have suggested that 12-80% of patients with a WPW pattern in the electrocardiogram may have paroxysmal tachycardias of some form or another. Chillingly, ventricular fibrillation may be the first and only presenting arrhythmia in these patients.

Additionally, WPW syndrome may be associated with a number of congenital cardiac defects. These are:

- Ebstein's anomaly of the tricuspid valve
- ventricular septal defect
- prolapsing mitral valve

The treatment of WPW found in the young diver consists of:

- cardiac referral
- 24-hour taping and exercise testing
- regular monitoring
- catheter or open ablation of the accessory pathway if necessary

Lown-Ganong-Levine Syndrome

This is another fast conducting atrioventricular disorder but this time characterised simply by a short P-R interval and a normal QRS complex. In normal sinus rhythm, the P-R interval is less than 120 msec in these patients. The same comments apply to this group as to the WPW group and specialist referral is indicated in most cases.

Abnormalities in Ventricular Conduction

Right bundle branch block is a common finding in up to 15% of the population. It is of no significance and is a normal variant.

Left bundle branch block is to be regarded as potentially pathological and certainly is if acquired later in life. Refer for further opinion before qualifying.

Abnormalities of Repolarisation

An inverted T wave in lead III, a VF and lead V1 may be normal. In III and a VF they should become less negative on inspiration. (Record on full inspiration and call it a IIIR). Isolated T wave abnormalities may be seen in V2 occasionally. The acid test is what happens on exercise testing.

Prolongation of the Q-T interval is associated with ventricular tachycardia if excessive but to measure needs to be corrected for the heart rate (corrected for QTc interval). Few practitioners would pick this up without computerised ECG. Two syndromes of familiar QT prolongation are seen, one associated with congenital deafness and the other not.

CARDIOLOGICAL INVESTIGATION AND ASSESSMENT
Dr. P.T. Wilmshurst

"Diving should be prohibited if the candidate has a medical condition which endangers him (or his buddy) by predisposing to in-water incapacity (e.g. unconsciousness, dizziness, dyspnoea, death) or predisposing to serious diving-related illness."

The problem is that many of the conditions we think predispose to incapacity probably do not, and many of the conditions that we don't consider predispose to diving-related illness do. For example, we worry about people having a few ventricular ectopics even though there is no good evidence that they are at risk of developing ventricular fibrillation, but we let people smoke 40 cigarettes a day and still be a professional diver even though common sense says that smoking must predispose to pulmonary barotrauma. I will show you some evidence later that supports this. So we have to be clear about what predisposes and by how much it predisposes.

Consider an individual who had been an amateur diver for many years, done many hundreds of dives without any problems and has had no cardiac symptoms whatever. He then decided that he wanted to become professional instructor and had a 12 ECG lead which showed that he has Wolf-Parkinson-White Syndrome (WPW). The theory is that he is at risk of ventricular fibrillation because we know that the accessory pathway can conduct very fast and so, if he goes to into something like atrial fibrillation with an atrial rate of 600, he could go into ventricular fibrillation. You and I are protected because we don't have an accessory pathway and we can't conduct that rapidly to the ventricle. Common sense would say that this chap should not dive because he is at risk of getting ventricular fibrillation. The problem is that he is entirely asymptomatic and he has, in a sense, proved himself as an amateur diver. We know that in fact lots of people have WPW and it's never diagnosed because they never have a 12-lead ECG. They don't die from it. If we exercised this particular chap you would see that, as his heart rate speeds up, the ECG characteristics of WPW disappear. He goes back into it as he slows down. So we know that this chap can't conduct quickly enough to go into ventricular fibrillation because in his case the accessory pathway cannot conduct above 150. So here is a chap with WPW who might be stopped from diving because, in theory, he could conduct fast and go into ventricular fibrillation and die suddenly, but in fact we know that his accessory pathway cannot conduct that rapidly and therefore he is not at risk.

So blanket rules should not apply, there should not be "tablets of stone".

Well, some people think that WPW occurs in 1% of the population but not all the time, people get it intermittently. So there should be a couple of people in this hall who have WPW and probably do not know about it, and luckily so. For those of you who have got it, it is not as malignant as most people think.

There are other associations with WPW that you should be aware of, such as congenital abnormalities and hypertrophic cardiomyopathy. Someone with athlete's heart might have hypertrophic cardiomyopathy with WPW. It would probably be wise to refer him to a cardiologist to make sure the heart is structurally sound but, having said that, I would allow someone to dive if they came out of the WPW on exercise, or did not conduct rapidly through the accessory pathway.

The accessory pathway does have a certain amount of variability in its conducting but it does not have so much variability that it will one day not conduct at 130 and the next day will conduct at 400. You may find that if it conducts at 200 it may conduct at 240 on another day when his adrenalin is up, or you may find that another conducts at 250 one day and 300 another day. But it is not going to present major differences. A cardiologist would not ablate this particular slow conducting pathway, because we would say that this person is not at risk of sudden death. So we would be happy to just pat him on the head and say "go away" if he was referred to us. The rate at which he conducts may vary a little but it will not vary considerably from his 150 maximum.

Would I allow someone who has medical treatment for WPW to dive? No, I probably would not, but that is more to do with concern about the treatment than the WPW. If WPW needs treatment, it is so easy to get it ablated with radio frequency now, that it should be ablated and then dive.

There is a small incidence of recurrence when it has not been ablated properly that is why I say 9 times out of 10, no problem. But you can test for this electrophysiologically.

Interjection

Douglas: I am just wondering if, with these ECG abnormalities, a distinction has to be drawn between sport divers and commercial divers. The sports diver is much more likely to be immersing his face in cold water and experiencing the vagal responses accorded to that, whereas the commercial diver is unlikely also to be breath-holding. There is an article in the most recent SPUMS journal about a case of atrial fibrillation presenting as decompression illness in those circumstances.

Wilmshurst: Well, I think professional divers may be in the same situation because many who are professional divers are actually using scuba-type gear. I accept that there are distinctions that one has to take into account and all I'm trying to do is just raise some questions so that people actually think about what the individual is going to do and what is the appropriate decision. They should not just say, as seems to be the case, "ventricular ectopic beats are a problem" when they are not a problem. Fifty per cent of the population have ventricular ectopic beats every day. One per cent of the population have WPW and do not know they have got it and will never know they have got it. I am just trying to put things into perspective.

I also think that it is pertinent that we have standards for commercial divers which say that people are banned from being a commercial diver, and yet people with the same condition will happily be allowed to fly you in a jet as the pilot. Either the standard is wrong for professional divers or it is wrong for commercial pilots, they cannot both be right.

VALVULAR DISEASE

In valvular disease, we have to look at the haemodynamic consequences of the disease because, for example, people with aortic stenosis and mitral stenosis cannot increase their cardiac output rapidly in response to stress. Significant stenosis of valves would be a contra-indication to diving. We have to look also at the short and long term risk of complications, for example in people with mitral stenosis there is a risk of developing atrial fibrillation, there is a risk of developing systemic emboli and strokes, and there is the consideration of the long term deterioration of valve function. If one is going to allow someone to dive now but are going to say to them in 5 years time "you have got to stop because the valve has deteriorated", is it fair to let them undertake the expense of training in the first place? We ought to consider these factors.

Those with aortic stenosis may get angina, syncope and heart failure. The problem with sclerosis and bicuspid valves is that they do progress to aortic stenosis although they are no real problem until they do. There is a slight risk of emboli but not very much with the bicuspid valve. Aortic regurgitation occurs but where do you draw the line? Colour-flow doppler shows that 25% of the population have some degree of aortic regurgitation. So it is a real problem to draw the line and say what is significant and what is not.

In terms of the mitral valve there could be stenosis which predisposes to pulmonary oedema particularly if fluid overload occurs or if central blood volume is high. These occur when immersed, so mitral stenosis is a real problem for divers. They should not be allowed to dive with mitral stenosis because of these risks. Mitral regurgitation? Well over 30% of the population have mitral regurgitation so again it is a matter of degree. Mitral prolapse - well I think that is a normal variant in 10% of the population. It is like being left-handed in my opinion. Complications are rarely associated with prolapse, but when they do occur, they are usually in the type of prolapse which is associated with other pathologies, for example the Marfan syndrome. To make the distinction may be the job of a cardiologist.

Mild stenosis or regurgitation of the pulmonary and tricuspid valves is not a problem. In fact, it is so common it is a question of whether the absence of tricuspid regurgitation is abnormal!

Problems come after valve surgery, and the cardiologist will assess residual valve dysfunction. Some have their original valve which has been cleaned up, or a valvotomy of some sort has been performed so it is no longer stenosed. Those people have the same sort of risks as someone with sclerosis of the valve, i.e. they do not have major risks if they do not have major haemodynamic problems, unless of course they had previously developed a large left atrium which would put them at risk of atrial fibrillation or emboli. Mild degrees of residual valve dysfunction after surgery are not, in themselves, a problem.

Valve replacement may present a problem. Certainly, if someone is on anti-coagulants because they have a metal or plastic valve, that presents a contra-indication. But what about the individual who has a tissue aortic valve? They are not on any treatment. What about the patient who has had their own pulmonary valve put in the aortic position so that they have actually got their own valve tissue in the aortic position and it is a normally functioning valve. Should they be allowed to dive? The valve will be functioning pretty normally. We have to consider associated problems such as chamber enlargement prior to the valve replacement or valve surgery, in which case they may still be at risk of emboli or arrythmia. Then there is the question of chest surgery, but some people will not have had any surgery. There is an increasing number of people who have had a percutaneous pulmonary valvotomy for pulmonary stenosis such that their valve has been dilated without any incision in the chest. Should they be allowed to dive? I cannot see any reason why they should not. Their valve has been dilated, it is nearly normal in function in most cases and all they have had is an incision in their leg. Each case obviously needs to be considered on its own merits.

ISCHAEMIC HEART DISEASE

Symptomatic ischaemic heart disease predisposes to in-water incapacity: they have angina, they die suddenly, they get arrhythmias or they get left ventricular failure. What about the 30% of people with ischaemic heart disease who have asymptomatic or silent ischaemic heart disease? By and large you will not pick it up on a 12-lead ECG. You might pick it up on a standard exercise test, but most exercise tests which are performed are unstandardised. With an unstandardised exercise test on healthy, asymptomatic persons showing significant changes on the ECG during exercise, Baye's theorem says that it is more likely to be a false positive than it is to be a true positive. That is why commercial pilots do not have exercise ECG's before they are 50, because all you will be doing is disqualifying people from flying when there is nothing the matter with them. If you do exercise tests on asymptomatic people, positive tests will usually be false positives.

But what about the people who have ischaemic heart disease? What about when you have dealt with it? Well, you could deal with it by coronary grafting, but that presents some problems. The first problem is that you rarely get complete revascularisation even if you use multiple grafts because those who need grafting usually have multiple narrowings throughout their coronaries. Graft survival is finite. Of vein grafts, 20% are occluded in one year so if you have 5 grafts, at the end of the year you may only have 4 left. After 10 years most of the vein grafts are not working anyway. But the interesting thing is that some people after coronary grafts are allowed to fly commercial aircraft, at least as a co-pilot.

Interjection

Unidentified speaker: One brief point, there are in aviation history extremely few recorded incidents due to myocardial infarction or cardiovascular disease and in fact there is one that is truly documented. So I think that bringing in aviation is not wholly analogous to diving as the two do not share the same set of environmental problems.

Wilmshurst: I sort of accept that, I mean the only one I know about that was documented to be due to myocardial infarction was the Staines aircrash which killed over a 100 people. All I am trying to do really is to get you thinking.

If a patient has had successful revascularisation of single vessel disease by angioplasty, there is a risk that he would get restenosis subsequently but this risk is really during the first 3 months and you can look for it prospectively. If he has not got restenosis then, he probably will not get restenosed in the short term and possibly not in the long term. Would you allow that chap to dive? We know now that he has got near normal coronary arteries, better I would guess than the majority of divers on whom you have not done a coronary angiogram.

HYPERTENSION

Hypertension is associated specifically in diving with pulmonary oedema. It is also associated with:

- stroke
- coronary artery disease
- infarcts
- angina
- aortic aneurysm
- peripheral vascular disease

Many of those complications could cause a sudden incapacity. One can screen for many of them at the physical examination. The problem with hypertension is defining a cut-off value. This would be entirely arbitrary which is why different countries have different blood pressure cut-off values.

The risk of these vascular events increases as hypertension becomes worse, so if anyone is slightly hypertensive there is a slightly increased risk for their future diving. What degree of risk should one accept to allow them to dive?

One example is that of a woman who ascended from a dive near Plymouth. She had acute pulmonary oedema, coughing up froth and blood, and was short of breath and cyanosed. The oedema was confirmed in the chest x-ray. This had cleared two weeks later. She had had no treatment in the interim and she had been entirely returned to normal.

DISCUSSION

Cross: Since you mention this case, I might just say that this particular lady was in her 40's. She was airlifted to the recompression centre with a diagnosis of pulmonary barotrauma and/or pneumothorax. She had surfaced acutely short of breath with chest pain and was a bit blue at the edges. She might well have ended up in the chamber but in fact she resolved very rapidly with a dose of intravenous Frusemide.

Wilmshurst: Of the first four people I saw with diving-induced pulmonary oedema, one of them was markedly hypertensive. The other three, with time, went on to develop hypertension. Indeed, that is the finding in subsequent cases and I now have about a dozen cases of amateurs who have developed diving-induced pulmonary oedema. The problem is that, at the time you screen for it, they are not necessarily hypertensive. They later go on to develop hypertension but the vascular and neural problems which predispose to hypertension and which predispose to pulmonary oedema pre-date the actual hypertension. So many of these would be allowed to dive commercially.

We studied their vascular resistance during a number of physiological interventions such as exercise. We used a modified cold pressor test and instead of putting the arm in iced water, we immersed the head in iced water while breathing oxygen from a regulator, as oxygen is also a mild constrictor in most people. These persons have a higher vascular resistance than controls at rest and it does not come down as much as do the controls on exercise. They have a greater pressor response to all pressor stimuli, pharmacological and physiological. To get forearm vascular resistance up to near 200 is very abnormal (with a phaeochromocytoma in crisis one might get up to 150). So these individuals form an interesting sub-group which is not fully understood. The problem is that, although they go on to get hypertension, the risk of heart failure pre-dates the development of hypertension. This presents a problem for screening.

Cross: Are you saying that you ought to do a cold pressor test as part of a diving medical?

Wilmshurst: No. It is too difficult. The reason we don't use the standard cold pressor test, ie by immersing the hand in ice, is that some persons vasodilate. There is a mixed response (partly a cold-mediated constrictor and partly a pain response) and so some people actually dilate. To do it reproducibly one would have to have the head in iced water.

Cross: Would your group of abnormals have shown an exercise-induced hypertension?

Wilmshurst: Their blood pressure does rise on exercise but there is certainly an overlap with the normal population.

Cross: If you did an exercise test on a diver and he put up his diastolic considerably during the exercise, would you say he was at risk of immersion pulmonary oedema?

Wilmshurst: I do not know the answer because nobody has studied it enough. I would be concerned if someone developed a diastolic of 150 during exercise.

Mebane: As regards athletic heart, in reading the standard exercise physiology texts, they make the point that the heart is indeed a large heart but it still remains within the bell-shape curve of normal heart size. It is not an abnormally large heart. So, do you gentlemen regard the hypertrophic athletic heart as out of the range of normal? In contrast, I have atrophic cardiac myopathy, where there is true left ventricular hypertrophy. This is definitely an abnormally enlarged heart with the risk of sudden death and so on.

As regards prosthetic valves, aside from anti-coagulation which concerns me considerably, there is some limitation on cardiac output and one can foresee that a diver could get into a problem with a current in the water which would demand in emergency an amount of cardiac output that he could not meet. There is no prosthetic valve that puts out the amount of cardiac output that a normal valve will. I would appreciate your comments on those matters.

Wilmshurst: It is very difficult actually. One says that an athlete's heart should fit within normal distribution but I happen to know many top Olympic athletes' hearts do not fit within the normal distribution. In fact, you can demonstrate that if they stop training, it returns to within the normal distribution. Many have very large hearts on chest x-ray and on echocardiography they have some features which could be difficult to distinguish from mild hypertrophic myocardiopathy.

Prosthetic valves vary in their ability to open and close but generally I am against those with such valves diving, because most prosthetic valves are slightly stenosed. A greater problem is those who have a tissue valve which is often normal in function, particularly early on if they have not started to calcify as may happen. Every case needs to be considered on its merits. It is too easy to lay down rules and say that no one with this condition should dive.

Cross: My experience is with the fit young diver. I have never seen a diver with a prosthetic valve and hope I never do. However, as a slob, I find the idea of an exercise induced cardiomyopathy rather satisfying, good luck to them - they deserve it. However, I do see a lot of very fit young men presenting to be professional diver trainees and when you echo them they have a very fat septum. One has to define it as a very fine "piece of steak". There is always the problem of the fit young man who has the big athletic heart: is this chap going to croak or is he not? I am afraid one finds really fit young men who do croak at the peak of their athletic performance, they just drop off their perches!

Lepawsky: I was interested in the concept of diving-induced pulmonary oedema and I wonder if you could develop that a bit further.

Wilmshurst: There is a group of people who get pulmonary oedema when they dive and this was described in the Lancet (Wilmshurst et al, 1989). The main thing that causes them to vasoconstrict is a pathological response to cold. The raised partial pressure of oxygen may contribute because it is a vaso-constrictor too and, coupled with the fact that they are immersed, so their filling pressures will be raised.

Having said that, we recognise that hypertensives get pulmonary oedema when they go out in the cold. We also recognise, for example, that all sorts of cardiac mortality are 50% more common in the winter in this country than in the summer. In most countries there is a seasonal variation of significant proportion but not necessarily the same magnitude. There is a significant increase in risk related largely to cold exposure and vaso-constriction. We also know that there are groups of people with normal coronaries, who get pulmonary oedema when they have other stimuli. Some of these persons we have catheterised and they have essentially normal hearts and normal coronary arteries in particular. They can be precipitated into a left ventricular failure despite normal coronaries and we have got others who are precipitated by other stress. For example, one man who reproducibly was going into pulmonary oedema during sexual intercourse, for him that was a stress. On vaso-dilator treatment he was fine until another doctor decided to stop it and he went back into pulmonary oedema on intercourse, and so he is now on the treatment again. There was a general practitioner who used to get into pulmonary oedema, twice requiring ventilation, when he argued with patients and we put him on treatment. So now he can argue with patients all the time! One other patient, who is a football club supporter, went into pulmonary oedema three times, once each time after Swindon Town had scored a goal. We debated about whether we should treat this because we doubted the chances of Swindon Town ever scoring another goal!

Cross: I have a comment which is more concerned with hyperbaric oxygen therapy. Oxygen is a vasoconstrictor and probably also a veno-constrictor. Anybody who does regular hyperbaric oxygen therapies on the sort of crumble that gets served up by the health service for HBO treatment, needs to watch the older person with a large heart. A number of them in the chamber for HBO end up with pulmonary oedema. I am sure that this is due to their central venous pressure shooting up and on several occasions I have had to go in and decongest them in some way.

Wilmshurst: In response I would just say that if you look at the venous tone in these people, it goes up in the same way as the arterial tone, so not only have they increased their afterload, they are increasing their preload.

Lepawsky: In following that up, how do you differentiate between diving-induced oedema and the manifestations of decompression illness?

Cross: For a time I did wonder whether diving-induced oedema might not be diagnosed as the chokes. In the good old days, until Peter wrote his paper, it was not something that I was recognising very often. I think if you are aware of it, you take a lot more care to identify it. In my experience as a diving doctor I have not seen a recent case of the "chokes", maybe one but it is very rare. Water-induced pulmonary oedema is probably a lot commoner, but could well be wrongly diagnosed as acute pulmonary decompression illness (chokes). This is a real problem in diving medicine for, whatever goes wrong with the diver, it is diving-induced, and so they get brought to the chamber. One could perhaps miss that diagnosis.

Elliott: The "chokes" is indeed rare. The only case to present with classic manifestations whom I have treated, followed a few hours after a dry dive in a warm chamber. He had no neurological manifestations. So, in making the diagnosis of pulmonary oedema after a wet dive, what delay is the maximum interval after surfacing before you would expect this to come on?

Wilmshurst: There's no interval. Many of these people actually were puffed at depth.

Elliott: So that would be diagnostic. For differential diagnosis, if a person does not have oedema upon arrival at the surface, can he get it later?

Wilmshurst: No. They rapidly get very much better as soon as you get them out of the water.

Cross: As a matter of interest, are you still recommending that they take a dose of Nifedipine before they dive?

Wilmshurst: Officially, I recommend that they don't dive. Some amateurs will say they are going to dive anyway so I say "well, if you insist you are going to dive then I will give you my best advice but it's not what I would recommend, I recommend that you don't every dive again." Those who ignore that advice take Nifedipine and that helps. Some of them have ACE inhibitors but I'm not recommending it.

Turner: I was particularly interested in the case of WPW syndrome which you described. A few weeks ago I had a young man who came to me for a commercial diving medical because he wanted to be a SCUBA instructor. He also wanted to have a PADI and a BSAC medical performed. I did the commercial diving medical and he seemed very fit until I looked at his

ECG which demonstrated WPW syndrome. On the basis of this, I failed him. I discussed the case with my local cardiologist who agreed with my decision that he was at risk of developing sudden blackouts and should not be passed. When I failed him I told him that if he could find a cardiologist who would support his application and state that he had no risk of these blackouts, I would reconsider the decision. He has, in fact, now told me that he has obtained such a letter. I would like to ask, if he produces this letter, do you think that I should pass him myself or should I defer a decision and insist that he appeals to the HSE?

Wilmshurst: Can I just go back a bit. Did the first cardiologist say to "this chap should not dive because he is at risk of blackouts?" That is what he said?

Turner: That's what he said, but he didn't do an exercise test. He just looked at the ECG.

Wilmshurst: Well, do you not think it is a bit odd if you are just going to say that you have got a young man who is at risk of dying? I think you have then got to investigate him. It is a moral imperative to assess him and, if he really is at risk, do something about it. You must think about ablation and think about medical treatment. If you do not believe it then you do not have to bother about that. There is a paradox here. A doctor cannot say that this chap has a treatable condition and he is at risk of dying but I am not going to do anything. So there is something wrong with the first statement. The second thing is, I think that if you have been given two conflicting views, you should find out why the second cardiologist feels that he is not really at risk. If the second cardiologist feels that he's really not at risk because he has done the test, such as an exercise test, and decides for those reasons he is not at risk, then I think it is perfectly reasonable to suggest that the chap should appeal to the HSE in order to find out an official answer.

Turner: Do you think any pressure should be brought to bear on sport diving associations to make ECG's compulsory?

Wilmshurst: I am not sure that they are really of great use. Twelve lead ECG's are not useful in picking up ischaemic heart disease so I am not sure that there is any great value in them.

Turner: I was really thinking in terms of picking up asymptomatic WPW.

Wilmshurst: If people are asymptomatic I do not think there is a problem. I would rather not know that I have got it.

Broome: With an asymptomatic diver in his mid-twenties and his first ECG has a right bundle branch block pattern, do you investigate, refer or ignore?

Wilmshurst: Right bundle branch block in a fit man with nothing else to find, I personally would not investigate.

Boonstra:** What can be said about a diver with hypertension without systemic complications (as evaluated by the specialist in internal medicine) who will be treated with ACE-inhibitors? Should this diver fail an initial examination? What is the timescale before he is stable on this type of medication (during which he might be unfit to dive)?

Reply from Wilmshurst: Unless blood pressure was controlled on a very low dose of ACE-inhibitor, I would suggest that he is unfit to dive.

REFERENCES

Wilmshurst, P.T., Treacher, D.F., Crowther, A., & Smith, S.E. *Br. Heart J.*, 1994; **71**: 229-231.

Wilmshurst, P.T., Nuri, M., Crowther, A. &, Webb-Peploe, M.M. Cold-induced pulmonary oedema in scuba divers and swimmers and subsequent development of hypertension. *Lancet* 1989; **1**: 62-65.

EXERCISE TOLERANCE TESTS FOR DIVERS
Dr. J. Madsen

The physical work capacity of man is limited by his maximal rate of oxygen uptake ($\dot{V}O_2$ max) which again is limited by his cardio-pulmonary function. It is obviously necessary to make sure that a diver will not be handicapped by a subnormal ability for physical work. As there is a linear relationship between protracted external work intensity and the rate of oxygen uptake, a man's $\dot{V}O_2$ max is also a measure for his capacity for sustained labour.

What is the lowest acceptable limit for $\dot{V}O_2$ max? For healthy, normal men between the ages 20 and 40 years the mean value decreases from 3.5 to 3 l/min (varying from 2.6 - 4.5 l/min). In older age it declines below 3 l/min (Åstrand & Rodahl, 1986; de Vries 1986). On this background a minimum $\dot{V}O_2$ max of about 3 l/min is often recommended. For young men this does not imply a high degree of fitness. Since the physical demands on divers do not decrease with age, it seems appropriate to maintain the same requirement for older divers, although for them it means better fitness than the average for the age. The oxygen consumption of 3 l/min corresponds to the cost of underwater swimming at a speed of about 2.2 km/h.

The Swedish Directorate for protection of workers have suggested, as the lower limit for divers below 40 years, the ability to perform 200 Watts for 6 minutes and 150 Watts after the age of forty. This corresponds to oxygen uptakes of only 2.75 and 2.13 l/min respectively.

Since big people have a higher $\dot{V}O_2$ max than small people, the $\dot{V}O_2$ max is often expressed per kg body weight. This figure is often given as a multiple of 3.5 ml/kg/min, which is taken as the resting oxygen consumption and called 1 MET (metabolic equivalents/measurement in exercise training).

The MET value indicates how many times the individual is able to increase his resting oxygen uptake. Bove (1987) recommends 13 MET's as lower limit. For a body weight of 70 kg, this corresponds to a $\dot{V}O_2$ max of 3.2 l/min. However, the MET score for a certain $\dot{V}O_2$ max decreases with increasing body weight (Table 17). Since the work demands are similar on small and big divers, it seems reasonable to state the $\dot{V}O_2$ max requirements in l/min rather than in ml/kg/min or MET's.

TABLE 17 - MET SCORE RELATED TO BODY WEIGHT

WEIGHT kg	$\dot{V}O_2$ MAX	
50	3.2 l/min	18 MET's
60	3.2 "	15 "
70	3.2 "	13 "
80	3.2 "	11 "
90	3.2 "	10 "
100	3.2 "	9 "

The $\dot{V}O_2$ max can be assessed in various ways:

1. It can be measured directly during graded exercise increasing to exhaustion on a bicycle ergometer or treadmill. This requires complicated equipment and experienced personnel, and implies a certain risk for the subject in case of incipient cardiac illness.

The $\dot{V}O_2$ max can also be extrapolated from heart rate and $\dot{V}O_2$ measurements at steady state submaximal work loads (Åstrand & Rodahl, 1986; deVries 1986). Extrapolation is done to the maximal heart rate corresponding to the age (which is 220 minus age). However, this is given with a certain inaccuracy (SD +/- 10 beats/min).

The oxygen uptake measurements can be omitted, since the ratio between external work and oxygen consumption (i.e. mechanical efficiency) is fairly constant for different persons (SD +/- 6%).

In this way the $\dot{V}O_2$ max is estimated with a SD of 15% (Åstrand & Rodahl, 1986).

3. A great number of maximal and submaximal step tests have been described. I shall only mention those I have seen recommended in connection with medical examination of divers. They have in common that the heart rate is not measured during exercise, but during recovery. The idea is, that a fit person in comparison with an unfit will have a small oxygen dept after a standardised exercise load, and that he will be able to repay more oxygen per heart beat during recovery.

The Harvard Physical Fitness Test (Brouha, 1943): the candidate is required to step up and down a 20 inch (50.8 cm) platform 30 times per minute for up to 5 minutes. The pulse is counted from 1 - 1.5, from 2 - 2.5 and from 3 - 3.5 minutes after stopping work. Fitness is read from an index relating duration of exercise to sum of pulse counts. An index above 80 is good.

The Army Physical Fitness Test (HSE, 1987) is the same, except that the platform is only 43 cm high and that the 5 minutes must be completed. The sum of pulse counts is required to be less than 190.

Various workers have studied the correlation between $\dot{V}O_2$ max and the Harvard Physical Fitness Test. DeVries and Klafs (1965) found a correlation coefficient of 0.77 and a standard error in predicting $\dot{V}O_2$ max from Harvard Physical Fitness Test of Ý 12.5%. However Hettinger (1961) found only a correlation coefficient of 0.41. Thus this type of test can only give a rough idea of $\dot{V}O_2$ max. More primitive are the following:

In the **Master's two-step test** (Ellestad, 1975) the subject has to walk up and over a 2 step device 18 inches high for 1½ mins a number of times depending on age, sex and body weight, after which the heart rate is determined. The load is very modest and the heart rate increases only to between 50 and 60% of the maximal for the age. The test has been shown to be a very poor predictor of $\dot{V}O_2$ max.

The "**5 step test**" is recommended in the British Underwater Association Code of Practice for Scientific Diving and in the statutory Danish Regulations for Medical Examination of Divers. A candidate must pass the following simple test: after stepping up onto a chair 5 times in 15 seconds, the pulse rate should return to the pre-exercise level in 45 seconds.

Ehm and Seeman (1965) have suggested a similar test. After 30 deep knee-bends in 30 seconds the pulse rate must return to resting level in 3 mins.

These tests say nothing of $\dot{V}O_2$ max, but may serve as a screen for the most unfit. I have found no comparison of their results with $\dot{V}O_2$ max determinations.

A high $\dot{V}O_2$ max is no guarantee that the diver is able to do strenuous work underwater. For the professional diver, the exercise tolerance test need only serve as a measure of cardiopulmonary function, since his physical proficiency underwater is checked in other ways. However, for the recreational diver, who may want to resume diving after a year's pause, a test that informs on his capacity for work in the water would be more useful.

At the Danish Navy Diving School, Ahrenkiel has compared $\dot{V}O_2$ max values with the time for swimming 1 km in a pool. The results for 19 diver candidates are shown in Fig. 2. It is no surprise that good swimmers have a high MET's, while high MET's may be seen in poor swimmers. The 4 candidates who dropped out of the course because of poor practical performance were all poor swimmers. It is finally seen that several passed the rather strenuous course with MET values of 11 and 12. The number of subjects is small, but the results suggest that a satisfactory swimming test indicates a satisfactory $\dot{V}O_2$ max and in addition gives information about the candidate's in-water skill.

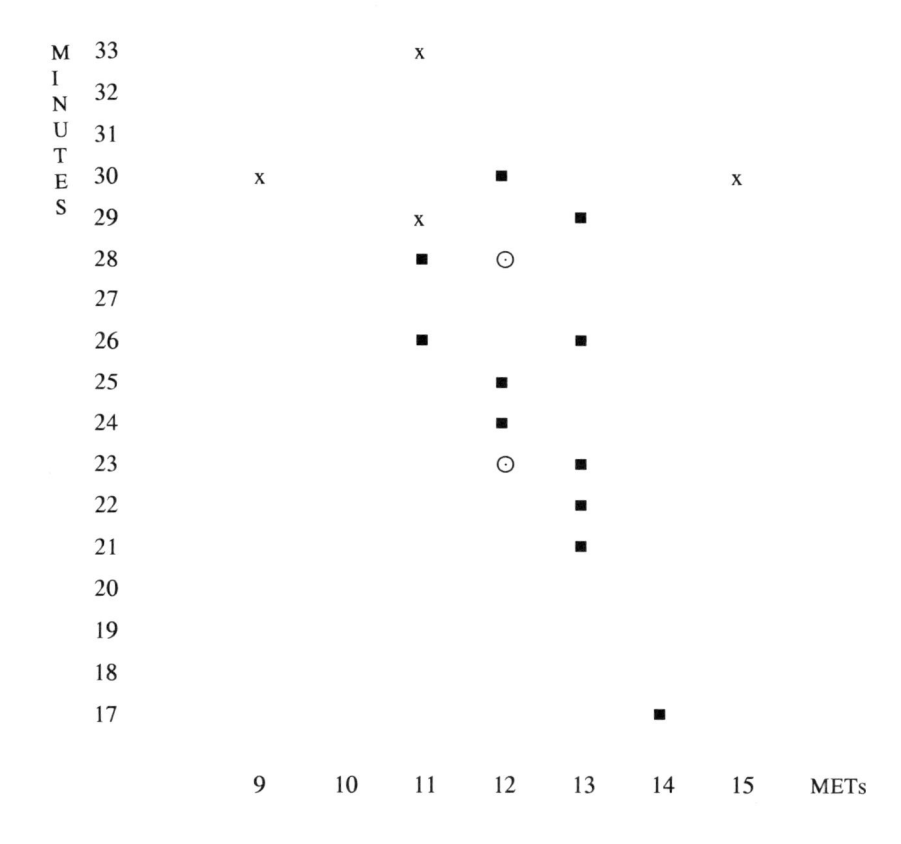

```
M   33                    x
I
N   32
U   31
T
E   30        x           ■           x
S
    29            x       ■
    28        ■   ⊙
    27
    26            ■       ■
    25            ■
    24            ■
    23            ⊙   ■
    22                ■
    21                ■
    20
    19
    18
    17                ■
         9   10   11  12  13   14  15   METs
```

Fig. 2: Time for swimming 1 km in pool plotted against METs values obtained by sub-maximal bicycle ergometry. Measurements from 19 diving school candidates at entry to the Danish Naval Diving School, Winter Class 1994.
x = Drop outs
⊙ = 2 subjects with identical values

The desirability of tests for fitness to particular types of exercise that are typical of diving has led the US Navy to identify a number of physically demanding tasks representative of fleet divers work and to design a test battery based on them (Marcinik et al, 1993). The test battery consists of:

1. lift of a 100 lbs descent line clump 3 feet up;
2. lift and carry an 83 lbs SCUBA bottle 100 feet, repeated 6 times;
3. in SCUBA gear with fins and breathing air, to swim and carry a 50 lbs tool bag a distance of 50 feet repeated 4 times;
4. in SCUBA gear with fins and breathing air, to tread water by fin kicking for 2 mins;
5. to pull a 100 lbs umbilical line a distance of 150 feet and
6. with MK-12 diving gear and breathing air, to descend and ascend a 14 foot vertical ladder.

These tests will serve as the basis for minimum entry and graduation level for physical standards for the US Navy fleet diver training.

CONCLUSIONS

1. The $\dot{V}O_2$ max limit should be stated in l/min, not in MET's or ml/kg/min.

2. The limit could probably be set somewhat below 3 l/min, maybe at 2.7 or 2.8 l/min.

3. The $\dot{V}O_2$ max requirement shall not be reduced with age.

4. A demanding swimming test or some underwater exercise test is probably more useful than the $\dot{V}O_2$ max determination.

REFERENCES

Åstrand, P.O. & Rodahl, K. *Textbook of work physiology*, 3rd Ed. McGraw-Hill: N.Y. 1986.

Bove, A.A. Pp 26-41, in PG Linaweaver & J Vorosmarti (Eds.). *Fitness to dive: 34th UHMS Workshop.* UHMS: Bethesda. 1987.

Brouha, L. *Res. Quart. Am. Assoc. Health* 1943; **14**: 31-35.

de Vries, H.A. *Physiology of exercise*, 4th Ed. Brown: Iowa. 1986.

de Vries, H.A. & Klafs, C.E. *J Sports Med. Phys. Fitness* 1965; **5**: 207-214.

Ehm, O.F., Seemann, K. *Sicher tauchen.* Albert Müller Verlag: Zurich 1965.

Ellestad, M. *Stress Testing, Principles and Practice.* Davis: Philadelphia 1975

Hettinger, T., Birkhead, N.C., Horvath, S.M., Issekutz, B. & Rodahl, K. *J. Appl. Physiol.* 1961; **16**: 153-156.

HSE, Health & Safety Executive, UK. *MA1, the medical examination of divers.* HSE Medical Division: London. 1987.

Marcinik, E.J., Hyde, D., Doubt, T.J. *Undersea & Hyperbaric Medicine* 1993; **20** (Suppl): 38-39.

DISCUSSION

Nome (Chairman): You focused on equipment for testing that can be easily made available in any doctor's surgery. One of the main requirements for testing is that it is reproducible, and this is the real basis for re-examining the same diver's performance when he comes back, year after year. We should aim for a set of tests that are standardised.

Broome: Bicycle ergometer $\dot{V}O_2$ max's tend to be some 10% below treadmill $\dot{V}O_2$ max's but they are both called $\dot{V}O_2$ max. Of course neither of them is. How do you reconcile that potential problem with the interpretation of what is really just an arbitrary figure which bears little relation to function?

Madsen: I would say that if you do treadmill testing with skiing poles you get even higher values. The concept of $\dot{V}O_2$ max depends on the technique used. It is not very important to have a precise value in comparison to a person's ability to perform in the water.

Grönkvist[**]**:** Dr. Madsen - what exercise tolerance testing is appropriate? In the Swedish Navy we use bicycle ECG to establish working capacity and to investigate the cardiac reaction to physical stress. One main problem with this method is that a lot of divers have difficulty to reach their maximum pulse rate due to the fact that their leg working capacity on a bicycle is not sufficient to reach maximum pulse rate. How do you deal with this problem?

Reply from Madsen: The problem of difficulty to reach maximum pulse rate is well known; particularly in well-trained individuals with large stroke volumes. Cardiologists here believe that for cardiac evaluation it is not necessary to reach the maximal heart rate (220 - age), if only the heart rate x blood pressure product increases by at least a factor 2.5. Moreover, higher heart rates can be obtained on a treadmill (particularly walking with ski poles) than can be reached on the bicycle ergometer.

INTRACARDIAC SHUNTS
Dr. P.T. Wilmshurst

I would like to speak about intracardiac shunts including what most people know as patent foramen ovale (PFO) in relation to diving decompression illness and fitness to dive.

Forty per cent of bends occur in divers who have adhered to tables. In different circumstances some people say the figures are higher or lower but a significant proportion of divers have adhered to accepted tables and most of those get neurological symptoms with onset soon after surfacing.

The first of these cases whom I saw had done a 100 previous dives. Then, at age 40, he did a single dive to 38 m for 15 mins. Two minutes after surfacing he had girdle pain and then unilateral paraesthesia, dizziness and syncope. When he woke up he was paraplegic. He was successfully recompressed, discovered to have a murmur afterwards and found to have an atrial septal defect which was subsequently repaired.

The next case was a man who, at the age of 23, had a cerebral embolus which occurred quite suddenly while straining at stool. He made a good recovery, he was not investigated for a PFO at that time and no cause for his stroke was found. He started diving and made 75 uneventful dives and then one day did a single dive, 29 m for 20 minutes and, 10 minutes after surfacing, became hemiplegic. He recovered and then did another 7 uneventful dives. He then dived to 26 m for 26 minutes and got another early neurological bend. That is when I saw him for the first time and did a contrast echocardiography which demonstrated a PFO.

Another case was that of a diver of 30 who had done over 900 dives, the deepest 46 m, and then he had done a seemingly innocent dive, 30 m for 18 minutes. After a 6 hour surface interval he did a second similar dive and, on surfacing, got tightness round the neck, dizziness, vomiting and hemiparesis. He was recompressed. He was later found to have a shunt.

So we decided we would look at the relationship between intra-cardiac shunts and decompression illness, which we discovered had previously been described in aviators.

In atrial septal defects there is bi-directional flow but usually with a PFO there is only uni-directional flow, right to left, because it is usually a true flap valve. We looked at the relationship between right to left interatrial shunts and decompression sickness in divers and, although most of them are PFO's, we cannot with this technique usually distinguish a small atrial septal defect from a PFO, but we will talk collectively about "PFO's".

The aim of this study was to investigate the relation between the different manifestations of decompression sickness and the presence of right to left interatrial shunts in a blind controlled trial. We had 97 divers with a history of decompression illness of whom 50 had early neurological (CNS) symptoms on 58 occasions. We had decided in advance that our cut-off between early and late CNS symptoms was 30 minutes on the basis of the 3 uncontrolled observations I have just described and 2 others. Thirty five divers had late onset neurological symptoms on 38 occasions and 20 divers had limb bends on 23 occasions. Fourteen divers had cutaneous decompression sickness on more than 29 occasions but some people could not give us details of the dives so we considered only those in which we only got the dive details. Twelve divers had cardiorespiratory symptoms on one occasion each. We compared them with divers who had never had decompression illness.

We considered the following dive-related risk factors for decompression sickness:

- missed stop
- rapid ascent
- post-dive ascent to altitude
- dives >50m
- repetitive deep diving (40m or deeper)
- frequent diving (>3/day to >10m)
- DCS in the companion

We felt that decompression sickness (DCS) in a companion indicated some problem with the decompression profile. In fact this was never the only factor. We never had 2 bent divers unless there was something else the matter with the dive and often there were 3 things wrong.

We conducted a blind controlled study with contrast echocardiography at rest, with a modified Valsalva (x 6) and with a cough (x 2). Both of these cause shunting, right to left. After one injection one finds shunts in 11% of the population, but after two injections one finds it in 22%, and it then starts to plateau out. So we think 5 or 6 injections are needed to be fairly certain a shunt will not be missed if an individual has one. Once a shunt was found we didn't go on and do the further procedures.

In the control group of 109 divers, we found that 24% had shunts. Of those with early neurological bends, 66% had shunts. Those who had late neurological bends and limb bends were 26% and 15%, not significantly different from the control group. Thus early neurological bends (66%), skin bends (86%) and cardio-respiratory symptoms (58%) were all significantly more often associated with PFO than in the control group.

When we looked at the number of episodes, rather than the number of divers, in relation to risk factors we found that in late neurological bends and limb bends the majority (about 80%) have risk factors in their dives. In the other groups, those with skins bends or those with early neurological symptoms, the minority had risk factors in their dives. Risk factors were present in about half those with cardio-respiratory symptoms, and this was significantly less than for late neurological and limb bends and higher than for early neurological and skin bends.

In those with early neurological symptoms a significantly higher proportion had done single dives compared with those with late neurological symptoms and limb bends. In those with shunts and early CNS bends there were 40 episodes of which 28% had risk factors. There were also 4 in this study who we found had lung disease, of whom none had risk factors. Of those who had early neurological symptoms but no pathology, the great majority had risk factors in their dives.

Those with shunts and lung disease had done intermediate depths of dives, about 30 m, but those with no pathology could be sub-divided into those with rather deeper dives and those with shallower dives, depending on whether there was a risk factor present. There was no pathology but risk factors present in deeper dives and no pathology and risk factors absent in shallower dives, but there was a higher incidence of smokers in the latter. This is not statistically significant because of small numbers, but it has got us thinking about those who had early neurological symptoms but had no risk factors, no overt lung disease and no shunts. If there were no risk factors in the dive, no shunt and no overt lung disease we wondered whether there might be occult lung disease. From this study we conclude that a large proportion of divers have potential inter-atrial shunts. These divers are at risk of decompression illness when performing dives which have a low morbidity risk in divers without shunts. Neurological symptoms and cutaneous decompression sickness soon after surfacing suggests the presence of a shunt.

We then studied further the role of cardiorespiratory abnormalities and dive characteristics in the manifestations of neurological decompression sickness, with the aim of determining the cause of bends arising inside the tables in those who do not have an intracardiac shunt and, in particular, to determine whether occult lung disease or smoking could be responsible.

The subjects were divers who had neurological symptoms with onset within 5 minutes of surfacing, referred during a 4 year period, but those with evidence of lung disease on chest x-ray were excluded.

The divers were divided into 3 groups (Fig. 3.). The first 2 groups were those who had neurological decompression illness after unprovocative dives. **Group 1** were those with intracardiac shunts on contrast echo and all of them had a large shunt. Only a very small proportion of divers have a large shunt using the accepted grading based on the number of bubbles, and a very small proportion of the normal population have large shunts. So to have a group of 13 divers with large shunts is unusual. Each of them had one episode of rapid onset neurological DCS but, in addition, there were in 2 of the divers 3 episodes in which similar symptoms occurred between 5 and 30 minutes after surfacing.

In the **Group 2**, who had no intracardiac shunts, there were 11 divers and 14 episodes of rapid onset neurological DCS following unprovocative dives.

The next group were those who had neurological decompression illness after provocative dives and we divided those into **Groups 3a, 3b and 3c**. There was one diver who fell into group 3a on one occasion and 3b on another occasion, that is to say he got one episode of neurological decompression illness after a rapid ascent and on another occasion he got it after missed stops. Group 3c consisted of 2 divers, 2 episodes, rapid ascents, missed stops and no shunts.

So you will note that in our 36 divers there were in fact 17 shunts.

UNPROVOCATIVE DIVES

GROUP 1: intracardiac shunt on contrast echo (all large)
- 13 divers
- 13 episodes (+3 episodes, 5-30 mins. post-surfacing)

GROUP 2: no intracardiac shunt
- 11 divers
- 14 episodes

PROVOCATIVE DIVES

GROUP 3a: rapid ascents
- 5 divers, 5 episodes
- 2 shunts (small)

GROUP 3b: missed decompression stops
- 6 divers, 6 episodes
- 2 shunts (large)

GROUP 3c: rapid ascents & missed stops
- 2 divers, 2 episodes
- 0 shunts

Fig. 3. - The grouping of divers with neurological symptoms

The primary end-point was the "blind" comparison of flow-volume loops for abnormalities in Groups 1 and 2. Secondarily there was a comparison of other lung function abnormalities and prevalence of smoking in Groups 1 and 2 and a comparison of dive characteristics and clinical manifestations in all three Groups.

The important thing is that in Group 1 where the divers had PFO's, none of those had abnormal flow-volume loops but 50% of those in Group 2, who had neurological symptoms after unprovocative dives, did have abnormal flow-volume loops. This is very unusual in a fit, healthy and young population. (One diver could not perform lung function tests because of residual high spinal paralysis and bullous lung disease visible on CT but not on plain chest x-ray). This difference was statistically significant (Fig. 4).

GROUP 1	-	0/13
		$p < 0.01$
GROUP 2	-	5/10*

* 1 diver could not perform lung function tests

Fig. 4. - Flow-volume loops (premature airway closure)

If we looked at the groups of divers and their smoking (Fig. 5) you will see that in Group 1, 2 out of 13 were smokers whereas 6 out of 11 in Group 2 were smokers. The difference just failed to achieve significance. In Group 3, 17% were smokers, which is similar to Group 1 and the British Sub-Aqua Club (BSAC) membership, 17% of whom are smokers. So in Group 1, 3 and the BSAC, 15-17% are smokers, but the incidence of smokers is nearly 4 times as high in group 2. If you add together smokers and evidence of gas trapping on lung function tests you will see that 15% of Group 1, that is to say two of them, were smokers but did not have evidence of gas trapping but in Group 2 you will see 8 out of 11 were either smokers or had evidence of gas trapping. That difference was significant.

	SMOKERS	SMOKERS AND/OR GAS TRAPPING
GROUP 1	2/13 (15%)	2/13 (15%)
GROUP 2	6/11 (55%)	8/11 (73%)
	$p < 0.1$	$p < 0.05$
GROUP 3	17%	
BSAC	17%	

Fig. 5. - Smokers in the groups of divers and in the BSAC

This led to the following conclusions:

1. neurological symptoms soon after unprovocative dives are related to (large) intracardiac shunts (Group 1) and to occult gas trapping (and possibly smoking) (Group 2).

2. dive characteristics & clinical manifestations in these groups generally differed.

3. pulmonary barotrauma & resulting gas embolism caused spinal injury when spinal tissues were able to amplify embolic gas.

We also conducted an investigation into the functional size of shunts in divers who had decompression illness after unprovocative dives.

CONCLUSIONS

1. Gas embolism due to pulmonary barotrauma causes early symptoms (within 5 minutes) after surfacing.

2. Symptoms are predominantly (but not exclusively) cerebral.

3. Paradoxical gas embolism can produce symptoms after unprovocative dives.

4. Neurological symptoms generally occur within 30 minutes of surfacing.

5. Spinal effects are more common than cerebral because the lag before peripheral bubble nucleation occurs has the effect that spinal >cerebral tissues and white >grey matter have greater tissue nitrogen loads and greater ability to amplify gas emboli.

6. Autochthonous bubbles and arterial gas embolism which occurs by pulmonary vascular transit of bubbles are only likely to be important aetiologies of decompression illness after extreme dives.

7. Arterial gas embolism due to pulmonary vascular transit of bubbles is likely to be associated with cardiorespiratory symptoms due to pulmonary artery obstruction, but similar symptoms could result from coronary artery embolism following paradoxical gas embolism and pulmonary barotrauma.

REFERENCE

Wilmshurst, P., Davidson, C., O'Connell, G. & Byrne, C. *Clinical Science* 1994; **86**: 297-303

DISCUSSION

Denison: Peter, your work is potentially very important but I have got two criticisms. One is that in your paper in Clinical Science, you really didn't have any controls. You made a comparison between those who had PFO's and those with respiratory defects but it was obvious in the paper, and I have read it carefully 2 or 3 times, that there were no controls. But the other worry I have is that you do not distinguish between cause and effect and, when you tell us that you could pick up PFO's better the greater number of times you tried, this could be interpreted as showing that you were maybe creating the PFO's with the bubbles. It could be that there is a high percentage of PFO's in divers who have had a decompression illness because the illness has created the PFO, it's opened the garden gate. What do you think about that?

Wilmshurst: I accept that it would be preferable to have better controls but the problem about doing contrast echo's is there is a small morbidity risk associated with it. We have looked at people who have not dived but are wishing to dive and want to have a contrast echo but we have not finished that yet because I have moved jobs. There are similar proportions of PFO's in divers who have not had the bends and in control subjects who have not dived. Autopsy studies show a similar percentage of PFO's somewhere between 25 and 30%.

Denison: I accept that but its the higher incidence in those who have surfaced with neurological symptoms where decompression illness may have opened a previously closed PFO and you do not discuss that in your paper.

Wilmshurst: No, we have not discussed that and I do accept it. One can only do that if you look at divers prospectively. Do their contrast echo's and follow them up throughout their career but do not tell them if they have got a PFO so they don't modify their diving habits. Then wait and see which one is going to bend. That is the only way to do it.

We are exactly analogous to the studies with smoking and lung cancer. No one disputes the evidence about smoking and lung cancer but, in fact, no one has ever taken two groups, made one group smoke and the other not smoke, then follow them prospectively and see if the smoking group gets more lung cancer. We are looking retrospectively and it does have that problem but I think it becomes more compelling particularly when you look at shunt size.

Nome: As Chairman, I need us to answer the specific questions. What are the cardiovascular contraindications to acceptance for diver training? It has been mentioned but not succinctly. Could you give a brief statement?

Wilmshurst: I think that the cardiovascular contraindications are those where there is a haemodynamic problem with valvular disease or a cardiomyopathy.

Nome: I would also like some comments about which of these examinations could be performed by family practitioners and which ought to be performed in specialist centres by consultants? This may be related to which components of the conventional cardiovascular examination are essential annually? The ECG?

Wilmshurst: As far as ECG's are concerned, I think that its not so much whether you do ECG's annually but whether you compare them annually. One can have one's ECG one year by one doctor and another doctor the second year and some other doctor the third year. It may remain normal each time and yet show evidence of significant disease because it is steadily changing. By the same token, an ECG could be "slightly abnormal" but really not be indicative of heart disease and if it did not change it would not matter. So you need to make sure that it is reviewed in the light of all the previous ECG's. It is not so important as to how frequently you do them but how you watch the changes.

Cross: Certainly the practice in our own unit has been that when you find that an "abnormal" is normal, this is written on the man's certificate. If we have a diver who has a murmur, we investigate it and if we find it to be not significant to his diving, the best thing is to write it on his certificate. We may also give them copies of their ECG's to take them to their next medical.

Nome: There would be benefit in having a central registry of this information which is available to doctors when they were seeing a diver for the first time.

Now, using validated procedures, what are the blood pressure limits on entry, when a person want to become a diver, and the subsequent thresholds in relation to age?

Wilmshurst: I have no idea. I think it is entirely arbitrary.

Cross: Much depends on your ability and willingness to sneak up on him. A lot of people, when threatened, have high blood pressure. There is the diver who comes and says "I always have high blood pressure doctor, they tell me every year" and that means that his normal response to stress is hypertensive. I think there is a great enthusiasm on the part of the medical profession, who do not like failing people, to regard "white coat hypertension", as it is sometimes called, as a normal finding when, in fact, the man is a labile hypertensive and a hypertensive responder.

If you want to get someone's normal blood pressure, exercise them, put them back on the bed, get them to relax, because there is nothing quite like the vasodilatation after exercise, tell them they have done fine and that they have probably passed. Then sneak up on them and take their blood pressure. Then, if you do not get a normal result, fail them.

Lewkowicz: Exercise tests are relevant, we can do them in the GP surgery. Should we be doing them annually?

Wilmshurst: The problem is with annual exercise tests they are a good way of assessing fitness but I am never too sure of how good they are for picking up heart disease. In asymptomatic people the value of the test is very low. What are you going to do next if a 25 year old man on exercise gets no pain, but his ST segments go down?

Lewkowicz: I am not talking about a treadmill ECG test I am asking about his ability to perform as a mark of cardiorespiratory fitness.

Cross: In my unit we don't do fitness exercise tests at all, what I do in fact is look at the man's logbook. If he comes to me as an active professional diver and his logbook is full of dives then I tend to say that the he is fit enough to continue diving. I have never found any value whatever in fitness testing for evaluating a diver. Exercise testing in divers has two functions. One is to elucidate or demonstrate something that you are suspicious of, such as hypertension or a murmur. The other is if you want to know if there is a reduced cardiorespiratory response to exercise. Perhaps another reason we do exercise testing is purely punitive: if I have got an obvious couch potato I stick him on the treadmill and flog him, so he goes away chastened and learning that he had better get himself fit. That is quite effective but we do not actually do it for assessment.

LeDez: I am very concerned about blood pressure, the limits seem to be arbitrary because the HSE in the UK say a diastolic of 80, some other countries are saying 90 or 100, and it seems to me we need more time to discuss this. A lot of young people coming for dive medical examinations do have some mild hypertension, say 160/90 or sometimes 160/95. What about the role of medication? Are we going to accept some divers on medications to control the blood pressure?

Elliott: Could I interject here because I can see ourselves running out of discussion time? The existing guidance says "the initial examination should not exceed 140/80" but it says nothing about a numeric limit at later examinations. Do our consultants agree with that, or do they say it is wrong? Is an appropriate conclusion that, after the initial medical, it is at the diving doctor's discretion?

Wilmshurst: Certainly a diastolic of 80 struck me as being rather too low. It is not hypertension and one would not consider treating it. So it is hard to stop someone doing a job because of a disease which they don't have.

Elliott: But this is only at the initial examination before they begin to be trained.

Wilmshurst: Yes, I accept that.

Nome: Could we please reach a conclusion on components of the conventional cardiovascular examination are essential annually?

Cross: Take a history. Listen to the chest, although I don't think you'll find much. I am against routine chest x-rays every year. I think a normal chest x-ray on starting and then I do not do them again until the age of 32 unless I have a reason to do it. Thereafter about every 3 years until about the age of 40 when it drops down, unless they are a bad smoker or something like that, I think the radiation risk is far greater than the health risk. An electrocardiogram because everybody has an ECG machine although I doubt very much that, after the initial examination, it is worth much.

Wilmshurst: I think people undoubtedly need a history and examination but I am not sure what tests need to be done. I agree people ought to have a chest x-ray on starting but not for some time after. I am not sure of the value of a 12-lead ECG. If people give no history of past cardiac symptoms or there is nothing to find on examination then the only reason is to have one for later reference once people are 40 and review its progress. I do not see that you need it annually.

Cross: When would you first do a lipid profile?

Wilmshurst: I would not.

Nome**:** a) This session did not provide enough guidance. Blood pressure levels are important, and a set maximum level must be established (e.g. 140/80 or 140/90).

b) Physical fitness test - I strongly recommend using bicycle ergometer testing and <u>not</u> using any step tests.

c) $\dot{V}O_2$ maximum level - For divers over 35 years, the minimum level should be 35 ml O_2/kg/min.

Reply from Wilmshurst: a) It is convenient for there to be a generally accepted level of blood pressure which is approved for professional divers, but the level chosen should ideally be based on scientific evidence. Unfortunately, such evidence does not exist, so any "cut-off" will be arbitrary and, hence, unfair to some prospective divers. However, it seems to me particularly unreasonable to set a level at which individuals who are normotensive by conventional criteria are excluded from diving because licensing authorities believe them to be hypertensive (cf. - HSE level of diastolic BP of 80 mm Hg).

b) Any test of physical fitness should be standardised to allow reproducibility, but the choice of protocol should be based on objective evidence of value.

c) Why?

Desola**: Your human experimental studies on bubble formation due to the presence of a foramen ovale, would have been much more interesting if they had included doppler bubble detection in those divers. Why did you not use this valuable technique, trying to correlate bubble degree with clinical symptoms and echocardiograms?

Reply from Wilmshurst: The divers were not studied at the time of their bends, so it was impossible to measure the degree of bubbling. Clearly it was not possible to subject them to the dive profile which caused their bends again, in order to correlate the degree of bubbling.

Welslau**: Would you recommend a standardised bicycle ergometer with 12 lead-ECG for recreational divers fitness certification? For the first examination, or also for every follow-up examinations? For every diver, or only for recreational divers over 40 years old?

Reply from Wilmshurst: I do not believe that there is any good evidence for performing exercise tests on asymptomatic recreational divers.

Örnhagen**: Decompression illness in professional divers is rare today. One of the differences in dive procedures between professional and sports divers is the ascent rate. Professionals usually ascent at 10 m/min. while sports divers ascent at 20-40 m/min. (especially from <20m depths). Could this difference in ascent rate be the explanation for the difference in decompression illness incidence?

Reply from Wilmshurst: I am not aware of any commonly used sport diving decompression tables which uses such rapid ascent rates. I assumed that the predominance of decompression illness in sports divers is the fact that there are considerably more dives by sports divers than by professional divers.

Lewkowicz**: Dr. Cross stated that he assesses a diver's fitness by looking in his log and if he has been busy diving in the last year then he considers that the diver is fit. I do not agree because being fit enough to make 200 routine dives does not necessarily render the diver fit enough for an emergency. I consider some sort of annual basic fitness test to be an essential part of a commercial diver's medical evaluation.

Elliott: I would remind you that we do have a form for supplementary questions on this particular topic and on aspects which have not been addressed, like the peripheral vascular disease. We have had a very good tour through the minefield of cardiology, which appears to confirm that we do require for referral highly trained cardiologists who understand diving. We do not have the good fortune to have universally available in this country consultants who are competent in diving, like those speaking to us today. They are both active divers themselves and they appreciate the special features of the diver's working environment. We also need to define the "specialist centre" but this will be addressed in the later session on training standards.

COMMENTARY

In this section there was time to cover the majority but not all of the items that needed to be reviewed. Dr Peter Wilmshurst has subsequently commented further on some of the paragraphs of guidance which are quoted at the beginning of this session, page 75. He has made the following proposals:

(b) any organic heart disease is a cause for rejection *unless it is considered by a cardiologist to be haemodynamically unimportant.*

(d) disorders of rhythm, except for sinus arrhythmia and ventricular extrasystoles *(OMIT "which disappear as the heart rate increases")*, should be referred for the opinion of a cardiologist. These should usually be a cause for rejection;

(f) any evidence of coronary insufficiency or myocardial ischaemia, clinical or electrocardiographic, is a cause for rejection *but bear in mind false positive exercise tests in young fit people.* Coronary artery bypass surgery will not render a person fit for diving, *though percutaneous transluminal coronary angioplasty (P.T.C.A.), if it produces revascularisation, should render a person fit.*

(h) the resting blood pressure at the **initial** examination should not exceed 140 systolic or 80 diastolic ... *This should be changed to 90 diastolic.*

Dr. Wilmshurst stressed that the problem with exercise testing is that the types of exercise tests recommended are not comparable. An individual would easily pass one but fail another. He also summarised his answers to some of the questions that were still outstanding:

The cardiovascular contraindications to acceptance for diver training are ischaemic heart disease, all types of cardiomyopathies, haemodynamically significant valvular disease (but not trivial valve lesions), cyanotic heart disease and other shunts, primary or secondary heart disease. Each valvular defect must be assessed on its own merits. Any rhythm disturbance which might cause in-water incapacity should disqualify, but individual assessment is required. Discussion of the case of a diver with a Wolf-Parkinson-White syndrome led to the conclusion that general rules cannot be applied.

There is better evidence for screening for PFO's in prospective divers than there is evidence for measuring BP or performing ECG's. Dr. Wilmshurst proposed three possible strategies:

1. screen all new professional divers for PFO's but not stop any from diving. Follow them all prospectively;

2. screen all new professional divers for PFO's and disqualify those with "large" PFO's (using our published criteria) which are seen on one or two contrast injections;

3. screen all divers who have had bends (or bends unexplained by their dive profile) and ban all those who have a PFO.

The consensus view at Edinburgh and Luxembourg did not accept Dr. Wilmshurst's options but supported the present HSE advice to screen divers by echocardiography only after two or more episodes of neurological manifestations.

Dr. Wilmshurst continued that there is no data published showing the value of the ECG in the evaluation of diver fitness. The consensus view was that the current recommendation, for an annual resting ECG to be carried out at each examination, should be discontinued.

The various indirect methods of estimating maximum oxygen uptake by exercise testing were reviewed. The results of the Step Tests were unreliable to the extent that a subject might pass one of them but might fail another and so should be used as only gross guidance. There is merit in considering a more functional test, such as the time taken to swim one kilometre, as an annual measure of continuing fitness but this could not be easily verified by the examining doctor. It was concluded that, rather than the indirect, the direct methods of measuring oxygen consumption are more appropriate for providing an indication of fitness but that these were possibly too complex or costly to be considered as an annual routine. It was considered as relatively unimportant that the treadmill test gives results 10% greater than those from bicycle ergometry. Thirteen METS (45.5 ml/kg/min) was generally considered to be a useful measure of individual fitness. A less specific proposal that a general standard of 2.8 litres/min oxygen consumption, regardless of weight or age, would provide a functional target, did not achieve consensus. The METS standard should be assessed at 3-yearly intervals or, at the doctor's discretion, more frequently.

Obesity may predispose to some type of bends and is inversely related to fitness. Body mass index [$BMI = Wt(kg).ht(m)^{-2}$] is the best way to measure it but is relatively arbitrary. Some degree of fatness can protect against the cold and that, as an indicator of fitness, exercise tolerance testing would seem to be more appropriate.

Peripheral vascular disease may predispose to cold injury. Each case should be assessed as a relative contraindication.

PULMONARY

Chairman : T.J.R. Francis

The recommendations from the Guidance Notes on "The Medical Examination of Divers" are:

26. There are two essential and inter-related aspects. These are:

    (a) to exclude as far as reasonably possible the presence of any respiratory condition which would be hazardous to individuals or their colleagues while employed in a diving operation;
    (b) the assessment of the respiratory function of divers to ensure that they are capable of meeting the demands of their occupation.

27. A review of the history of the respiratory system should be taken at **the initial statutory medical examination** and brought up to date as necessary as subsequent examinations. Clinical examination of the chest must be carried out at each medical examination and any abnormality investigated. The diver must be able to breathe freely through each nostril. The finding of an abnormality may require that the individual be referred to a specialist unit for detailed investigation. Full sized PA and lateral chest radiograph are essential at the **initial statutory medical examination** and thereafter full sized PA annually.

28. Ongoing respiratory conditions which preclude diving are:

    (a) any respiratory infection such as pneumonia, tuberculosis, sarcoidosis or pneumonitis;
    (b) the presence of lung cysts, emphysematous blebs or bullae, poorly aerated areas of lung, a pneumothorax, pleural effusion, lung fistula, bronchiectasis, fibrosis or neoplasm;
    (c) a history of spontaneous pneumothorax (but see (g) below);
    (d) chronic bronchitis/emphysema or asthma;
    (e) functional evidence of generalised or localised air trapping in the lungs;
    (f) any evidence of chronic or recurrent sinusitis, rhinitis, nasal congestion or severe allergic conditions of the upper respiratory tract.

    There are also conditions requiring individual assessment but which may be allowable. These are:

    (g) history of pneumothorax, if provoked by unusual respiratory stress or following surgery where there has been sufficient time (at least 3 months) for the rupture to heal and where detailed respiratory functional investigation by a specialist laboratory shows no evidence of local or generalised airflow obstruction;
    (h) history of asthma or broncho-constriction after early childhood provided that there is now normal lung function and no evidence demonstrable of increased bronchial reactivity;
    (i) thoracic trauma, provided the injury has healed and there is evidence of normal lung function.

29. Spirometry is essential at each examination. The forced vital capacity and forced expired volume in one second must be recorded (see also Appendix 2).

    APPENDIX 2 (Paragraph 29)

    It is recommended that the following prediction formulae be used for interpreting the measurements *made from the spirometric trace:*

(a) Forced Vital Capacity - (FVC)
    Males   = $(0.052 \times ht) - (0.022 \times A) - 3.60$ [SD 0.58]
    Females   = $(0.041 \times ht) - (0.018 \times A) - 2.69$ [SD 0.37]

(b) Forced Expired Volume in one second - (FEV_1)
    Males   = $(0.032 \times ht) - (0.028 \times A) - 1.59$ [SD 0.52]
    Females   = $(0.028 \times ht) - (0.021 \times A) - 0.87$ [SD 0.33]

where ht = height in cm
A = age in years

A value below 1 SD of the mean should be investigated by a pulmonary physician. When interpreting the value FEV_1 /FEVC %, allowance should be made when the FVC is greater than 100% of the predicted value calculated from (a). This assessment can be made using the relationship expressed in the linear regression equation:

$$Y = -0.177 \times 0.177 X + 102.1$$

where Y is the FEV_1 / FVC % and X is the FVC expressed as a percentage of the predicted value noted in (a)

A range 2SD from the mean is suggested as defining the limit of normal distribution of FEV_1 /FVC. The SD of the correlation coefficient is 0.03, hence the X value should be multiplied by 0.237 to obtain the lower limit, and by 0.117 for the upper limit of the range.

HSE "Health Notes" : RADIOGRAPHY OF THE CHEST AND LUNG FUNCTION TESTING IN COMMERCIAL DIVERS

As a result of discussion within HSE and consultation with external diving medical experts we feel it appropriate to recommend a change in the current guidance relating to radiography of the chest and lung function testing.

It has hitherto been advised that commercial divers have an initial PA and lateral chest radiograph at commencement of employment and that the PA film be repeated an annual intervals. We have also indicated the need for annual assessment of lung function by spirometry. Experience has shown that whilst chest radiographs do reveal otherwise undetected abnormalities of the heart and lungs at initial examination they do not, in isolation, identify significant pathology at subsequent annual examinations.

In view of our wish to reduce overall radiation exposure we are, therefore, amending our guidance on the examination of divers. From now on we recommend that:

(i) PA and lateral chest film should continue to be obtained at the first commercial diving medical examination;
(ii) thereafter chest radiography should not be carried out as a routine;
(iii) the need for chest radiography should be assessed by the examining doctor in the light of the divers medical history, a clinical examination of the chest and the assessment of lung function;
(iv) lung function should continue to be assessed by spirometry;
(v) we shall be issuing revised forms MS80 with boxes in which the examiner will be asked to enter the values for FEV_1 and FVC obtained. This will provide a "fallback" source of information for future examiners in the event that the diver does not attend the same examiner on successive occasions.

PULMONARY FITNESS - AN INTRODUCTION
Surgeon Commander T.J.R. Francis, R.N.

I am grateful to Hans Örnhagen who yesterday suggested that our objective should be to look at criteria for the exclusion of divers from diving. This will be a difficult task because we require knowledge to make such decisions. Setting standards presupposes that we know what is going wrong in the diving accidents that we are trying to prevent and secondly that we know what predisposes to the sequence of events.

This morning we will try and address both of these issues. In the first part we will look at the effects of lung function on diving. After that we will look at the effects of diving on lung function. In conclusion we will try and answer the following questions:

- What are the pulmonary contraindications to acceptance for diver training?

- How significant is a history of chronic obstructive airway disease? How is this defined and how can it be assessed?

- What is the role of provocation testing for asthma? Indeed, how is asthma defined, and is it proven to be a risk factor in diving safety?

- What are the mechanisms of pulmonary barotrauma and are there pulmonary risk factors which can be assessed and controlled?

- Is a history of spontaneous pneumothorax always disqualifying? What is the evidence that transthoracic surgery *per se* or traumatic pneumothorax is a risk factor?

- Many divers dive with a recent cold, what is the evidence that a recent acute 'chest infection' is indeed a reason for temporary disqualification?

- What are the pass/fail criteria for the initial chest x-ray?

- What pulmonary function tests are needed? Have the current pass/fail criteria for FVC and FEV_1 been effective? To what should they be changed? What is the role of flow-volume loops?

- What is the significance of a diminishing TLCO? At what value does it warrant further investigation? Is a low value, *per se*, ever disqualifying?

- What are the effects of age on pulmonary function?

- How frequently are the components of a physical examination needed? What components of the routine pulmonary examination may be unnecessary annually? Are there components that require less frequent examination, at least until some specified age?

- To what extent is the examination focused on in-water safety and to what extent on the avoidance of diving-related disorders?

MECHANICS OF PULMONARY BAROTRAUMA
Professor D.M. Denison

When Oscar Wilde first went through U.S. Customs he said "I have nothing to declare by my genius", which roughly translates into "I have very few slides". Similarly his description of a group of intellectuals "earning a precarious living taking in each others washing" signifies "I am largely going to talk about other peoples' work".

The lungs contain very flimsy alveoli and even flimsier airways. On breathing out, these airways collapse before the alveoli are empty, creating the "residual volume" typical of the lungs of all terrestrial mammals. Even when the lungs of such a mammal are breath-hold dived to a depth of 1000 ft (300 metres) they contain alveolar air trapped by the collapsed airways, remaining in contact with pulmonary capillary blood. Common sense suggests that on rapid decompression, the obstructed parts of the lung will have the greatest difficulty in emptying and that it is therefore these parts that will be at the greatest risk of lung rupture. This prejudice has led to the belief that the purpose of doing lung function tests on divers is to identify obstructive elements in the lung that would predispose to lung rupture. Yet the evidence in favour of this belief is itself flimsy.

When you expire forcibly, the harder you blow the emptier you get and the less flow becomes, until eventually you reach residual volume, still with one or two litres of air in the lungs but despite all the pressing, none coming out. At this stage all the airways are closed but the moment you take a breath in the airways open up and air can sweep inwards very easily. There is no doubt that in severely damaged lungs where many airways are damaged, lung emptying can be dangerously impaired in the event of rapid decompression but such degrees of damage would preclude people from swimming safely in any case, i.e. they would not be fit to go to sea.

However there is much evidence from submarine escape training and from the rapid decompression of aircrew in training that reasonably healthy lungs can vent very freely indeed. What is required to burst a lung? It is known from wartime experiments and from the studies of Malhotra and Wright (1961) that healthy lungs burst at a transmural pressure of about 75 mm Hg (10 kPa). Calculations suggest that lungs must have a time constant of emptying of 0.4 seconds to prevent such an overpressure developing during an ascent at a rate of 10 ft/sec (2 to 3 metres/sec) as in submarine-escape training. This is considerably faster than the 0.8 seconds seen in a voluntary forced expiration which is of course a totally different and inappropriate comparison. In other words, on rapid decompressions healthy lungs empty at surprising speeds.

Instinctively one expects that when the lungs tear it will be the flimsy alveoli that rupture, but such tears are probably of little significance because of the small dimensions involved, and the high pressures that are required from Laplace's Law to force air through small but moist apertures. On taking a deep breath the elastic tissue of the lung is stretched longitudinally and, by stress concentration, it is the medium to moderately small airways that are most likely to rupture and release significant quantities of gas into the moist mediastinum. Malhotra and Wright found that lungs that were allowed to expand freely would burst on the outside, leading to a pneumothorax, but those that were pressurised but prevented from expanding burst within, leading to a pneumomediastinum.

There are two groups of people in whom lung rupture is common but the patterns of presentation are quite different. In one group, patients on ventilators, lung rupture leads to pneumothoraces and quite often to pneumomediastinum, but cerebral arterial gas emboli are rare. In the other group, divers and submariners, pneumothoraces are rare, pneumomediastinums are common and cerebral arterial gas embolisms almost equally so. The explanation for the difference springs from Malhotra and Wright's studies. The patients are usually given muscle relaxants so that they do not "fight the ventilator". When they are over-pressurised the lung expands unopposed and bursts on the outside, hence the pneumothoraces. When divers are over-pressurised they are trained and struggle to breath out, inhibiting the expansion, so that the lung bursts on the inside leading to the pneumomediastinums and to gas embolism.

Nevertheless there is still some mystery about gas embolism. In the lungs the arteries run extremely close to the airways. When the lung ruptures internally the escaped air is believed to travel along the peri-arterial sheaths. It might have sufficient pressure to burst into the pulmonary arterial system and get swept into the alveolar capillaries and trapped, doing little harm and being slowly resorbed. However the gas also gets milked up towards the hilum where it can break into pulmonary veins and from this systemic gas emboli arise.

There is little objective evidence to date that obstructive lung disease increases the risk of lung rupture in divers. Also it is known that very many people with severe obstructive disease have flown commercially and none has come to harm from lung rupture. What is odd is the observation by Colebatch et al (1976) that rupture occurs more frequently in people whose lungs are small and stiff. This has been confirmed more recently by the Royal Navy in an important study on trainee submariners and Peter Benton will talk about this later.

Also, more recently, in studying many divers and submariners thought to be at risk of lung rupture, I have seen several cases of spontaneous pneumomediastinum in which the lung has ruptured when the subject has simply taken a deep breath. This has led me to think that internal lung rupture is a normal event that usually passes unnoticed, but should it occur due to deep breathing at depth it will lead to gas embolism even on a well-controlled and slow ascent. So, although there is no doubt that uncontrolled ascents and breath-holding on ascent are important causes of lung rupture, best prevented by careful training, there is another and significant preventable cause which is that of "skip-breathing", i.e. the deliberate practice of taking deep breaths and holding the lungs at full capacity underwater, to economise on air. Therefore I believe all divers and submariners should be trained to avoid taking deep breaths under any circumstances when under pressure.

REFERENCES

Colebatch, H.J.H., Smith, M.M. & Ng, C.K.Y. *Resp. Physiol.* 1976; **26**: 55-65.

Malhotra, M.C. & Wright, H.C. *J. Pathol. Bacteriol.* 1961; **82**: 198-202.

CURRENT CRITERIA OF PULMONARY FITNESS TO DIVE
Dr. S.J. Watt

What does a diver need in terms of lung function in order to dive safely? In order to provide adequate alveolar gas exchange there must be adequate lung function and no impairment of exercise tolerance. A person with inadequate respiratory function is on the surface is unlikely to be fit underwater because of the dense gas and the limitations of using breathing apparatus. Inherent in that requirement is the need to be able to tolerate breathing apparatus. Some persons for example are happy to use oronasal masks underwater but are unhappy with a nose clip and mouthpiece.

Professor Denison has already discussed some of the issues concerning the risk of barotrauma. Clearly the diver's lung function must be adequate to leave him with an acceptably low risk of barotrauma. We know that there is a population of sports divers with asthma who dive regularly and we also know that there are some commercial divers who have evidence of air-flow obstruction who can dive successfully. Are we screening for the wrong reason? There is evidence that asthmatics are over-represented in the statistics from both diving fatalities and from the DAN data on diving accidents. However, they appear not to be the victims of pulmonary barotrauma. The implication is that they have increased risk of decompression sickness. We are therefore using pulmonary screening perhaps to screen out the risk of decompression sickness. Finally, what are the risks of the early dives? Australian data suggests that among those who die at a very early stage in their diving activity, there is a disproportionately high number of asthmatics and there are anecdotal reports of persons with mild asthma who have got into serious difficulty in the early part of their diver training.

The problem of the candidate who possibly has asthma is determined by pulmonary function, can he exercise adequately when in the water? First in most circumstances this means that the diver will have normal lung function when he is not suffering from the acute effects of his condition. Secondly, one needs to be sure they will not get into any difficulty when in the water. The diver also has to be able to tolerate breathing cold gas and not get therefore exercise induced asthma. The exercise test therefore is an essential step. Those who have a significant broncho constriction on exercise should not dive. In fact there is experience of sports divers who have quite marked impairment on exercise and yet who never have problems in the water but this may be because the level of exercise in the water never the achieves the level of ventilation necessary to trigger exercise-induced asthma. However it might arise in an extreme rescue situation. Other challenge tests are much less useful. Bronchial hyperactivity in response to histamine does not seem to be a relevant test. At the beginning of the challenge test when one has to do a control inhalation of nebulised normal saline, one diver who had a history strongly suggestive of asthma dropped his FEV_1 by 30% and I did not bother to proceed further. If he could do that with saline then a few drops of sea water would create a real problem.

I have no difficulties with what Professor Denison has just said about airway obstruction but we must remember that asthma can cause other problems. One such problem is spontaneous collapse of a lobe in a young person with asthma. Asthma must be considered in a wider sense since mucus can plug significant airways.

In the existing guidance there is no difficulty with the recommendation that those with acute infections are not to dive. The problem is much more so with the chronic disorders. Whatever the risk of barotrauma for such persons they are in any case going to fail on the basis of inadequate ventilatory capacity. It gets a bit more difficult with those whose pulmonary function is entirely normal but who may have a lung cyst. There is also the problem of previous spontaneous pneumothorax of which a recurrence is likely. If it occurs underwater this could be fatal. Whether it is reasonable to allow those who have had some kind of pleural fixation to return to diving is another question. In my opinion a pleurectomy would be the only possible acceptable procedure because with all others there still remains the possibility of a recurrence. We do not know enough about interstitial lung disorders or upper zone fibrosis. We do not know if conditions which produce areas in the lung of different compliance represent a potential risk factor for barotrauma. It is suggested, anecdotally, that pleural adhesions may also be a risk factor for barotrauma.

A traumatic pneumothorax, whether from a road traffic accident or from an underwater explosion, should make a complete recovery and diving is then allowable.

Acute sarcoidosis may reveal clear lung fields on chest x-ray but patchy interstitial change can be demonstrated by CT. This is an acute condition which tends to be self-limiting and there appears to be no evidence that this is a risk factor. In reviewing the case for annual chest x-rays for divers, we found that acute sarcoidosis was the commonest finding but, as a transient condition it is likely to have been and gone between annual examinations. This implies that many many more cases have been missed between x-rays. So it seems most unlikely that this carries any particular hazard.

Finally, the lung also protects the diver from decompression sickness by acting as a filter for bubbles so if there is an intrapulmonary shunt e.g. a-v malformations in the lung he is potentially at risk from decompression illness.

The current situation is that the criteria that we are using at present are based on theoretical risks. We have not had much scientific information to sort out these disorders. The FEV_1 and the chest x-ray are very crude tests of lung function while pulmonary barotrauma and other disorders of pulmonary dysfunction are extremely rare in the commercial diving industry. Therefore it is reasonable to conclude that what we are doing is reasonably effective indeed it may be even over-restrictive. Those who fall into a borderline position deserve to have a detailed investigation.

DISCUSSION

Challenor: Could you please tell us, what is the value of the lateral chest x-ray in the first examination of divers?

Watt: The increase in yield from carrying out an additional x-ray on a person who is asymptomatic and the chances of picking up an abnormality are negligible, if the PA is normal.

Broome: Please comment on spontaneous pneumothorax.

Watt: For the young fit diver who may develop pneumothorax the test we use for looking at pulmonary function will not offer any way of picking up such a person at risk. A tall "Marfanoid" shape is associated with an increased risk so, apart from that, I do not think there is any way that we can screen out anybody who might have a spontaneous pneumothorax.

If one has had a spontaneous pneumothorax I do not think there is any hard evidence that such a diver is at increased risk. Medical practice has based its disqualification upon theoretical risk and therefore such persons have not been exposed to the hazard. Whatever such a person does, they have a very high chance of having a recurrence within the next two or three years and the decision that they should not dive has been based on that theoretical risk.

Broome: Then this is similar to obstructive airways disease in that some of the recommendations which we have been making are perhaps over restrictive? We may have to revise our view of such things and if the Americans with Disabilities Act in the United States is a precedent, the onus of proof will be upon the medical profession to show that the disqualification from diving of an individual is based upon a certain risk to the individual's safety. For most conditions we do not have that information.

Le Dez: You did not mention much about smoking. I know a number of divers who have had pulmonary function tests sufficiently bad that the laboratory refused to do a histamine challenge test because the individuals fell below the limits. Is there any hope that can be held out for these people that, if they stop smoking for a year or two, that they will return to normal function?

Watt: There is a small population of heavy smokers whose lung function does improve when they stop smoking. These are probably people with very reactive airways disease, it is possible that they would then be able to be passed as fit.

Knessl**: 1) Should a professional (30 year old) diver with a history of unilateral right spontaneous pneumothorax resume diving activity after ipsilateral pleurodesis or pleurectomy? 2) Is a contralateral (prophylactic) pleurodesis or pleurectomy recommended? 3) Is there any increased risk of air trapping with consequent risk of barotrauma/embolism after such procedure? 4) The diver wants to dive at any price.

Reply from Watt: 1) The risk of a further episode of pneumothorax occurring on the same side is 30-40% and on the contralateral side 10-15% after spontaneous pneumothorax. 2) Pleuradesis is not a satisfactory treatment for pneumothorax, with a high recurrence rate. Therefore only pleurectomy should be considered as a potential prophylactic measure. Because of the risk of contralateral disease this would require to be carried out on both sides. 3) The risk of air trapping after pleurectomy is unknown. 4) I personally do not believe that it would be appropriate to advise a diver in this position to undergo extensive surgical procedures, with peri operative risks and risk of post thoracotomy pain, as a prophylactic procedure when the risks of diving after this procedure remain unknown. The risks of a further spontaneous pneumothorax are known, the risks of operative morbidity and mortality are known, but the risks of diving after a bilateral pleuradesis are not.

Lockett**: Following traumatic pneumothorax, a diver may be allowed to dive. Are these people still not at higher risk to diving because of the risk of having pleural adhesions, particularly if there was blood in the pleural cavity at the time of injury?

Reply from Watt: We really do not have sufficient experience to answer this question definitively. Pleural adhesions may represent a risk of pulmonary barotrauma and Dr. Calder's studies certainly suggested this. We have no method of examining for pleural adhesions.

I have taken the view that provided lung function returns to normal, the chest x-ray returns to normal (i.e. without significant pleural thickening) and CT scan shows no evidence of bulla formation as a result of lung injury, it is reasonable to return to diving. We have experience of 8 or so such cases over the last 10 years all of whom have returned to diving uneventfully. I continue to regard them to some extent as "guinea pigs" and it is important that the unknown potential risk is fully explained to them.

Professor Elliott has also described a case in the past in which recovery from surgery involving the chest was followed by recovery of lung function but not of chest x-ray appearances which continued to show pleural abnormality. Some time after returning to diving this man suffered an episode of pulmonary barotrauma.

Grönkvist**: Are there any figures about acute asthma and diving? Breathing dense, ice-cold and dry gases ought *per se* trigger effort-induced asthma? This may be the main reason for us not to allow asthmatics to dive. Someone during the morning said that asthmatics are more common among diving accidents than expected?

Reply from Watt: I agree entirely with this comment. We should exclude from diving those people whose lung function does not enable them to undertake the work or environmental exposure associated with diving. In relation to diving, breathing cold gas may well induce bronchospasm sufficient to incapacitate the diver, or at least make it difficult to cope with breathing through a demand valve.

The mortality studies carried out in Australia, New Zealand and Canada have all suggested that asthma appears as a potentially important medical contributory factor to an accident more frequently than one might expect. This may relate particularly to early open water dives which I suspect are the most dangerous experience for the "asthmatic trainee diver". However, not all asthmatics experience cold or exertion induced episodes and some asthmatics are able to dive without this problem.

The other potentially important consideration is whether asthmatics may be at increased risk of decompression sickness as a result of ventilation perfusion disturbances causing intrapulmonary shunting of bubbles.

Nome, Norway**: Experience from offshore (top side) installations in dealing with acute "status asthmaticus" in situations of fog or in helicopters, indicate that asthma should not be allowed. A "stable asthma" may change because of stresses due to diving.

VITALOGRAPHY AS A PREDICTOR FOR PULMONARY BAROTRAUMA
Surgeon Commander P.J. Benton, R.N.

This is a review of spirometry from submarine escape training, a situation which exposes the trainee to the risk of pulmonary barotrauma. Ascents are made from air locks at 9, 18 and 30 metres and from a simulated one-man submarine escape tower (SET) at 28 metres. Between 1954 and the end of 1993 a total of 277,147 ascents have been made by trainees. The 30 metre ascent was abandoned in 1974 on the grounds that the incident rate associated with this ascent was unacceptably high. At the same time the 18 metre ascent for requalifiers was removed from the training schedule.

An analysis of the 193 incidents which have occurred over the years, from 9, 18, 28 and 30 metre ascents at about 2 metres/sec, suggests that the appropriate policy of "when in doubt, recompress" is likely to give an over-estimate of the true number of cases of barotrauma that have occurred. Previous reviews of SET incidents have assumed that the mechanism involved in all "true accidents" has been one of pulmonary barotrauma with or without subsequent air embolism. Pearson in 1981 formulated a set of criteria which were to be met if such a diagnosis was to be made.

THE PEARSON CRITERIA (1981)

A. PULMONARY BAROTRAUMA WITHOUT ARTERIAL GAS EMBOLISM

1. X-ray evidence of extra-alveolar gas in the lung parenchyma, mediastinum or other sites to which mediastinal gas may track.
2. X-ray evidence of pneumothorax with or without other evidence of extra-alveolar gas.
3. Clinical evidence of subcutaneous or sub-mucous emphysema in the neck, lower face or upper chest wall.
4. Symptomatic evidence in the form of frothy blood stained sputum, other symptoms of pulmonary over-inflation are well recognised such as chest pain, cough and dyspnoea. However they are not in themselves thought to be sufficiently reliable diagnostic criteria when unaccompanied by any of the criteria listed above.

B. CEREBRAL ARTERIAL GAS EMBOLISM

1. Central nervous system signs and symptoms which can be attributed to cerebral dysfunction and which occur *de novo* within 10 minutes of the training ascent.
2. Full or partial response of central nervous system signs and symptoms to recompression therapy.
3. Confirmation of cerebral involvement by post-recompression therapy, clinical investigations and a failure of these investigations to provide alternative diagnosis for the presenting neurological signs and symptoms.
4. Signs and symptoms of neurological dysfunction in association with radiographic or clinical evidence of extra-alveolar gas.

In light of recent work the criteria for cerebral arterial gas embolism are no longer considered rational because:

(1) similar neurological signs and symptoms can occur in the same timescale as those of inert gas disease;
(2) a full or partial response on recompression would be expected whether it was due to gas embolism or due to inert gas disease;
(3) no investigation is currently known that will reliably confirm neurological involvement post-incident;
(4) extra-alveolar gas does confirm pulmonary barotrauma but does not exclude concurrent inert gas ("decompression sickness; DCS") disease.

Because of the difficulties of distinguishing between air embolism and inert gas disease, the decompression disorders have been reclassified using a descriptive terminology which makes no assumptions of the mechanism of causes.

The records of the 193 reported SET incidents were examined and each incident placed into one of 14 mutually exclusive categories. The criteria for inclusion into these categories make no assumption as to the mechanism, relying purely on the objective descriptive information contained within the incident reports. For the diagnosis of pulmonary barotrauma (PBT) to be made, there had to be x-ray evidence of extra-alveolar gas or palpable sub-cutaneous emphysema. In all cases where there was palpable sub-cutaneous emphysema there was x-ray evidence also. Neurological decompression illness was diagnosed only when there was a hard physical sign. Those persons who had symptoms only prior to recompression were put down as possible neurological decompression illness (DCI). Included in this were categories in which there was a combination of possible diagnoses.

Barotrauma Alone

a) Pulmonary barotrauma without DCI
b) Pulmonary barotrauma with syncope
c) ENT or dental barotrauma with syncope
d) ENT or dental barotrauma alone

Decompression Illness Alone

e) Neurological DCI
f) Possible neurological DCI
g) Limb-pain DCI

Barotrauma and Decompression Illness

h) Pulmonary barotrauma with neurological DCI
i) Pulmonary barotrauma with possible neurological DCI

Non-specific Symptoms

j) Chest symptoms only
k) Pain other than of chest, limb, ENT or dental origin
l) Syncope
m) Dizziness
n) Recompressed for no obvious reason

By applying the Pearson criteria to the SET incidents, 130 (67%) of 193 incidents are diagnosed as having been the result of pulmonary barotrauma. By comparison, this study revealed only 29 (15%) of the 193 incidents to have unequivocal evidence of PBT, with a further 70 with definite neurological or limb pain DCI. This gives a total of only 99 (51%) of incidents in which there is unequivocal evidence of PBT or DCI.

The reason for dividing into pre- and post-1975 is that, since 1975, spirometry has been performed upon all of the 34,472 trainees who have between them completed 104,497 training ascents. In 1988, Brooks & Pethybridge, using the Pearson criteria to identify cases of pulmonary barotrauma (PBT), noted an association between low FVC and PBT amongst these 34,472 SET trainees. As has already been illustrated, the use of objective diagnostic criteria results in a much smaller number of the incidents being identified as due to PBT. Between 1975 and 1993, only 5 cases of PBT can be identified compared to 33 if the Pearson criteria are applied. An additional 3 cases were identified in which confirmed neurological DCI developed following insignificant inert gas loads. Although PBT cannot be confirmed in these cases, it is difficult to envisage any alternative mechanism.

In an attempt to discover whether the association between low FVC and PBT still held true, the 50 incidents which have occurred between 1975 and 1993 following 104,497 ascents by 34,472 trainees were placed into five categories ranging from DEFINITE PBT to DEFINITELY NOT PBT.

CATEGORY 1: DEFINITE Pulmonary Barotrauma; n = 5, where there was x-ray evidence of pulmonary barotrauma.

CATEGORY 2: PROBABLE Pulmonary Barotrauma; n = 3, where there was confirmed neurological DCI of short latency, less than 10 minutes, with very low inert gas burden.

CATEGORY 3: POSSIBLE Pulmonary Barotrauma; n = 33, where AGE from PBT cannot be excluded or confirmed, i.e. where there was definite OR possible neurological DCI with significant gas burden, syncope, or dizziness etc.

CATEGORY 4: IMPROBABLE Pulmonary Barotrauma; n = 3, where there is a significant inert gas burden with long latency (90 - 210 mins).

CATEGORY 5: DEFINITELY NOT Pulmonary Barotrauma; n = 6, cases of ENT or dental barotrauma and cases where recompression was for no obvious reason.

The standardised residual of FVC for each of the 50 cases was calculated using data from Brooks & Pethybridge's 1988 study of 3,788 RN submariners to obtain predicted values:

$$\text{STANDARDISED RESIDUAL} = \frac{\text{OBSERVED} - \text{PREDICTED}}{1 \text{ S.D. OF PREDICTED}}$$

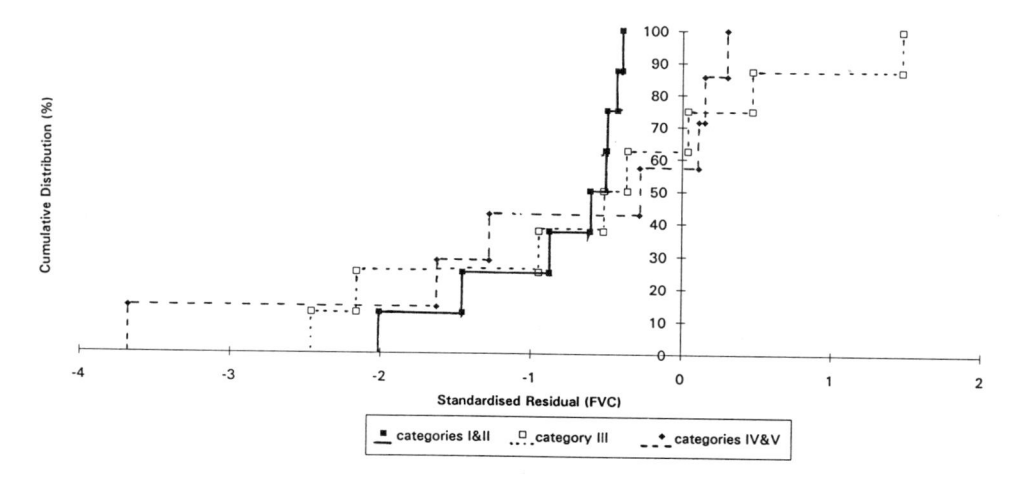

Fig. 6
Cumulative distribution of standardised residual of FVC by category

Assuming that values of FVC are distributed normally within each of these groups, it would be expected that there would be an equal number of -ve and +ve values of standardised residual of FVC in each group. This is not the case. In this graph (Fig. 6.) it can be seen that all of both category 1 & 2 cases have -ve values. The probability of all 8 cases in a random sample having -ve values is only 0.4% (p =0.004).

This final graph, by plotting the cumulative distribution of standardised residuals of categories 1 & 2, 3 and 4 & 5 is an attempt to display a biological gradient. The question to be answered is where on this graph should the line be drawn between acceptable FVC and unacceptable, as regards SET training? If -ve 2SD is chosen, then by excluding 2.5% of potential trainees, 20% of incidents would be prevented. However, only one case of confirmed PBT would have been prevented. If a value of -ve 0.5 SD is chosen then, although 48% of incidents would have been prevented including 6 (75%) of categories 1 & 2, this would have been at the expense of excluding approximately one-third of all trainees.

REFERENCE

Brooks, G.J., Pethybridge, R.J. & Pearson, R.R.: *Lung Function Reference Values for FEV_1, FVC, FEV_1 / FVC ratio and FEF 75-85 Derived from the Results of Screening 3788 Royal Navy Submariners and Royal Navy Submarine candidates by spirometry.* Proceedings of the Annual Scientific meeting of the European Undersea Biomedical Society. Aberdeen, EUBS 1988.

DISCUSSION

Reed: When you say a small vital capacity, do you mean small in absolute terms or smaller than predicted?

Benton: Smaller than predicted.

Reed: At what sort of magnitude?

Benton: That was the purpose of the last graph, the question being where do you draw the line? All the people with definite pulmonary barotrauma had smaller vital capacities than predicted. However that is still within the range classed as normal. If you look at abnormal, generally taken to be 2 standard deviations, that would be about 20% of the population incidents.

Ramaswami: Was any note made of where exactly in the sequence of trainees the casualty made his ascent? If they were first out they would not have much of a gas load but perhaps some cases were among the last to escape.

Benton: Unfortunately that was not recorded.

Zachariedes: What percentage of those with a low vital capacity develop pulmonary barotrauma?

Benton: Two and half per cent of the divers had vital capacities below -2 standardised residuals and the number of cases in that group were 8 times those you would expect in the normal distribution.

Denison: There will have been 7,000 who would have been below 2 standard deviations there, the implication is that only at worst 9 out of 7,000 would have been affected and therefore the rest would have been okay.

Grönkvist:** A few years ago, the Dutch Navy claimed that since they started with provocation test (metacholine/histamine) and excluded all persons with "hyper-reactive airways" from training free ascent, they have not seen any PBT. Is there any recent report on this?

Reply from Benton: I am unaware of any report on the use of histamine challenge to identify and exclude submarine escape trainees with hyper-reactive airways. The current Royal Navy policy is to screen all trainees by questionnaire, clinical examination and spirometry. If this screening reveals any suspicion of abnormal lung function, including hyper-reactivity, then the trainee is referred for full lung function screening. This includes an exercise challenge but not a metacholine/histamine test. To date no individual who has been passed as fit following full lung function testing has been involved in a SET incident. With the large number of trainees involved, 34,472 in the past 18 years, it would be impracticable to perform full lung function testing on every trainee.

LUNG FUNCTION TESTING OF DIVERS
Professor D.M. Denison

Those of us who have spoken at this meeting agreed that when we are testing the lungs of divers we are not doing it to test their liability to pulmonary barotrauma but to find out whether or not they are fit to be in the water at all. The ultimate test would be to ask the diver to exercise maximally in water and then to sample his arterial blood and see whether it was fully saturated with oxygen and had an acceptably low carbon dioxide tension. Unfortunately this test is thought to be too invasive to apply routinely. All our non-invasive tests are surrogates for this. Three measures are widely used:

1. spirometry
2. absolute lung size (by radiography or whole-body plethysmography)
3. carbon monoxide transfer as a measure of lung blood volume (TLCO)

On the basis of such measurements made on some 100,000 patients and healthy volunteers, we know that all three tests have roughly the same degree of variability in healthy populations, that is a standard deviation of $^+/-7.5\%$, i.e. the range of normality is about $^+/-15\%$. This means that even people in the middle of the normal range have to lose a very significant proportion of their capacity before they can be recognised as impaired. It follows that these tests are very poor at detecting whether disease is present. From that point of view the chest radiograph is a much more sensitive guide. Often, changes in the radiograph can be seen when lung function tests are "completely normal". Those patients who were previously at the top of the normal range would have to lose as much as 30% of their lung function before they would be diagnosed as functionally abnormal. On the other hand the reproducibility of these tests within an individual is around $^+/-3.5\%$. For this reason the initial lung function tests can set a baseline for the individual and subsequent tests can be used as very effective monitors of the progress or resolution of disease.

In the context of diving, we use such tests as screens to discover whether or not, from a respiratory viewpoint, the person is fit enough to survive in rough water and fast currents.

The single most valuable measurement that can be made is the "maximal flow volume loop". Its normal form is shown in Figure 7. From the start of a maximal inspiration, there is a sharp rise of expiratory flow to a peak (PEF), and then a smooth linear fall towards residual volume (RV), and a smooth inspiratory return to a full lung (Total Lung Capacity or TLC). It so happens that peak expiratory flow should be about two predicted Forced Vital Capacities per second, and peak inspiratory flow should be around one and a half such measures. There are many cottage industries devoted to the over-interpretation of the maximal flow volume loop. The only things you need to know about the flow volume loop are:

1. peak expiratory flow;
2. the forced expiratory volume in one second (FEV_1), which is typically 60% to 80% of the way along the path from total lung capacity to residual volume;
3. the total traverse of the volume axis, which is the forced vital capacity;
4. peak inspiratory flow;
5. most importantly, you should look at its shape.

There are seven basic patterns of lung function impairment associated with chest disease. They are shown in Figures 8-13. (These are taken with permission from Denison, 1995).

With the weakening of elastic tissue with age, airways become floppier and tend to close off earlier in expiration, leading to a mild scooping out of the expiratory limb of the loop. This is a normal variant. Small variations in the later part of the expiratory limb are liable to over-interpretation. Such changes, sometimes attributed to small airways disease, are rarely of functional significance.

On first visits to our laboratory, all three tests are done, but we have found in a study of many repeat measurements in 6,000 patients, that it was extremely rare to get a change in lung volume without a change in spirometry (1 in 1,000). In about 1 in 10 cases however, there was a change in carbon monoxide transfer without a change in lung volume. So, the policy at the Lung Function Unit in the Royal Brompton Hospital is to make all three measurements on the first visit, but thereafter to only measure lung volumes if there is a significant change in the other two measurements because we know that, unless there is a change in spirometry there will not be a change in lung volume. A chest film taken in full inspiration can be a measure of lung volume ($+/-3\%$). Unless there is gross disease which can be seen on a radiograph there will not be a low carbon monoxide transfer. From a screening point of view therefore the most useful test is spirometry, but like any other clinical measurement it is only as useful as the quality control that supports it, and this is where many measurements fall down.

The advantage of the maximum flow-volume loop is that it is easy to look at it and see that it is normal or abnormal, in a flash, without using a calculator. It is important to look at the inspiratory limb as well because, for example, as with phrenic nerve paralysis, loss of inspiratory capacity is important to in-water survival.

During exercise, ventilation will rise to a maximum of about 35 FEV_1 per minute and this gives one good guide to the limits of maximum swimming abilities.

In summary, lung function tests, especially spirometry, are good guides to swimming abilities but are of very limited value in assessing liability to lung rupture.

REFERENCE

Denison, D.M. Clinical Physiology of the Lung and Chest Wall. In: Goldstraw, P. (Ed.) *A Textbook of Thoracic Surgery*. Butterworth Heinemann. Oxford 1995.

Fig. 7.

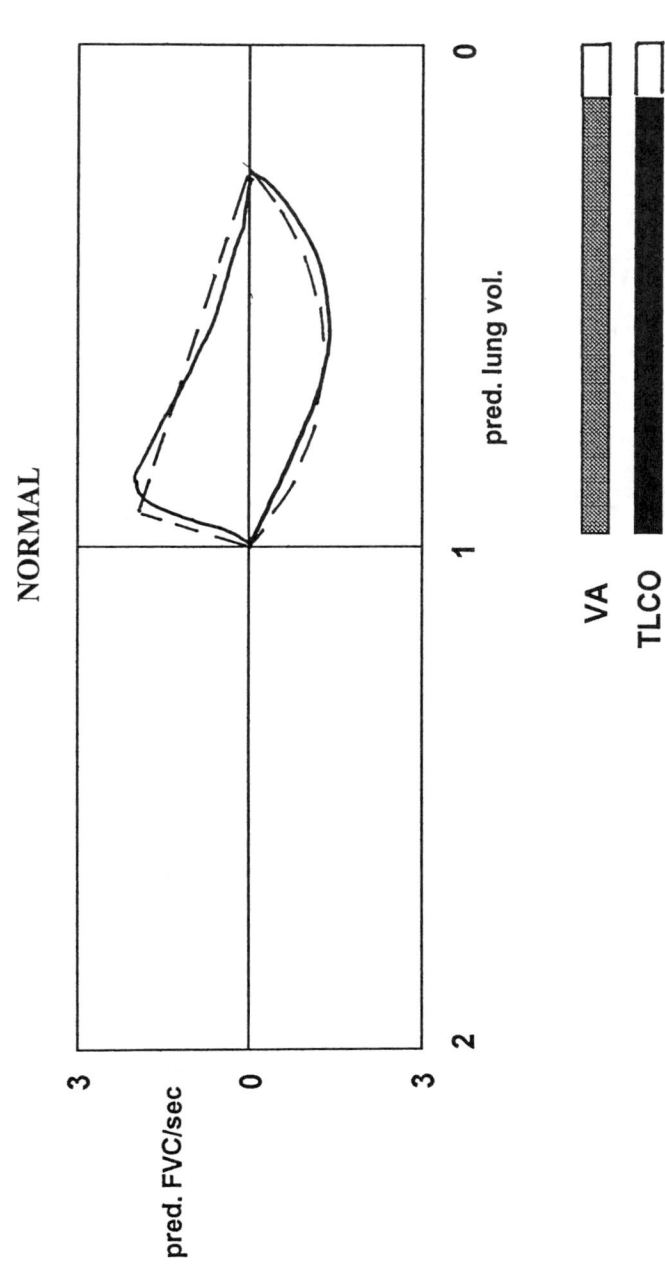

This graph is a plot of predicted lung capacity (as judged by the subject's age, sex and height) travelling antidromically along the abscissa, and of respired flows on the ordinate. Expiratory flows are above the line, and inspiratory flows below it. The maximal flow volume loop starts at its left-most point, in this case at the centre of the graph. Note that the maximal flow-volume loop shows a sharp rise to peak expiratory flow and a linear fall to residual volume, then a smooth return to total lung capacity. The accessible gas volume of the lung (VA) is about 90% of lung capacity. The amount of accessible haemoglobin in the lung (TLCO) is exactly proportionate to its accessible volume.

EMPHYSEMA

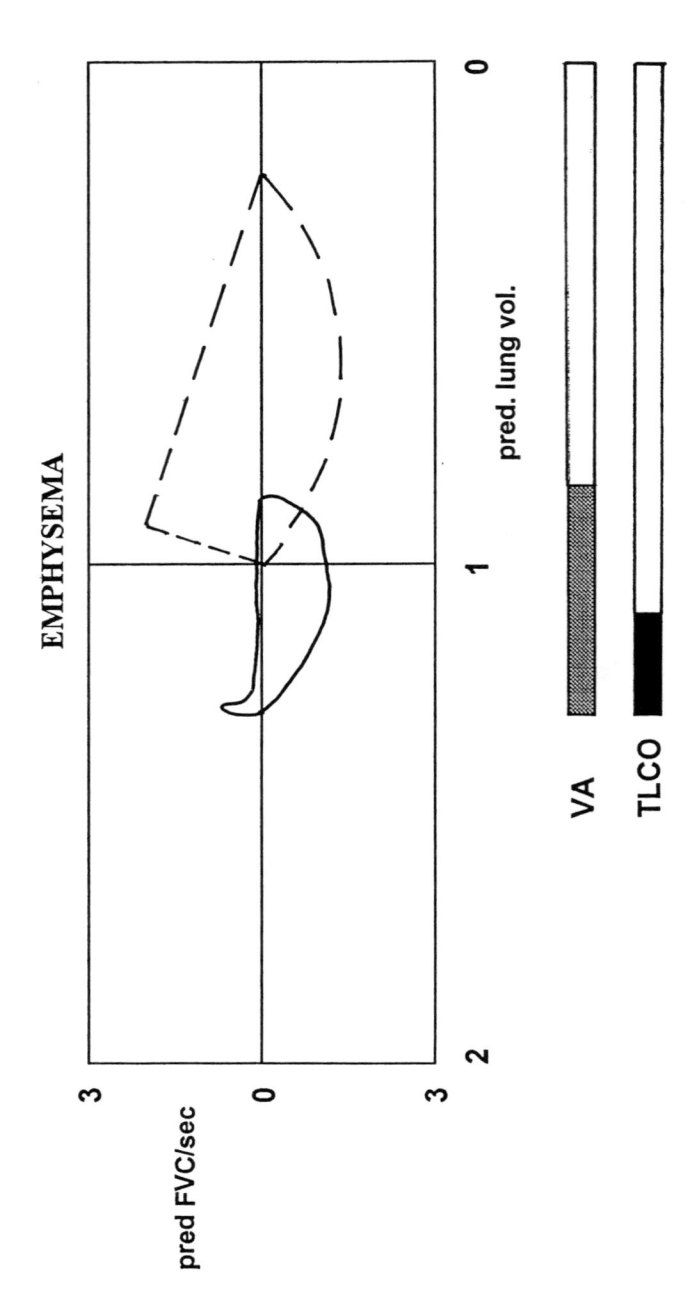

Fig. 8.

In emphysema, where there is destruction of lung elastin in airways and alveolar walls, the lung is big because it is easily stretched and needs to be expanded to keep its airways open, the alveoli collapse very early in expiration because they are floppy, and the alveolar walls contain disproportionately little blood because they are damaged.

ASTHMA

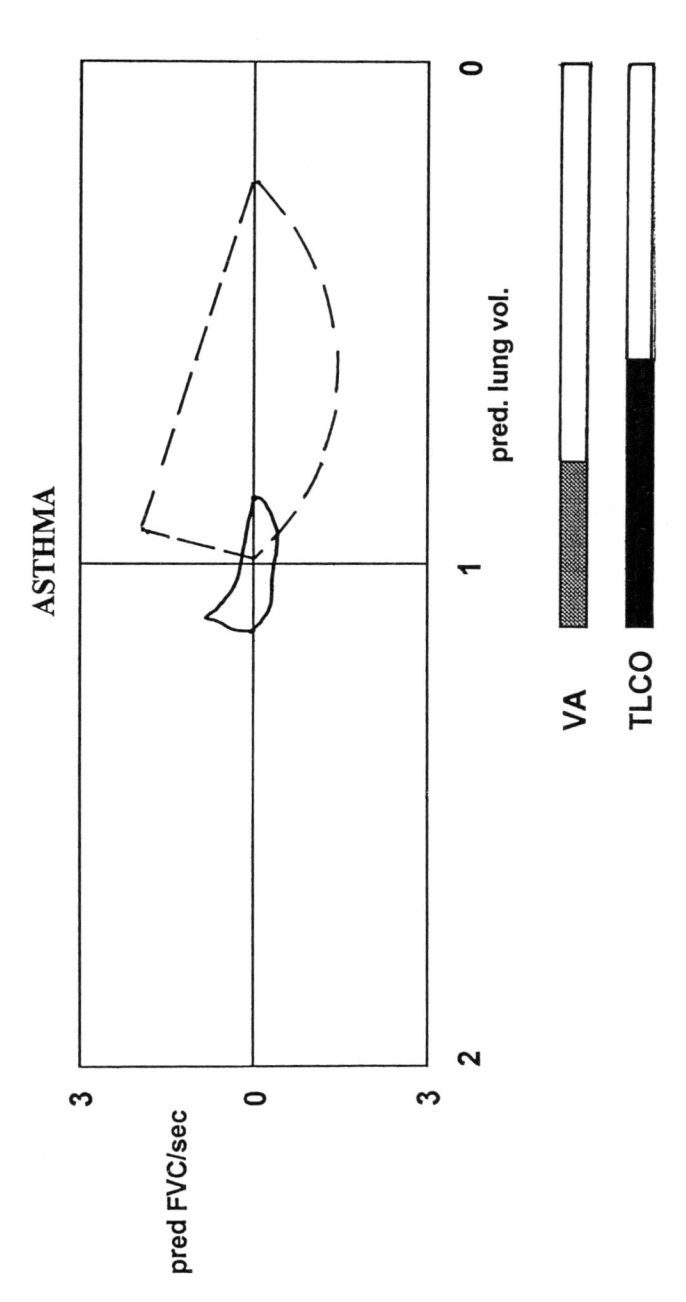

Fig. 9.
In asthma where there is inflammation and obstruction of airways but the alveoli are intact, the oedematous, constricted and obstructed airways block off prematurely and there is also some limitation of airflow on inspiration, but there is, if anything, too much blood in the accessible alveolar walls because of diversion from poorly ventilated to well ventilated parts by hypoxic pulmonary vasoconstriction and because of congestion by inspiratory effort.

TRACHEAL STENOSIS WITHOUT LUNG DAMAGE

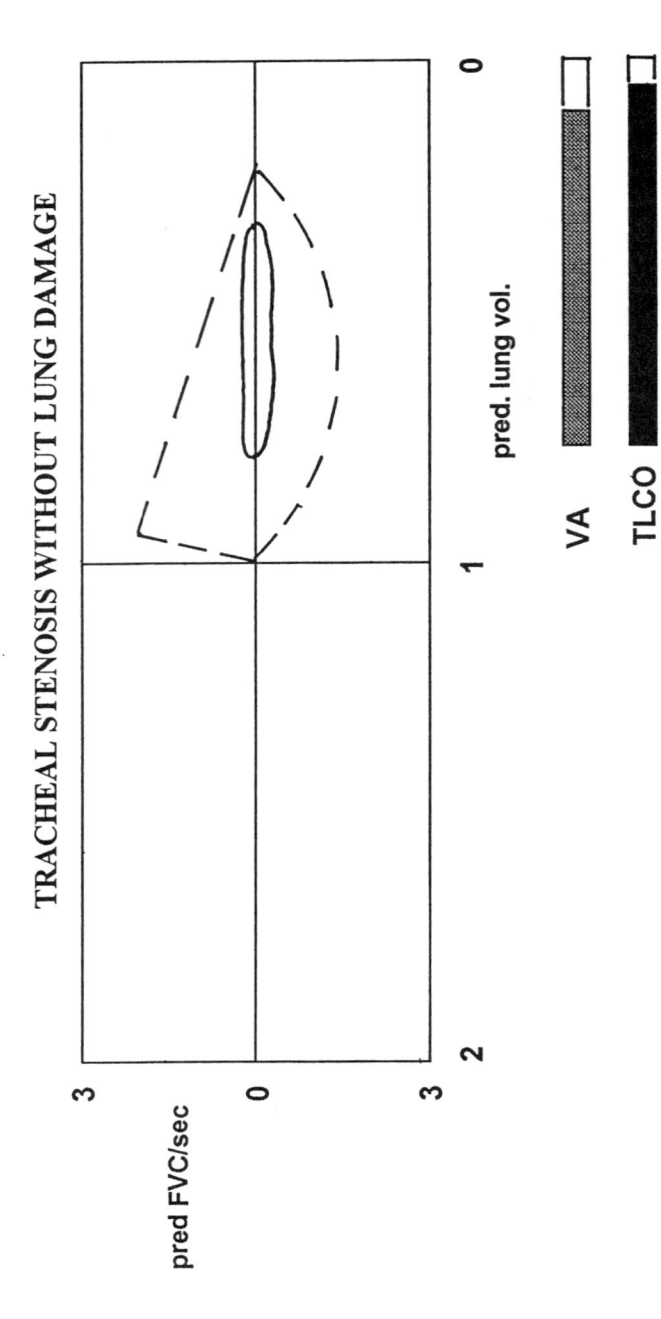

Fig. 10(a).

In pure tracheal stenosis inspiration and expiration are limited and may prevent real total lung capacities and residual volumes being reached but the distal airways and alveoli are undamaged so the accessible gas volume (VA) is a good 90% of the whole, and that accessible part of the lung is somewhat over-stuffed with blood due to inward suction by inspiratory effort.

TRACHEAL STENOSIS WITH LUNG DAMAGE

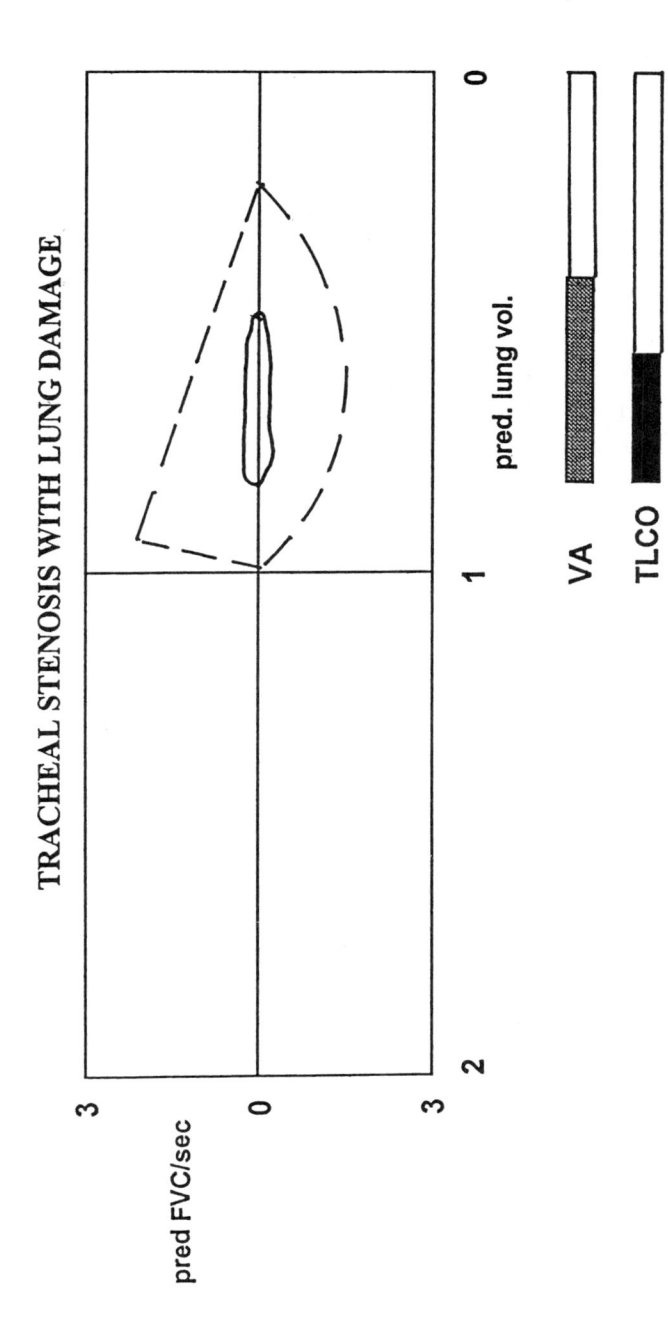

Fig. 10(b).

When tracheal stenosis is complicated by the presence of other lung damage as in, for example, the stenosis following tracheal intubation for profound pneumonia, the flow-volume loop is dominated by the effects of the stenosis, as in Fig. 4, but the accessible gas volume (VA), reveals substantial gas trapping and the whole lung carbon monoxide transfer is reduced by loss of alveolar capillary blood volume.

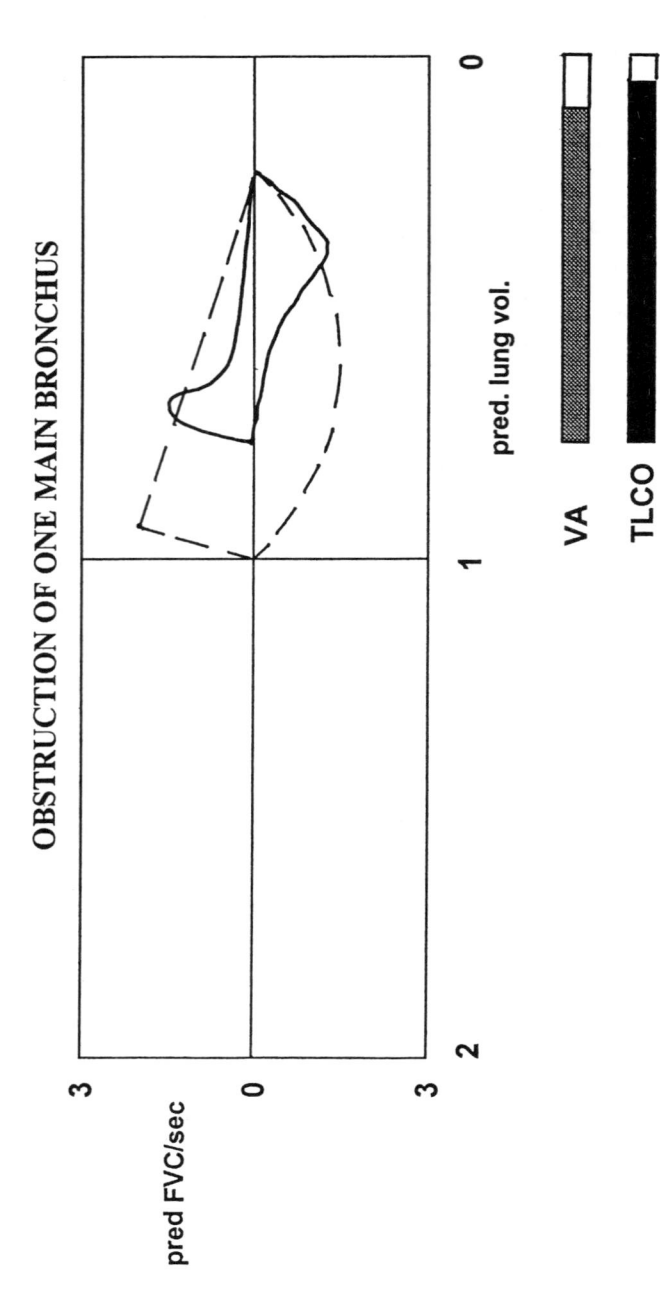

OBSTRUCTION OF ONE MAIN BRONCHUS

Fig. 11.
When one main bronchus is obstructed and the other is not, the inspiratory and expiratory limbs of the maximal flow volume loop have a peculiar shape in which the unobstructed lung fills and empties quickly while the obstructed lung takes much longer to do so.

RESTRICTION FROM WITHOUT

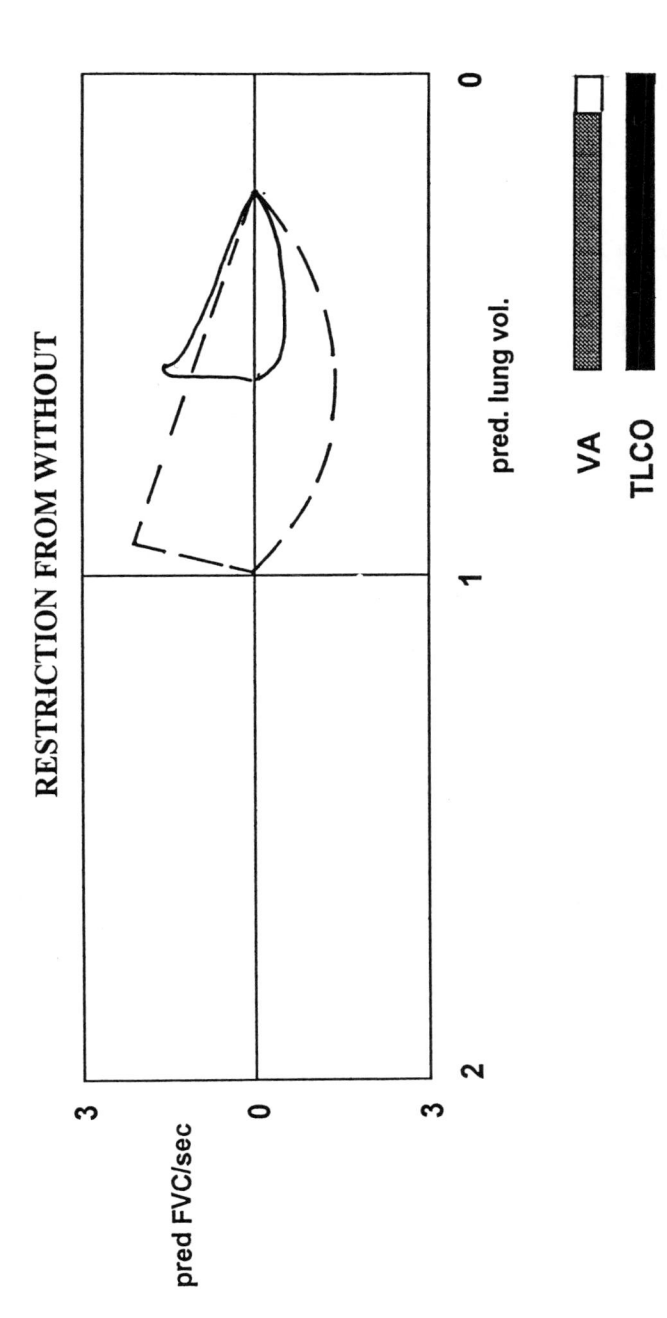

Fig. 12.
When the healthy lung is caged in a small prison as in pleural effusion, pneumothorax, ankylosing spondylitis, phrenic palsy or scoliosis, it has a small capacity, and a reasonably normal residual volume. Because its alveoli are essentially normal they are if anything over-stuffed with blood for the space they occupy.

RESTRICTION FROM WITHIN

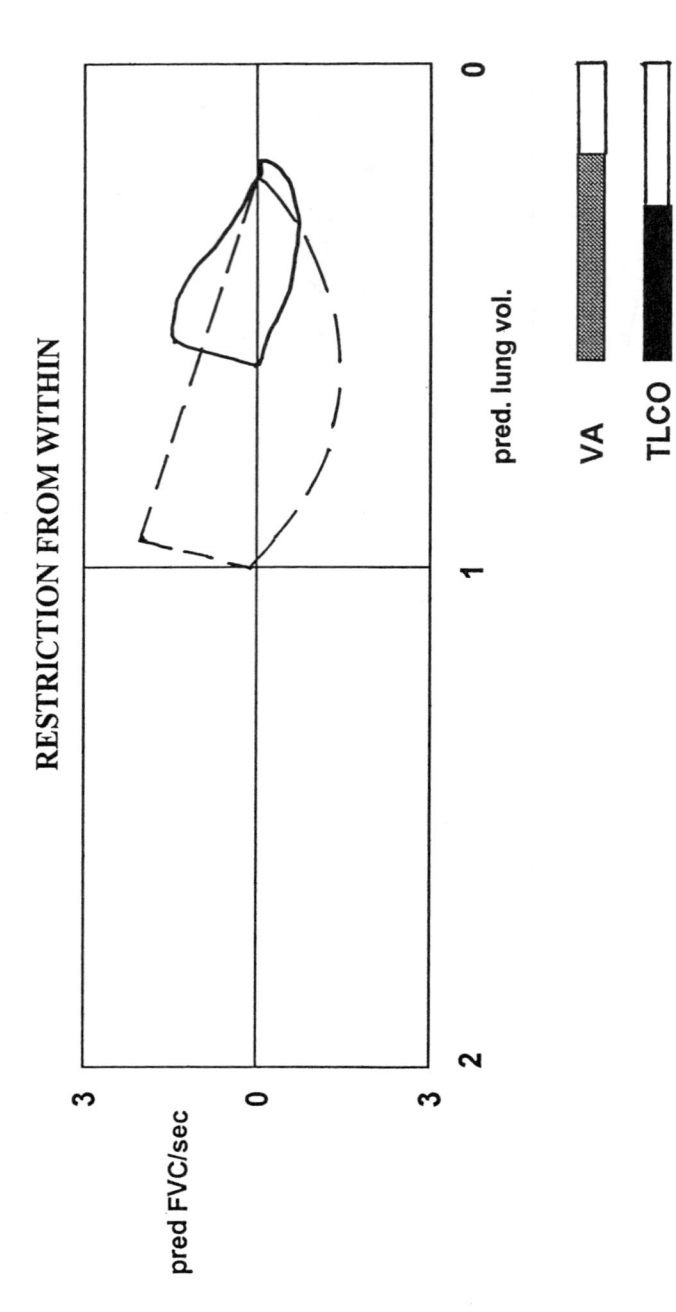

Fig. 13.
When the lung is constricted by scarring within, as in fibrosing alveolitis, it has a surprisingly well-preserved expiratory limb to the flow-volume loop because the fibrosis holds the airways open unnaturally long, the inspiratory limb is limited by the stiffness of the lung and the accessible alveoli contain too little blood because they are fibrosed.

DISCUSSION

Wendling: Is there an indication for a cold test among those suffering from allergy?

Denison: Yes, that is an important question but of course when one is examining a person whom you know is not normal, that is a different question. Asthmatics have normal lung function tests most of the time but a good guide to unsuspected asthma is that they have a relatively high TLCO. That is how we pick out asthmatics in remission. Once you have established somebody as being asthmatic you want to know how stable they and how severe it is, and certainly cold testing would be part of that evaluation.

However, spontaneous pneumomediastinum is asymptomatic and is seen quite frequently in asthmatics. I would like to comment on something said by Peter Benton: surgical emphysema is a common complication of childbirth. When it occurs it is a reflection of the forced straining and the stress that results is not so much in the lungs but from the airways in the root of the neck and upwards. This can also be seen in trumpet players, including one who had a tooth removed and perhaps that is how the air got in, so the important point is that one cannot always take surgical emphysema of the neck as diagnostic of pulmonary barotrauma.

Milne:** I understand that, rarely, the FVC is markedly less than the VC, reflecting "flap-valve" closure of airways and therefore airways obstruction on forced expiration. Therefore:

i) should there be emphasis on obtaining VC as well as FVC?
ii) would an FVC "markedly" lower than VC suggest unfitness to dive? If so, can "markedly" be quantified?

Lagercrantz:** FVC is increasing by years of diving as FEV_1 gets lower, so FEV_1 / FVC % decreases. When should one stop the diver?

Boonstra:** If burst lung in divers is due to tears in the middle size airways (as is claimed by the speaker), is it then still useful to screen for obstruction in small airways (closing) and small airways disease? At our institute we also take into account the MEF values, especially the MEF 25% (after 75% expiration) is to be above 1.5 l/min in our divers. Do you think the inclusion of such a parameter (as a measurement of the condition of the small airways) is still useful? If not, what parameters are necessary in your opinion?

Reply from Denison: These three questions have in common the use of indices as potential determinants of fitness for diving but they should be used as only part of a wider assessment. Thus there should be no pass/fail numerical threshold for a borderline value of the MEF 25, VC & FVC or the FEV_1/FVC ratio. Such results should merely alert the examiner to a possible pulmonary problem which needs further investigation.

LUNG FUNCTION CHANGES ASSOCIATED WITH DIVING
Dr. J.W. Reed

It is now widely accepted that divers have large lungs, partly but not wholly as a reflection of body size. Both vital capacity (FVC) and the forced expiratory volume in 1 second (FEV_1) are significantly greater than reference values. The fact that the FVC seems to be more affected than the FEV_1 has given rise to difficulties in the interpretation of the recommendations that in divers the FEV_1/FVC ratio should exceed 75%. It was also probably in the past the cause of some reporting of the highest FEV_1 and the lowest FVC from a series of measurements, a practice which has hopefully now stopped.

The question remains as to why they have very large lungs, and what is the significance.

TABLE 18
Mean results from seven men showing the increase and subsequent recovery of forced vital capacity (FVC) associated with a single saturation dive to 300 m for 3 weeks.

	Index	Pre	Post-1 (1 week)	Post-2 (4 weeks)	Post-3 (52 weeks)
Lung Function	FEV_1 (l)	4.35	4.59 *	4.49	4.27
	FVC (l)	5.90	6.32 *	6.12 *	5.75
	PEFR ($l.s^{-1}$)	11.9	12.6 *	12.3 *	12.0
	MEF-50 ($l.s^{-1}$)	5.42	4.95 *	5.23	5.30
	MEF-25 ($l.s^{-1}$)	1.76	1.69 *	1.73	1.92
	TLCO ($mmol.min^{-1} kPa^{-1}$)	13.9	12.6 *	13.1	12.9

* Significant change from pre-dive values ($p < 0.05$)

It is not difficult to demonstrate that diving will increase some lung volumes. Table 18 shows data from 7 divers who took part in a test saturation dive to 300 m over approximately 21 days. One week after the end of the dive both the FVC and FEV_1 were significantly increased, as was the peak expiratory flow rate (PEFR). These changes can best be explained as a consequence of a training effect on the respiratory muscles, although in this case there was no evidence of an increase in respiratory muscle strength. This effect would normally be accepted as a positive adaptation; however, it has been suggested that the increase in volume could be indicative of an over-distension of the lung and therefore an increased risk of damage. If this were the case, then one might expect to see changes in those indices of lung function which reflect the status of the small airways (MEF-25, MEF-50), and also possibly gas exchange (TLCO). In these seven subjects, the small airways do indeed show evidence of narrowing immediately post-dive, the MEF-50 still being reduced, though not significantly so, after one year. The gas exchange index TLCO was initially reduced by an average of 10%, and although the subsequent values were not significantly lower than pre-dive, did not recover fully. This was mainly due to three individuals who showed no signs of improvement at one year.

It is of interest here to note that both the FEV_1 and the FVC, whilst still being somewhat elevated at one month, were below pre-dive values at one year. Is this a real decrement? Subsequent experiments at the Norwegian Underwater Technology Centre (NUTEC) would suggest that this is so (Fig. 14.)

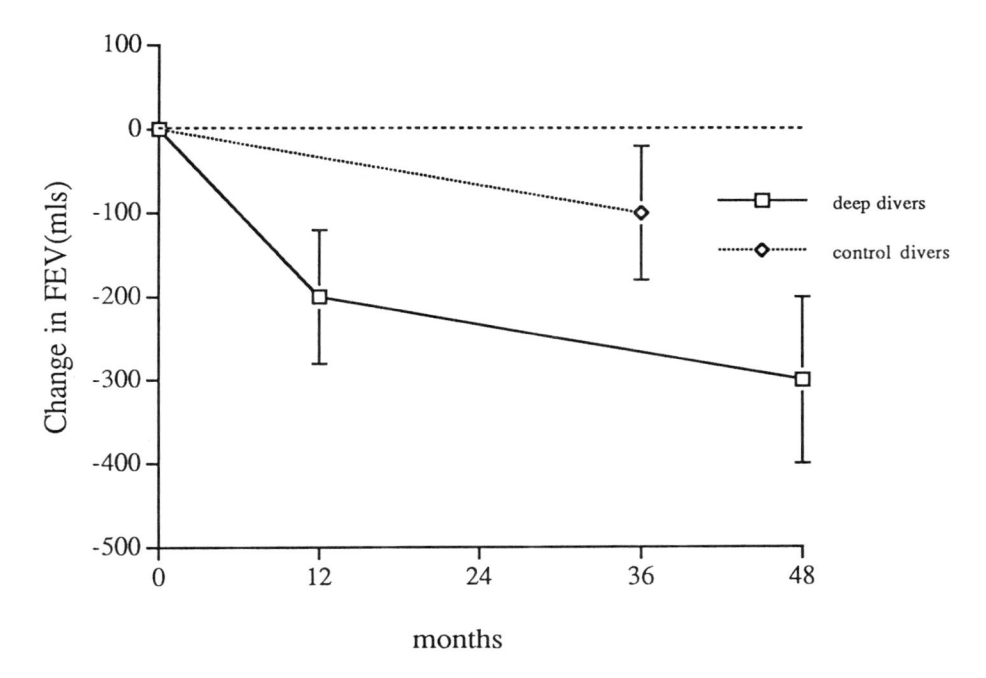

Fig. 14.
Reduction in FEV following a deep saturation dive

A group of divers who had undertaken a deep experimental dive (>250 m) were assessed at 12 months and then again at 48 months after the dive. The effect of the deep dive is very marked, the FEV_1 falling by on average 200 mls over the first year. Thereafter, when they continued normal operational diving, the FEV_1 continued to fall but at a much slower rate. This reduced rate of change is in fact comparable to that seen in a control group of divers who had not taken part in any experimental dives and whose usual operational dives had not exceeded 150 m.

A similar picture is seen for the gas exchange index (Fig. 15). The subjects are the same as previously and were studied at the same time intervals. There was again a marked fall after the deep dive which continued, although at not quite the same rate, over the subsequent months. In contrast the control divers showed no such diminution. Additional material is now available from NUTEC and elsewhere which relates the decrement in TLCO with depth (Fig. 16). There appears to be a linear relationship between the loss of gas exchanging capacity and the depth of the experimental dive.

There is little doubt that single, deep experimental dives such as these do result in changes in lung function, changes which are indicative of peripheral lesions affecting gas exchange. However, the relevance of these studies can legitimately be questioned. Are these simply one-off effects, with function subsequently returning to normal? The majority of divers never dive to such depths, so is there any evidence that normal operational diving can induce such changes?

The data from Fig. 14. and Fig. 16. would suggest that long lasting changes can occur, and that exposure to normal operational depths can affect lung function. The decrement in FEV_1 (Fig. 14.) evident at 12 months was not recovered, the FEV_1 of the "deep" divers continued to decline at the same rate as the control divers but from a much lower level. In a longitudinal study like this the rate of decline of the control divers, and the secondary decline seen in the "deep" divers was significantly greater than might be expected in a non-diving healthy population.

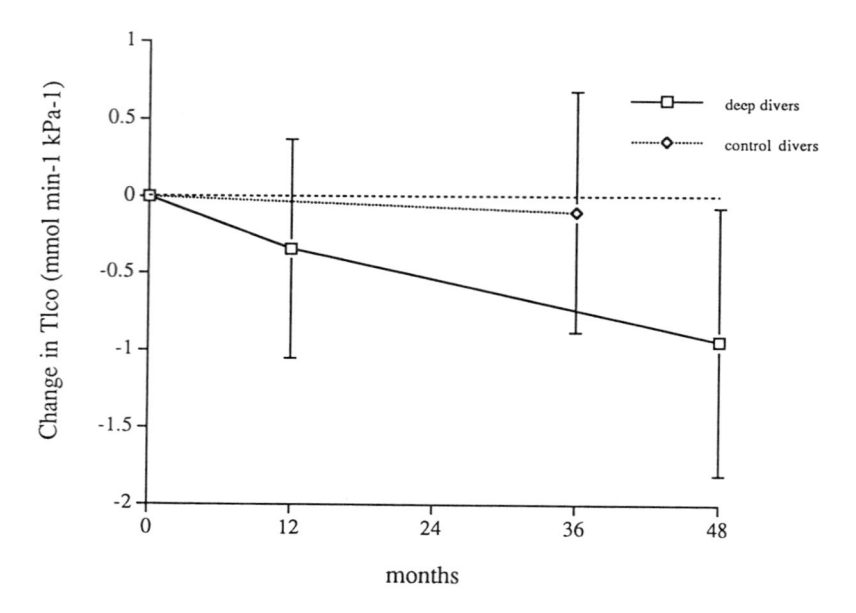

Fig. 15.
Reduction in TLCO following a deep saturation dive

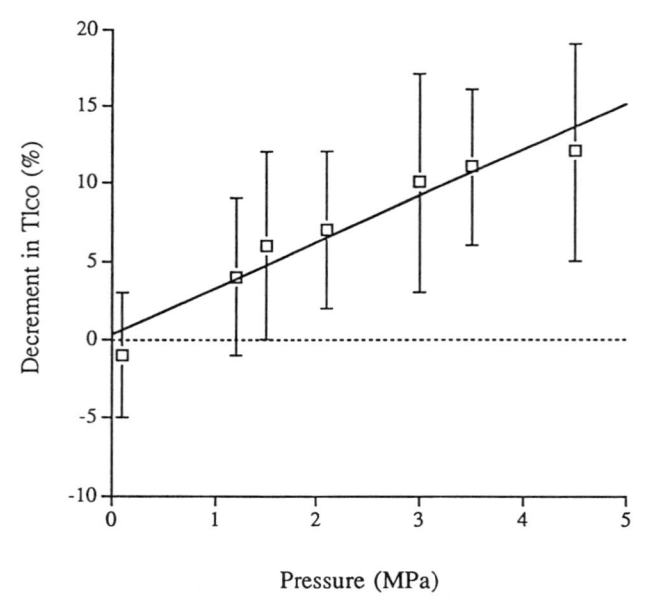

Fig. 16.
Association between acute decline in TLCO and maximal depth

in these shallow operational dives does lie on the same regression line as the deeper dive series.

The question remains therefore as to whether the effects of single dives may accumulate to produce significant changes in function over the course of several years of diving exposure. Table 19 summarises the findings of some cross-sectional and longitudinal studies of lung function which have been undertaken at the Respiration and Exercise Laboratory, University of Newcastle. In a cross sectional study of the logbook data held on 858 divers (Study 1), there was a significant correlation between FVC and the maximal depth they had ever dived. Of these individuals, 255 had 5 years or more of records (Study 2). In these persons the **changes** in FVC, not the absolute values, were significantly related to the maximal depth. Within this group those who had continued to dive progressively deeper had the greater changes in FVC, whereas for those who remained at roughly the same depth, there was little change and in some, a tendency to a decrease in FVC.

TABLE 19
Lung function association with diving exposure
Newcastle data

STUDY	SUBJECTS	STUDY TYPE	INDEX	MAX. DEPTH ■	YEARS DIVING ■
1	858 *	Cross sectional	FVC	0.0013	
			FEV/FVC	- 0.15	0.16
2	255 *	Longitudinal	FVC	0.0012	
3	81 †	Cross sectional	MEF25 ‡		
4	115 †	Cross sectional	FEV	0.0015	
			MEF-25		- 0.032

* logbook data ‡ reduced compared to controls
† laboratory data ■ partial regression coefficient

If the increases in FVC are related to respiratory muscle training, then the changes observed in the latter group must be influenced by the reduction in the training effect. These changes could then be interpreted as being the result of a progressive training effect of the deeper dives. The implication of such an interpretation is that divers who have stopped diving will lose lung volume at a fast rate than those who are still active.

In a further study of 81 (Study 3), the maximal expiratory flow index was found to be significantly lower than in a control group of firemen with similar sized lungs. This reduction in MEF-25 was confirmed in a second group of 115 (Study 4), and was found to be significantly correlated with diving exposure. In this group there was in addition, a positive correlation of FEV_1 with maximum depth.

There are, therefore, changes in lung function associated with diving, both acutely and long term. Vital capacity does increase with increasing diving exposure, but a respiratory muscle training effect may conceal a progressive loss of lung volume. There is in addition evidence of small airway narrowing which is related to the number of years diving. The mechanisms underlying the changes have yet to be clarified, it is not yet known whether these changes are reversible or progressive. More data is needed, particularly from longitudinal studies and from retired divers.

Finally, and possibly most pertinently, does it matter? The changes may be correlated with diving exposure, but they are small, and maximal expiratory flow rates seem to have little prognostic value in patients. Even so, as was suggested by Dr. Wilmshurst earlier, occult lung disease may increase the risk of decompression illness even after unprovocative dives.

DISCUSSION

Denison: Firstly, your finding of changes late in the flow volume loop are the sort that Peter Wilmshurst implied in his paper and draws attention to the fact that what he may have been looking at were not causes, but effects.

My second point is that you spoke of small airway narrowing and that implies some kind of physical obstruction when in fact it is possibly just an increase in the collapsibility of airways and there may not be anything to be seen physically, they are merely more floppy.

Reed: I agree absolutely with what you say but it makes no difference to the final conclusions. It merely means that they are narrowing while under the conditions of the test and that is consistent with the increased stretching of the lung associated with the increased forced vital capacity.

CHANGES IN PULMONARY FUNCTION : NORWEGIAN EXPERIENCE
Dr. E. Thorsen

Last year there was a meeting in Norway with the objective of determining a consensus view on long term health effects from diving. The Godøysund conference agreed that:

> "there is evidence that changes in bone, the central nervous system and lung can be demonstrated in some divers who have not experienced a diving accident or other established environmental hazard. The changes are in most cases minor and do not influence the divers' quality of life. However, the changes are of a nature that may influence the divers' future health."

The pulmonary specialist group reported that:

> "extensive studies have shown that professional diving has no marked lasting influences on the lung. However, there is good evidence that deep diving has slight but definite long term effects. These would become increasingly obvious in retirement and with age.
>
> The long term effects are:
>
> - increases in total lung capacity;
> - reductions in small airways conductance;
> - reductions in gas transfer capacity;
>
> There is independent evidence that these changes should limit maximum exercise ability and therefore ought to be considered as clinical effects."

The lungs are exposed to several potentially harmful agents during diving. The exposure takes place with all forms of diving, but is quantitatively dependent on the method of diving. Agents known to have pulmonary toxic effects are hyperoxia and venous gas microemboli filtered in the pulmonary circulation during stressful decompressions. Pressure *per se* affects pulmonary mechanical function indirectly as increased density of the breathing gas results in increased airways resistance and work of breathing. The visco-elastic properties of the lungs are probably not changed by pressure *per se*. Contaminants which are toxic to the lungs may accumulate in the confined space of hyperbaric chambers and of welding habitats, and during in-water activity exposure to cold and dry breathing gas may induce a bronchomotor response.

Our approach to studies of effects of diving on pulmonary function includes measurements of acute effects of a single operational saturation dive over the range of pressures from 1.1 to 4.6 MPa, and two experimental saturation dives to pressures of 0.15 and 0.25 MPa (Thorsen *et al*, 1990a, 1990b, 1993a), a cross-sectional study of divers' lung function (Thorsen *et al*, 1990c), and a longitudinal follow-up of Norwegian divers who have performed an experimental deep saturation dive to a pressure of 3.1 - 4.6 MPa (Thorsen *et al*, 1993b).

A reduction in pulmonary diffusion capacity and an increase in static lung volumes immediately after saturation dives were demonstrated. Hyperoxia contributed significantly to this effect. Independent of the effect of hyperoxia, venous gas microemboli were also shown to affect diffusion capacity and maximal oxygen uptake. The changes in static lung volumes could be a mechanical effect of increased gas density.

The dive at only 0.25 MPa, which corresponds to a depth of 15m, was with an oxygen profile that corresponded to a deep dive to 3.7 MPa. The results did show that immediately after the shallow dive there was a significant reduction in diffusion capacity (TLCO) comparable to the reduction following the deep dive with a similar oxygen exposure. The 28-day dive to a depth of 5 m was a normoxic isolation study for the European Space Agency, and showed no changes whatsoever in lung function.

In the cross-sectional study of saturation divers, a low FEV_1 and a low FEV_1 / FVC ratio was found. The reduction in maximal expiratory flow rates was shown to correlate with cumulative diving exposure, and a longitudinal follow-up of pulmonary function after deep saturation dives and a shallow saturation dive with an equivalent oxygen exposure showed development of changes consistent with airways limitation (Figs. 14 & 17).

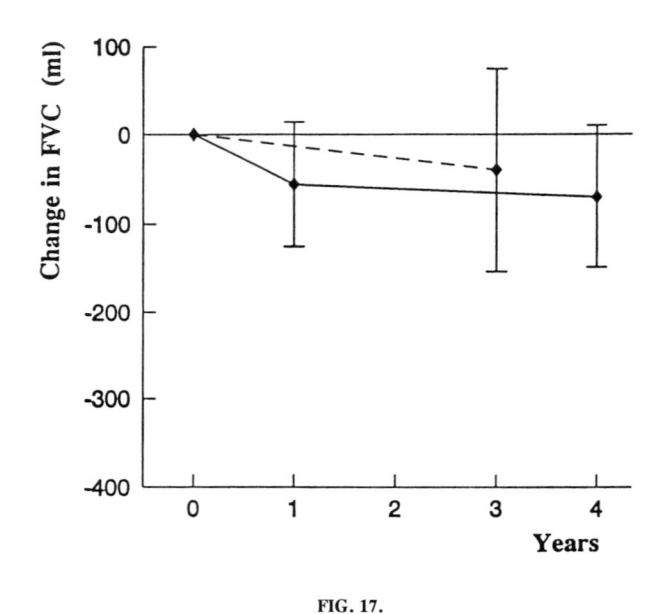

FIG. 17.

Change in forced vital capacity (FVC) one and four years after a deep saturation dive to a pressure of 3.1 - 4.6 MPa (—), compared with a group of professional saturation divers doing ordinary saturation diving in the North Sea to pressures of 0.6 - 1.6 MPa (--). The changes in forced expiratory volume in one second ($FEV_{1.0}$) are shown in Fig. 14. The mean reductions in FVC and $FEV_{1.0}$ and their standard deviations are shown. (Thorsen et al, Scand. J. Work Environ. Health 1993; 19: 115-120).

A major problem in the studies of acute effects of a saturation dive, and in epidemiological surveys of divers is how to quantitate diving exposure. Diving exposure is multifactorial. However, the studies of acute effects of saturation dives indicate that hyperoxia, venous gas microembolism and hyperbaria contribute to the changes by different mechanisms. A new approach to the quantification of cumulative hyperoxic exposure is necessary since the Unit Pulmonary Toxic Dose (UPTD) and Cumulative Pulmonary Toxic Dose (CPTD) concepts are not applicable within the range of oxygen partial pressures used in saturation diving. Further work is necessary to better quantify the decompression stress and load of venous gas microemboli. Nevertheless, diving exposure must in some way be based on the basic physical characteristics of a dive; pressure, time and gas mixture.

GODØYSUND RECOMMENDATIONS

On the basis of this and many other studies the Godøysund consensus conference made the following recommendations for routine surveillance of working divers:

- *improved selection of divers;*
- *baseline measurements at entrance of diving career;*
- *collect better data at periodic medical examinations;*
- *define proper indices for diving exposure. This must at least include pressure, time and breathing gas composition, if possible using continuous recordings;*
- *establishment of a registry for complete confidential data on divers as an epidemiological tool.*

Finally, considering what examinations should be in the periodical medical we agreed upon a maximum flow-volume loop annually and we also suggested diffusion capacity (TLCO) every third year.

A prospective longitudinal study of divers from the start of their professional career at the diving school will start in Norway this year. Every third year they will be followed up with measurements of flow-volume loops and diffusion capacity, and with registration of cumulative diving exposure based on the pressure, time and gas mixture profiles of their diving activity.

REFERENCES

Hope, A., Lund, T., Elliott, D.H., Halsey, M.J. & Wiig, H. (Editors). *Long-term health effects of diving; an international consensus conference, Godøysund.* NUTEC: Bergen 1994.

Thorsen, E., Segadal, K., Myrseth, E., Påsche, A. & Gulsvik, A.. *Br. J. Med.* 1990a; **47**: 242-247.

Thorsen, E., Hjelle, J.O., Segadal, K. & Gulsvik, A. *J. Appl. Physiol.* 1990b; **68**: 1809 - 1814.

Thorsen, E., Segadal, K., Kambestad, B. & Gulsvik, A. *Br. J. Ind. Med.* 1990c; **47**: 519 - 523.

Thorsen, E. et al. *Scand. J. Work Environ. Health* 1993; **19**: 115-120.

Thorsen, E., Segadal, K., Reed, J.W., Elliott, C., Gulsvik, A. & Hjelle, J.O. *J. Appl. Physiol.* 1993a; **75**: 657 - 662.

Thorsen, E., Segadal, K., Kambestad, B. & Gulsvik, A. *Scand. J. Work Environ. Health* 1993b; **19**: 115 - 120.

DISCUSSION

Chairman (Francis): We need first to discuss the questions which are for review and then take the general discussion after that.

The first question is "what are the pulmonary contraindications to acceptance for diver training?" I would like to divide them into 3 categories: one where we justify excluding people from diving, a middle category which will be a pending tray which I fear may be quite large and thirdly, a few in which we feel there is no reason for medical disqualification. The reason for a having pending tray is because at present we do not have sufficient information. We may now have a wonderful opportunity to set up a registry in order to gather this information then, as the years go by, we should be able to whittle away the pending tray until we are down to a very few residual problems. So first, Steven Watt, what are the contraindications to diver training.

Watt: We have no disagreement about acute pulmonary conditions; those are on the list of absolute exclusions.

Francis: Are there any dissenting views? *(Pause)* No objections to that, good.

Watt: Going on to chronic conditions I think the first thing on the list would be evidence of large air spaces within the lungs, i.e. bullous lung disease would be an automatic exclusion.

Francis: Any dissent to that? David do you have any views on that?

Denison: I do not think there is good objective evidence to support that. I have seen many divers with severe bullous disease, in fact it is difficult to see how a bulla would not empty normally during decompression if it contained pressurised gas. It cannot empty when you breathe out under normal circumstances because it will compress the airways. But were it to retain gas at a higher pressure than the rest of the lung it will open that airway and empty. If any part of the lung is seriously obstructed then there would be absorption atelectasis. The fact that a cyst contains gas means that there must be a way for the air to get in, and therefore for it to get out.

Watt: With most of these conditions we are going to be in the same position where we cannot turn to a reasonable epidemiological survey and say that there is proper evidence that they are a risk factor. There are a number of case reports of pulmonary barotrauma in association with underlying lung disease and there are several in association with localised bullae within the lung. I still have some reservations. Is it not perhaps like a tooth cavity where gas can get in and out easily under normal circumstances but given the extremes of pressure in some teeth, there is an explosion? This is just a theoretical consideration, but we do have to take these sort of things into account.

Francis: If I can summarise then, we have theoretical reasons for saying that bullous disease should be excluded but we do not have enough hard information. The next on your list is lung cysts.

Watt: I do not really see any difference between that and a bulla.

Francis: Spontaneous pneumothorax comes next.

Watt: Here we are in a worse situation as far as evidence is concerned because, having excluded them all from diving, we now have no evidence. I repeat that persons who have had one pneumothorax have a high risk of another and should that recurrence occur while under pressure, it is likely to have a serious potential. I will step back from the issue of whether or not they could be made fit to dive by having a surgical procedure because if one pursues that line, then one is getting into an area which has ethical difficulties. One is submitting a person to one if not two operations, each of which carries risk, simply to maintain them in employment.

Francis: Can I ask the Panel to tell us if they consider that somebody whose been pleurectomised is fit to dive?

Denison: What we do know about spontaneous pneumothorax is first, there is a 50% recurrence rate on the same side and 10% recurrence on the opposite side, but it is extremely rare for a recurrence after 4 years. In contrast, with traumatic pneumothoraces and chest surgery, it is very rare for a pneumothorax to recur. So the algorithm that I use is that if somebody has had a spontaneous pneumothorax within the last 4 years then they should either have surgery or not dive again until the 4 clear years have elapsed. One surgical procedure that is available is a pleurodesis which is not that satisfactory because there is a high recurrence rate after that. The most effective is talc pleurodesis but even that has a recurrence rate of 8% which is really unacceptable in diving. Recurrences after pleurectomy are rare.

Somebody who presents with a spontaneous pneumothorax, should you do a unilateral or a bilateral pleurectomy? Invariably pneumothoraces are associated with blebs which are most common at the apex of the lung. These are very rarely apparent on a conventional chest x-ray. If you want to find them you must do a CT scan. It is not necessary to expose people to a lot of radiation, you just do a few slices near the apex. There you can detect blebs as small as half a centimetre and possibly less. If you don't find them on the contralateral side you have a reasonable basis for confining it to an ipsilateral pleurectomy but if you do find them on the other side you should do both.

As far as ethics are concerned, all treatments carry a risk and providing you have explained this to the individual then he or she should make their own informed decision.

Francis: Thankyou. Stephen, are there any other conditions which we need to discuss?

Watt: The next conditions are where lung function is impaired sufficiently to affect exercise capacity, so the next thing to discuss is how it would be appropriate to make that assessment. The start point would be any evidence of lung disease or history associated with symptoms or pulmonary function testing abnormalities.

Francis: Are we therefore going to exclude people on the basis of pulmonary function findings? Do we have an algorithm for testing a person who gives some sort of history of "wheeze"?

Denison: Asthma is just a convenient label which is applied because there is continuum between normality and severe asthma. Childhood asthma is very common but usually can disappear completely. If there is no history of recurrence since the early teens then there seems no reason why they should not dive with normal lung function. If there is a history of occasional wheezing present in the last year or so then this may be a good idea and if lung functions are normal you may decide to try a challenge test. The other way of picking that up is by carbon monoxide transfer.

Francis: So, by way of tests, you would do spirometry and transfer factor?

Denison: If there was a history of wheezing I think its worth going to a challenge test, histamine or metacoline.

Francis: Would you use exercise?

Denison: This is essentially the same as a cold air test and that can be done with a small refrigeration unit and no need for the exercise.

Francis: How much airways lability are you going to accept as normal and what would you consider to be abnormal to the extent of excluding somebody from diving?

Denison: It is very difficult to specify any specific threshold. A significant change would be a drop in the order of 20% of FEV_1. Otherwise you are risking cutting out a lot of people who are perfectly normal. If we relax our standards very slightly, not too far, and then just sit and wait we will slowly gather the information which may enable us to relax them one step further. The justification is that by doing this we will no longer be stopping persons from work who have a valid reason to work in this field.

Watt: If somebody has a history of asthma, has intermittent coughing and wheezing, and whose lung function is never normal, then that is a criteria for exclusion. If people are having frequent episodes of acute wheeze to the extent that they need to take regular broncho-dilator therapy then that's another factor for exclusion. I think that we do have some difficulty in the middle ground. If they just have one or two episodes of wheezing in the year or some response to a substance at work then these persons should be studied further. I think the exercise test is useful and it doesn't matter whether you do it with cold air. You can do it quite successfully by sending the patient out to run up and down the road for a few minutes and a 20% reduction in peak flow after 5 - 6 minutes exercise is quite a satisfactory positive response. Persons with that evidence of lability should not be permitted to dive.

Francis: Why are we going to exclude people with labile airways from diving? Is it because of barotrauma or is it because these people are not sufficiently fit?

Watt: These persons have a condition which puts them at risk from not being able to perform adequately.

O'Kane: I asked a meeting with 130 experienced divers in the room and 15% of them had wheeze at sometime in their life. Eight per cent had regular wheeze but they had 3,500 dives between them. Carl Edmonds suggests that some 8% of deaths are associated with asthma but we have shown that 8% of our divers are asthmatic, this could therefore be no more than by chance. I would appreciate some guidance on this.

Denison: Evidence for the professional diver does come from the amateur community. My instincts are that if mild asthma is controlled by broncho-dilators and even steroids and is well controlled, and has been stable for a long time, that may be a circumstance when one can say that they are fit to dive. It was argued in the past that if they are using steroids they must have severe asthma and therefore that would be a contraindication to diving but now the therapeutic tendency is to get steroids in as early as possible. Therefore the use of steroids does not indicate that the asthma is one that would impair ventilatory capacity at depth.

Francis: Therefore, is an asthmatic, who takes medication in order to dive, fit?

Denison: Providing he is stable and he has the evidence from a peak flow chart that he is stable, then one should not pre-empt him from working.

Francis: Does anyone have a contrary view?

Lepawsky: I think the question was referenced to whether these divers should enter diver training for commercial diving, would your candidate qualify?

Denison: I agree that is a more important consideration because you are looking at the person's entire future. I believe that you must have evidence that they are abnormal in a relevant aspect. There are two problems: he might get barotrauma or he might get into difficulties in the water. If you can show that on medication he has a normal peak flow and he has been stable for a month, what evidence do you have to stop him from working?

Lepawsky: We had evidence yesterday that people with overt lung disease are more likely to get decompression illness, surely that is evidence?

Denison: That is a very tricky area. You heard one viewpoint on that but my standpoint is that you do not have objective evidence. The moment it puts lung function outside normal limits, then you have the evidence for that individual.

Watt: We also have to consider some of the practical implications of the decision which makes somebody fit under these conditions. I have some concerns about what the diver will do having been told he is fit to dive. A study by Farrell and Glanvill (1990) on amateur divers revealed that, although they were diving successfully, each of them had a very different idea of when it was safe for them to dive in relation to their symptoms. We have also heard that a number of commercial divers are lazy individuals who do not like keeping themselves fit. I think there are a lot of practical reasons for not having people who wheeze in this working environment as they may not behave in a way which is necessarily conducive to their health and safety.

Hickish: Bronchial reactivity testing has been shown in longitudinal studies to have no great relationship to an individual's asthma. You could not really use it to decide whether a person had bronchial asthma or labile airways.

Watt: You are quite correct. One can have bronchial hyperactivity and not be an asthmatic. In a person with no symptoms, normal pulmonary function and who is functionally able to perform normally, but who has a positive histamine challenge test, that test is irrelevant. The question is do they produce wheezing in a functional setting? I would move in the direction of the exercise test as being more suitable.

Moore: I do know asthma is unpredictable. Based on two recent case histories, I do not know what you mean by normal respiratory function tests. One case was a 25 year old physically fit person with an FVC and FEV well above average but the FVC/FEV_1 about 12% lower than anticipated, a chap who had asthma up to the age of 13 or 14 but no signs or symptoms since and certainly no auscultatory wheeze, should I let that chap dive? I sent him out for an exercise test and the FEV_1/FVC ratios remained the same. Can you please comment on that?

Watt: If this chap is symptom-free with a normal FEV_1 then his vital capacity is neither here nor there, he is probably fit to dive. If you want to be particularly careful, then you do an exercise test which, if normal, is fine. I would have no difficulty with that one.

Moore: The second case was a police officer who wanted to dive. He had exactly the same story when he entered diving and has dived without any problem for the last 10 years. Recently he got a chest infection and his asthma re-lit after 15 years in abeyance. He's had his diving certificate withdrawn which is a reminder that this condition of childhood wheeze may well come back later in their career. We may be sued if we say that they are unfit when they are fit, but equally we can be sued if we say they are fit and later are unfit. What is the answer?

Watt: There is a well established recurrence rate amongst people who have been childhood asthmatics. The question is whether you should use that as a history to stop them from a life as a diver? Personally I would not stop anyone from diving for that, but I would inform them that they may have a small risk of developing symptoms later which will stop them during their career. But the risk is about 1 : 7.

Moore: I agree with that, I think we have to inform the subject of the risk.

Nome: I want to make a strong point here about a tendency at this meeting. We are solely concentrating on the pure medical and scientific factors for evaluating and their implications for the safety of a diver. We are to a large extent forgetting that we are talking about the extremes of occupational health. We must not forget the liabilities, the responsibilities that we take upon ourselves when we declare a person fit. For instance, consider an asthmatic who has been stable for a time under medication who may be in saturation for weeks during which the stability may disappear. I would not wish to be responsible for a diver in that situation. So many of these decisions on medical fitness had some justification when they came in. Now we are getting more and more sophisticated knowledge and we are starting to doubt those earlier restrictions. We must not throw them away too quickly because there are practical implications to the working diver.

Francis: I think that is a good point and nobody up here is suggesting throwing away what we have. David Denison's point was that we could gradually retreat and sit back and wait for the evidence. To adopt this approach, however, we must collect the necessary data..

Watt: From our growing experience of problems arising during diving operations, for example 10 or 15 years ago we might all have been concerned about the man who suffered from asthma during a saturation dive we have now got experience of 4 or 5 divers who have had some serious episodes of asthma during saturation and all have been decompressed without any difficulty whatsoever. So I have become slightly less concerned about that possibility. Another example is the recurrent episode of renal colic which 10 years ago would have disqualified a diver but now we realise it is no longer a real problem.

Douglas: The reason for the re-adjustment of the criteria for allowing mild asthmatics, but certainly not those with exercise-induced asthma, to dive within the Scottish Sub Aqua Club is based upon several things. Firstly, the increasing incidence of asthma in the general population, also treatment has improved greatly, especially with the wider availability of inhaled steroids, so that we are more confident in deciding what is stable and what is not. If an asthmatic is allowed to dive after a very full investigation including exercise testing, then we give advice that they should not dive if they have had to use an inhaler within the previous 48 hours. The sports diver can say that he does not wish to dive but this is not true for the commercial diver.

Another simple practical point is, how would one take a pressurised aerosol can into a saturation chamber? Can one use the dry powder varieties? But what is the lung deposition of such substances when mixed with helium at different densities?

Watt: I don't think that we know enough about the deposition of inhaled steroids or broncho-dilators in raised environmental pressure. I would personally be unhappy about persons who required inhaled steroids being in saturation. I am unhappy about people who require regular bronchodilators diving at all. The diver is under an obligation to declare any problem with his health which might affect his diving and if he became wheezy he should certainly do that, but of course if he does that and tells his supervisor that he is unfit to dive, the end result is that he would be off the job and not re-employed. So the pressures upon the individual are enormous.

Griffin: The concept of persons with controlled asthma being fit to dive if one had a month long of peak flow charts, what is the utility of doing a saline challenge on them? I assume the person knows how much they can exercise, but if they get a significant drop of lung function following a saline challenge, then this is something that is likely to happen to anybody when they are wet diving. Do you think that would be an appropriate test before they go off on a dive?

Denison: That is a very good idea.

O'Sullivan: We must also consider different categories of job, for instance the police diver who will never go into saturation. We must also consider the difference between pre-employment medicals and the review of somebody who is trained and well experienced. But I think we should also look at the effect of our decision upon the mental health of that individual if we make him unfit to earn his living. It's not quite as simple as whether they are fit or unfit physically according to the various criteria, we must use our judgement on the whole equation for the individual as a member of the working community.

Mawdsley: The initial examination should be perhaps the most comprehensive one. Now that we are looking at contraindications for certifying these men, I am concerned about spontaneous pneumothorax being in the pending tray and I think it should be a definite contraindication. We have heard sufficient concern here.

Francis: I feel that it is up to the individual to decide, when he has been told what the risks and benefits are.

Örnhagen: Last night I was surprised to find that diabetic divers were allowed to go sports diving in order to find out whether or not diabetic sports diving is safe, outside a normal scientific programme *(see page 73)*. It might be possible to launch two scientific programmes, one for asthmatic divers and one for diabetic divers. Those who wish to dive with such disabilities could be supervised formally and covered by normal scientific procedures and ethical approval for such a project. This would take away some of the problems that Dr. Nome proposed earlier. I strongly recommend that.

Francis: The diabetics will be discussed later but the approach to asthma, if we are slowly going to withdraw from our exclusion criteria then, with the collection of data, the issue could indeed be addressed in a suitably scientific manner. I think we had better move on.

Question number two is, "how significant is a history of chronic obstructive airway disease? How is this defined and how can it be assessed?"

Watt: My definition of chronic obstructive airway disease or chronic bronchitis is one that is associated with chronic cough and abnormal pulmonary function. Such people by definition will fall into the group who have abnormal pulmonary function and will have symptoms associated with it. These will result in impaired exercise tolerance and therefore they are unfit.

Francis: Is there any dissenting view to that?

Broome: Could we cover the exercise tolerance tests then?

Watt: In the session yesterday, we discussed oxygen uptake and exercise testing, the pulse rate and so forth which ought to be achievable. If people can achieve those levels satisfactorily then clearly their pulmonary function is not impaired. What is important is that if their limit to exercise performance is pulmonary, they are on a slippery slope. If somebody has a minor abnormality of pulmonary function testing, then the correct way to assess that is to look at their oxygen saturation during the exercise test.

Denison: There are published normal ranges for $\dot{V}O_2$ max. and when one comes to diving one is already quite tightly restricted. One's normal buoyancy, deep breath in, is 5 pounds positively buoyant, and deep breath out is 5 pounds negatively buoyant. The maximum thrust one can develop with one's legs with good fins is just 10 pounds. The implication of that is that on occasions one might use one's total aerobic capacity to "get by". We need a safety margin in aerobic capacity and if anybody is below the normal limit of aerobic capacity then that is sufficient to say that they are not fit to dive.

Francis: Question number three is asthma which we have dealt with, so I shall move onto number four on pulmonary barotrauma. David, you had a pneumothorax algorithm.

Denison: Yes, that is the four year period without a recurrence which we discussed this morning but I did forget to mention that after a traumatic pneumothorax due to surgery, the lay-off should be 3 months.

Francis: Many divers dive with a recent cold, what is the evidence that a recent acute chest infection is indeed a reason for temporary disqualification? We had no objecting view to question one, so maybe we have really answered that. The question here is about colds and whether divers should not dive, but they do.

Griffin: How soon after they stop coughing up phlegm do they get to go back into the water and how long is it going to be before they probably no longer have a mucus plug?

Denison: I am not sure the mucus plug matters but the basic question is are they at risk from lung rupture?

Griffin: I have a colleague who has 3 cases that occurred last winter where people had a chest infection and had just died coming up on dives. He attributes these to a chest infection. He sees no other reason for it. On autopsy they didn't die of anything, possibly perhaps gas embolism. They were witnessed on their ascent, they had all the classical symptoms of air gas embolism and they did not drown.

Denison: It is important for him to publish that data.

Griffin: That's my point, if one cannot dive within 3 weeks of a cold, that is a lot of not diving.

Francis: If that was a big problem, I think we would know about it by now and certainly DAN would know about it also.

Galway: Could I just mention the problem as an anaesthetist, if you cough up a plug and go into laryngospasm, how would the Panel cope with that? Secondly, if you have a chest infection you often also would have ENT problems and I think that should be considered also.

Francis: What are the pass/fail criteria for the initial chest x-ray?

Watt: I would accept small scars, e.g. old tuberculous disease, of limited size. Essentially I am expecting to see a normal vascular pattern throughout the lung fields without any major abnormality.

Denison: Distinguishing between the initial and subsequent examinations I believe that expiratory films are also valuable. Inspiratory films have been used to look for abnormal shadows and defects. Expiratory films are to show abnormal lucencies. One striking case was when an inspiratory film was entirely normal and the expiratory film showed that one lung was more lucent than the other and subsequently the person had bilateral pneumothoraces and gas embolism. For diving, expiratory films are surprisingly useful. It may be worth considering that in the more detailed initial examination. It is very rare subsequently to get x-ray change without the presence of respiratory symptoms.

Elliott: Is that in addition to, or an alternative?

Denison: At the initial examination one should have both.

Francis: What pulmonary function tests are needed? Have the current pass/fail criteria for FVC and FEV_1 been effective? To what should they be changed? What is the role of flow-volume loops? Perhaps Dr. Thorsen would like to comment on what tests he thinks would be appropriate?

Thorsen: As I said earlier I really do believe in the flow-volume loop but I think we should consider adding TLCO perhaps once every 3 years. Exercise testing should be done at the examination and we need to discuss with a cardiologist what should be the maximum $\dot{V}O_2$ which should be obtained to get a certificate.

Francis: The next question is "what is the significance of a diminishing TLCO? At what value does it warrant further investigation? Is a low value, *per se*, ever disqualifying?"

Thorsen: That's the same problem, one should use exercise capacity. The TLCO measurement alone does not provide a pass/fail threshold. TLCO is very useful for longitudinal studies to tell you what is happening to lung function with time, that's why it should be done.

Denison: Remember that you have two clinical responsibilities as a diving medical examiner. One is ordinary clinical care, the opportunity to see a patient and see if they have anything wrong. Anything found that may be wrong should be followed up, clinically. The other duty is to decide are they fit to go in the water? It is important to keep these two apart. For example, with a diminished TLCO, I would be interested in that clinically but since it might impair only their maximum aerobic capacity, I would not let it interfere with their fitness to dive.

Reed: I would like to discuss the lung function findings of a 35 year old diver who we saw in our laboratory just a few weeks ago. We had first seen him 9 years ago but not during the intervening period while he has been working as a saturation diver (Table 20).

TABLE 20.

		Results 11.2.94	Reference 11.2.94	Previous Results 12.2.85	Predicted change	Actual change ■
FEV_1	(l)	3.12	4.55	3.45	-0.04	-0.73
FVC	(l)	6.34	5.73	6.56	-0.17	-0.22
FEV/FVC	(%)	49.0	82.0	58.7	-3.3	-9.7
PEFR	$(l.s^{-1})$	7.50	11.11	8.80	-0.11 ‡	-1.3
MEF_{30}	$(l.s^{-1})$	1.90	4.87	2.70	-0.34 ‡	-0.80
MEF_{25}	$(l.s^{-1})$	0.80	2.01	1.40	-0.27 ‡	-0.60
TLCO	$(mmol.min^{-1}.m.kPa^{-1})$	14.1	13.0			
KCO	(TL/VA)	1.57	1.76			

■ Longitudinal reference value
‡ Cross sectional reference values

He is physically fit, asymptomatic, he smoked fairly heavily up to the age of 22 and has passed his fit to dive medicals annually during this interval. He was aged 22 in 1989, in 1985 he had been in saturation diving for about 4 years, at that time his FEV was already significantly lower than the reference value and his vital capacity was significantly higher so he had a low peak expiratory flow rate and significantly lower indices of maximum flow at lower lung volumes. He was passed as fit to dive then and every year since. We saw him in March 1994 and his vital capacity has fallen by 220 cc, his FEV ratio is down to 49%, his peak flow has decreased further and the end-expiratory peak flows have also diminished. His transfer capacity, which had not been done in 1985, is still greater than predicted. The KCO, which is the transfer per unit lung volume, is significantly reduced at this time. He was passed as medically fit to dive on this data but I would draw your attention to the fact that his forced expiratory volume is decreasing at many multiples of what one would expect from a normal non-diving population. His vital capacity is decreasing significantly faster, his FEV/FVC is also diminishing rapidly. Peak flow rates are going down as roughly as one would expect but the mid-expiratory flow rates which reflect the smaller airways are going down again at a rate greater than one would expect in the normal population. The results are reported as being a significant respiratory impairment. In fact this man is still diving, but should he be? With that rate of decline I would predict that he is heading for a miserable old age.

Watt: Does this chap have any reversibility? It might be that if he were on inhaled steroids he might be a lot better.

Reed: No, no medication because nobody regards him as unfit.

Broome: Does he regard himself as being worse than he was previously?

Reed: No, he is asymptomatic. He regularly takes exercise and does not get particularly out of breath.

Broome: One must not automatically assume that these changes in lung function are due to his occupation. This may be the early stage of some other medical condition surely. If he is physically fit and if we wish to have some objective measurement, we must agree on some form of exercise testing?

Reed: Whether or not the changes are due to diving is irrelevant, the fact is that his lung function is indicative of respiratory impairment and this is being ignored by the diving doctors. This is an individual whose livelihood depends upon the doctor's assessment of his fitness to dive. There seems to be more emphasis on the man's subjective assessment of his own abilities than on objective measures of function. These people do not yet get the kind of objective test that is necessary to identify these types of impairment.

Hawson: In the consulting room we need to know what exercise test would be acceptable. Are the Panel able to agree what this should be? Several were discussed yesterday, the simplest and quickest seem to be the 5-step test, is this still acceptable or would the Panel recommend a different one?

Denison: What one needs is a test which will demonstrate the ability to exercise for a reasonable length of time. There are several such tests. For the consulting room rather than the laboratory, sending him for a 20-minute run, but then this needs to be established as a standard. If one wants to retain the stepping standards, then these must continue for 20 minutes if one wishes to demonstrate aerobic capacity.

Thorsen: I would suggest we do laboratory testing of maximal oxygen uptake perhaps every third year. We heard yesterday about a lot of healthy, fit, young divers with "athletic" hearts but have there been any measurements of maximum oxygen uptake on them? Are they really that athletic? On average, Norwegian divers are not more fit than anyone else in the community.

Reed: Most of these step tests and so forth are based upon heart rate responses. It is extremely easy for the subject in such a test to manipulate his heart rate to produce a much better result than in fact he deserved.

Francis: Yes, but we still have the problem of what should be done in the consulting room.

Robinson: I am a general practitioner who looks at a lot of divers at the diving school in Fort William. A recent diving medical changed my practice. A fit professional sports diver turned up from America for his medical and declared no past relevant history. I did a standard exercise test for his fitness and heard a wheeze. I then did a peak flow and vitalography. This chap went for a full pulmonary workup, he was failed and had to go back to America. So I suggest peak flows before and after the exercise.

Watt: We often return to this question of what is the right exercise test but one reason why we are stumbling is maybe that we do not know what the oxygen requirements of the job are. We have information about what oxygen consumption is required for swimming at particular velocities in the water but what is the oxygen consumption required to do a life-saving rescue?

Elliott: Can you not assume that they are maximal?

Watt: No, I do not think one can, one cannot sustain maximal levels of exercise for the period that we know some of these rescue divers might have to take.

Elliott: I think we are ducking the question for a wrong reason. We do know that a diver, on occasion must work maximally to save his own or somebody else's life. That is what we need to measure.

Watt: Turn that question back to front, it may be that if you put two divers with different levels of fitness in the water to undertake a rescue operation they may both complete the job in the same time. I therefore believe that we should not penalise the less fit individual if he can be equally effective.

Francis: The other objective of an exercise test is to estimate lung function.

Denison: There is a really important point in all these discussions about measuring lung function or exercise. It is vital that one's equipment is calibrated. There are many peripheral lung function measuring locations where the maintenance of equipment is not up to scratch. In order to do what we want to do we must have equipment that can be relied on and is properly calibrated.

Mawdsley: Could you please answer the question - what sort of exercise test is suitable? (*Applause*)

Reed: I do not think that one can give an absolute answer. There are differing requirements. If the question is "what exercise test is required to determine the suitability or otherwise of an individual for a particular piece of work", then, as Dr. Watt has said, one needs to know the energy requirements of that task. If the individual can attain an oxygen uptake equal to, or preferably greater than that then, given the necessary skills, he should be able to successfully complete that task. There is, however, the problem of the percentage of his maximal oxygen uptake that he has to operate at and the length of time necessary to do the job. Consider two individuals, one is large, has a big muscle mass but is not very fit. The second is smaller with less body muscle but is very fit. Both can perform a given task, operating near to maximal levels. In an emergency situation the second individual will be able to operate near maximally for an appreciable time, whereas the first individual will tire quickly and not only lose working capacity but may even lose coordination and fail completely with potentially disastrous consequences. If you do actually want to estimate the maximal working capacity of a diver, and there may be good reason to do so, then I would say that there is no good alternative to a metabolic exercise test with direct estimation of maximal oxygen uptake. One would then have not only the exercise capacity in absolute terms but also the sub-maximal indices from which can be derived estimates of endurance. At the moment this level of sophistication can only be achieved satisfactorily in an exercise laboratory.

Elliott: If I'm correct the Norwegian requirement is 47 ml O_2 uptake kg/min. Is that a standard which we could apply to everybody or would you be equally critical of that?

Thorsen: The average in this age group is 40 ml/kg/min. Yes, I accept that as a pass/fail criterion.

Challenor: We are talking about the pragmatic approach to testing in a surgery or an occupational health department. The Home Office test for firefighters requires an indirect test of $\dot{V}O_2$ max. which would be around 45 ml per kg per minute. This is done on a 5-minute step test at 45 steps per minute. Using that test with tables gives a reasonable indication of indirect $\dot{V}O_2$ max. Combining that with observation perhaps of peak flow before and after, plus "clinical acumen", would be a reasonable basis for the clinical test.

Madsen: I would like to show again an overhead from yesterday (Fig. 2). This is a study of the time taken to swim 1 km compared, in 19 individuals, with maximum ∇O_2 in METS which had been measured in sub-maximal work rates. It shows that the METS score is a poor predictor of performance in the water. Whereas if they have a good performance in the water this is a predictor of a good METS score.

Örnhagen (to Madsen): Are you suggesting that we bring back the old test of absolute muscular strength in some particular movement?

Reed (to Örnhagen): Are you suggesting that we substitute a test of absolute muscle strength for exercise testing? The two are not strongly linked.

Örnhagen: No, but we could add a test of absolute muscular strength to respiratory tests.

Reed: We are talking about fitness to work, not necessarily about physical fitness. There are skill factors, muscle coordination and many other factors. A person who is skilled will require less energy to do the same job.

Örnhagen: You are recommending that we should not have that as an additional test?

Francis: It is yet one more arbitrary test.

Broome: Most of the exercise tests are in fact arbitrary because they do not answer the question that we are all trying to answer. "How would he function in an emergency?" and "is he fit to be in the water?" are separate but very related issues. The functional tests such as moving weights around underwater deserve a comment from the Panel. Could something be devised along those lines?

Francis: I think that I will pre-empt this issue by saying that the subject of functional physical testing requires a separate assessment. I accept that we have not found a satisfactory answer to exercise testing and the subject will need to be re-addressed.

REFERENCE

Farrell, P.J.S. & Glanvill, P. *Br. Med. J.* 1990; **300**: 166.

COMMENTARY

As emerged clearly from these discussions, there is no great disagreement with most of the existing pulmonary guidelines. There is no evidence that use of the current criteria (page 109) are causing any conditions that might diminish safety to be missed. Indeed, it is probable that they may be excluding healthy potential divers by being too restrictive.

Thus the emphasis of discussion was upon the possibility of relaxing the guidance for one or two medical conditions in a manner which should be without significant risk. It would be necessary to analyse the relevant medical and diving exposure data in order to validate the change before any further step is considered. For example, contrary to the traditional view, it was proposed that stable asthmatics who are not triggered by provocation testing could be considered fit provided that they demonstrate normal pulmonary function on hard exercise. Indeed it was suggested that the use of steroids to maintain stability in a person with good peak flow was not *per se* an absolute contraindication to diving. However to allow this there must be a meticulous collection and analysis of data. This is the type of data that will need to be more readily available in order to justify a decision of unfitness, once laws such as the "Americans with Disabilities Act" are passed in more countries.

Considerable debate on the selection of suitable exercise testing procedures led to no firm consensus. Peak flows, before and after high stepping sustained for 20 mins, might be adequate for a simple pulmonary assessment but, for accurate testing which is of value also to cardiologists, a direct measure is needed of $\dot{V}O_2$ on bicycle or treadmill. The difficulties in assessing the results from such tests are not so much clinical as functional. An older and more skilled diver may need to use less effort during an in-water emergency that a younger and fitter individual. Thus once again the focus is away from pass/fail criteria and onto the importance of individual assessment by a doctor with appropriate skills and experience.

There were many other proposals in the Edinburgh session. For instance that the lateral chest x-ray has no value and should be discontinued but, for the detection of lucencies at the initial examination, an expiratory film is an important addition to the conventional inspiratory view. Other techniques such as the flow volume loop are important but the use of the FEV_1/FVC ratio to provide a numerical threshold for pass/fail should be discontinued although it remains an important indicator for referral.

The session illustrated well the need by the examining doctor for assessment of trends, particularly those still within the range of normality for the general population but revealed only by comparison with an individual's own previous records.

Another important feature of both the Edinburgh and Luxembourg meetings was the emphasis on the need for longitudinal pulmonary health surveillance and the need to coordinate this with records of occupational exposure. Epidemiological review of such data would be relatively easy though it would take many years to collect. A probable limiting factor will be a lack of sponsors to fund such work.

E.N.T., VISION AND ENDOCRINOLOGY

Chairman: Professor H. Örnhagen

The E.N.T. recommendations from the Guidance Notes are:

OTORHINOLARYNGOLOGY

24. *The diver should be able to clear his ears. Complications of otitis media such as glue ear, deafness, perforation and persistent discharge are causes for rejection. Mastoiditis would also debar.*

25. *The following points should be covered during examination:*

    (a) *Meati should appear normal. If wax is present, it is not necessary to disturb it unless it is excessive or obstructing the canal. Acute or chronic otitis externa is a bar to diving.*
    Exostoses are not harmful unless the canal is occluded, when the diver should be referred for their removal.

    (b) *The drum should be seen: well healed scars are acceptable. New entrants must demonstrate the ability to clear their ears. This may also be indicated after infection or barotrauma.*

    (c) *Hearing - The diver must be able to hear and understand normal conversation.*

    (d) *Audiometric examination must be carried out at each annual examination using equipment covering the frequencies 0.25 kHz - 8 kHz and according to prescribed procedures. Particular attention should be paid to divers who have only unilateral hearing, and the risks of further hearing damage should be discussed with such divers.*

OTORHINOLARYNGOLOGY
Mr. W.D. McNicoll

Are there any other E.N.T. surgeons here in the audience? No? Well, that shows how much interest E.N.T. surgeons have in diving medicine. In general, E.N.T. surgeons know very little about the problems related to diving. The E.N.T. side of diving is basically quite simple and practical. We are looking today at the specific contraindications to prevent an individual training as a diver.

THE EAR

External Auditory Canal

Otitis externa does not exclude an individual from diving however one should be concerned about individuals who suffer recurrent bouts of otitis externa. It is generally thought that otitis externa is due to recurring bacterial infection. In my opinion, this is not the primary cause, I think that bacterial infection is secondary to an initial fungal infection by Candida albicans.

The otitis externa usually presents with irritation in the ear canal followed by a discharge. The condition does not usually present as a discharge (otorrhoea). Usually the discharge is clear in colour but once secondary bacterial invasion occurs, the discharge becomes coloured and may be foul smelling. The secondary pathogens may be staphylococci, pseudomonas etc. Almost invariably the otorrhoea is treated with antibiotic drops which will eliminate the bacteria, but leave the fungi untouched which will result in recurrent infections. The precipitating cause of the otitis externa is a change in the pH of the skin which becomes less acid. Therefore the treatment of otitis externa is to make the skin more acid, by the use of 2% Boric Acid in 70% Industrial Spirit ear drops, 5% Acetic Acid in 70% Industrial Spirit ear drops, Aluminium Acetate ear drops etc. These drops are to be used by the individual whenever he thinks that the otitis externa is about to start, i.e., if there is any irritation in the ear. In those subjects prone to recurrent otitis externa, the ears should be dried using industrial spirit drops after each dive, or whenever the ears have become wet. This helps to prevent a recurrence of the infection. Chronic otitis externa is associated with a thickening of the skin leading to a narrowed external canal.

Psoriasis, when it affects the external auditory meatus is in effect like a chronic otitis externa and precludes the subject from diving. Seborrhoeic dermatitis prevents a similar problem. Psychocutaneous dermatitis is primarily a pruritus and the sufferers tend to scratch their ears all the time and also when they are asleep. This recurrent scratching debrades the skin and can become secondarily infected.

Ivory exostoses, are usually found in individuals who swim a great deal. The exostoses do not present a problem, until they become large enough to prevent wax being extruded from the ear. When this occurs, the subject is liable to get bouts of otitis externa. The treatment for this condition, once they start causing problems, is to remove them surgically. Occasionally one finds a solitary exostoses, looking like a ball on a long stalk, this is a cancellous osteoma and usually does not present a problem.

Tympanic Membrane

The tympanic membranes should be examined on an annual basis, as an individual may perforate an eardrum and be unaware of it. Divers are usually well motivated to carry on working unless the drums are inspected and found to be intact. Ninety-five per cent of traumatic perforations heal spontaneously. If closure of the perforation does not occur spontaneously, then repair of the drum (Type 1 tympanoplasty or myringoplasty) can be performed. The perforation can be repaired by use of temporalis fascia graft, fat graft or by using tragal cartilage and perichondrium. The operation takes between 20 and 60 minutes to perform with an overall 80% closure after one year.

A repaired perforation does not preclude an individual from becoming a diver. However the presence of an attic perforation in the tympanic membrane indicates the presence of middle ear disease, as do posterior marginal perforations of the drum. Such perforations preclude an individual from taking up a career in diving.

An atticotomy, modified radical mastoidectomy or radical mastoidectomy are not compatible with a career in diving. Simple mastoidectomy for acute mastoiditis is not a contra-indication to diving.

A patulous or atelectatic tympanic membrane is usually a result of previous middle ear disease and is also an indicator of poor eustachian tube dysfunction. Individuals with this type of ear drum are not fit to dive.

Calcium deposition within the layers of the tympanic membrane present as white plaques and are an indication of previous middle ear disease. If the drum is mobile on performing the valsalva manoeuvre and assuming that the individual can equilibrate a dynamic pressure change equivalent to 1 bar, then the subject is fit to dive.

A featureless tympanic membrane is also an indicator of previous middle ear disease and precludes the candidate from taking up a career in diving.

Middle Ear Problems

One attack of otitis media is not a contra-indication of diving. However recurrent attacks of otitis media or chronic suppurative otitis media is a bar to diving. A pink or red tympanic membrane on otoscopy is not pathognomonic of middle ear infection. Crying, sneezing, coughing, blowing your nose can all result in an injection of the tympanic membrane. Otitis media due to infection is painful! The pain is usually throbbing in type and the individual does not usually feel well.

Chronic suppurative otitis media is usually of two types: tubo-tympanic disease, usually the perforation is anterior and is as a result of poor eustachian tube function, the discharge is usually mucoid; or the chronic otitis media is as a result of attic disease, usually cholesteatoma. The discharge is often scanty and foul smelling as a result of associated osteitis. Chronic suppurative otitis media is a bar to diving, even when quiescent.

Labyrinthine fistulae are usually as a result of chronic middle ear disease and demonstrated by carrying out the fistula test which causes an affected individual to feel vertiginous.

Stapes surgery results in the individual being unfit for diving. The subject may swim on the surface, but on no account should he or she swim underwater. The reason for this being that the stapes prosthesis can be driven inwards thus destroying the hearing.

Inner Ear Problems

Perilymph leak via the round or oval window results in deafness, vertigo and tinnitus. Round window fistulae are more common than oval window fistulae and the subject usually has transient vertigo which is not severe, tinnitus and deafness which is sensorinueral in type and the deafness may be mild or severe. This condition is an E.N.T. emergency. If the affected ear is operated on within a week of the rupture the hearing can be regained. Seventy-five per cent of E.N.T. surgeons have never dealt with a perilymph leak. After successful repair of a round window rupture it is my policy to allow the diver to resume diving.

Meniere's disease, known as endolymphatic hydrops or episodic vertigo, is a bar to diving. Cupulolithiasis and benign paroxysmal vertigo is also a contra-indication.

Vertigo post head injury is usually as a result of a skull base fracture with the fracture lying transversely across the petrous temporal bone, and is usually associated with a facial palsy and a sensorineural hearing loss. Longitudinal fractures of the skull base usually result in a conductive hearing loss and blood in the tympanic cavity.

NOSE AND PARANASAL SINUSES

Unilateral nasal polypi are not a bar to diving. Do not remove these polypi without first sampling the fluid contained in the polyp and testing the fluid for glucose. Fluid positive for glucose confirms that it is a meningocele and not a simple polyp. Multiple polypi in the nose should be referred to an E.N.T. facility. They tend to recur after treatment and are therefore a bar to diving.

Nasal septal deformity may result in difficulties in breathing, epistaxis and also eustachian tube dysfunction.

Recurrent sinusitis is a bar to diving, whereas recurrent vacuum headache can be remedied by surgery and is not necessarily a bar to diving. A history of repeated nasal surgery (other than cosmetic) is a bar to diving.

Recurrent nasal furunculosis, usually due to a staphlococus aureus, is a contra-indication.

Hypertrophy of the inferior and middle turbinates causing nasal obstruction will ultimately lead to sinus problems.

ARE DIVERS DEAF?
Surgeon Commander P.J. Benton, R.N.

INTRODUCTION

"Divers have always been deaf, so the story goes", commented Bornmann in 1979 during a symposium on what was then known as Decompression Sickness. However the association between diving and hearing damage dates back to 300 BC when Aristotle asked the question "why is it that the ear drums of divers burst in the sea?" During the 19th Century with the introduction and use of caissons in mining and civil engineering plus the advent of compressed air diving it was noted that exposure to hyperbaric environments appeared to be associated with hearing loss. Paul Bert in his classic text "La Pression Barometric" commented on this in 1878 whilst Boot in 1913 first used the term "caisson workers deafness".

Moving to more recent times, in 1961 Coles and Knight studied a group of 62 Royal Navy divers and Submarine Escape Training instructors. Examination revealed that all of these men had evidence of a high frequency hearing loss. Unfortunately all of these men had also been exposed to noise, including gunfire and machinery noise during their naval careers and so the possibility of noise being the causative mechanism could not be excluded.

In an attempt to remove noise exposure from the equation, Edmonds in 1985 studied a group of 28 abalone divers, who with one exception had no history of noise exposure. All of these divers were found to have marked high frequency hearing loss with 40% failing to meet the Australian Standards Association hearing standards for divers and compressed air workers. These are very liberal standards, which accept a 35 dB loss at 1 and 2 kHz, 45 dB at 4 kHz and 50 dB at 6 and 8 kHz.

Finally, Molvaer in 1985 examined 164 professional divers. The results of his study revealing an apparent increase in the rate of hearing loss with increasing age. In 1990 116 divers from the original group of 164 were traced and re-examined. The results of this second study confirming the earlier findings.

Four possible mechanisms of hearing loss in divers have been suggested.

1. **Noise Induced Hearing Loss (NIHL):** Divers are exposed to a wide range of noise sources, both in and out of the water. Underwater tools have been recorded as producing levels of 140 dBA or more, whilst breathing gas passing into diving helmets can be responsible for noise levels of over 100 dBA. Divers are also exposed to machinery noise on the surface, including that of the helicopters used for transport to offshore platforms.
2. **Barotrauma:** Trauma to both the middle and inner ear can occur if the diver fails to equalise the pressure of the middle ear with that of ambient. This can lead to permanent hearing loss and it is of note that Edmonds commented on the fact that many of the abalone divers he studied linked their hearing loss to episodes of barotrauma.
3. **Decompression Illness (DCI):** The inner ear can be affected by DCI and if not treated promptly this may result in permanent hearing loss.
4. **Cochlear degeneration:** Animal experiments have revealed cochlear degeneration in animals which have been subjected to accepted compression / decompression schedules.

METHOD

To investigate the hypothesis that diving is associated with hearing loss, the audiometric records were inspected of a group of U.K. professional divers, all of whom had been examined by a single HSE approved medical examiner. Each year this one doctor sees between 14-18% of all U.K. professional divers. The selection criteria for entry into the study were as follows:

- all had had a recent audiometric examination, recent being defined as between January 1989 and March 1992, and
- all had a minimum of five years diving experience. This was to enable the rate of loss, if any, over a period of time to be calculated.

The 281 divers who met these criteria were placed into seven, five year age groups ranging from >25 <30 to >55 <60. The mean age was 37.7 years (SD 6.0), median age 37 years (range 26 to 56 years), and the mode was 36 years (in 17 divers). There were no divers under 25 years of age as the selection criteria, by specifying a minimum of five years follow-up excluded any younger divers. The minimum age to commence professional dive training in the United Kingdom is eighteen years of age.

RESULTS

The Median Hearing Level Thresholds for each age group were compared to the predicted values for otologically normal individuals, these being obtained from BS 6951 (British Standards Institute 1988). This comparison revealed that the divers median hearing threshold values lay between the predicted median and predicted upper quartile values. Within the older age groups, >40 years, the divers median values and the predicted median values for otologically normal persons were very similar. This is contrary to Molvaer's findings in which the hearing level thresholds of the older divers were in excess of the predicted values for otologically normal non-divers.

In an attempt to discover whether the rate of loss over a period of time was in excess of that which would be expected as a result of age alone in a normal non-diving population, two sub-groups were extracted from the main study group. Sub-group A (n = 220) comprised those divers whose records revealed the results of audiometry carried out five years prior to their most recent examination. Sub-group B (n = 127) comprised those divers whose records revealed the results of audiometry carried out ten years prior to their most recent examination.

Following correction for the hearing threshold loss expected due to age, calculated using BS 6951, no statistically significant change in hearing threshold level could be detected over either the 5 or 10 year periods.

Otitic barotrauma has already been suggested as a cause of hearing loss in divers. Thirty two divers (11.3%) in this study were recorded as having suffered otitic barotrauma during their careers and of these, 8 (2.8%) were found to have evidence of permanent hearing loss, defined as greater than 30 dB in two or more frequencies.

Of interest is the fact that half of the divers who developed permanent hearing loss following barotrauma were smokers, compared to only a little over one fifth of both the main study group, and those who suffered barotrauma in the absence of permanent hearing loss. Thus, although smoking does not seem to increase the risk of otitic barotrauma, which might be expected as a result of excess mucous secretion and hence increased difficulty in equalising middle ear pressure, it does appear to be associated with an increased risk of developing permanent hearing loss following such barotrauma.

Smoking has been implicated as a possible contributing factor to increased rate of hearing loss, due possibly to the ototoxic effects of nicotine, amongst both aviators (Thomas 1981), and divers (Molvaer 1985). However, in both of these studies the increased rate of loss was over a period of time, whereas in this case the hearing loss appeared to follow an acute event, otitic barotrauma. It is difficult to envisage why smoking should lead to an increased risk of developing permanent hearing loss following otitic barotrauma, although one possible explanation could be that smoking impairs the microvascular blood supply to the cochlea with the result that the ability of the cochlea to repair itself following damage is impaired.

CONCLUSION

In conclusion, contrary to previous studies, this study revealed no increase in hearing threshold loss associated with diving, except in the small number of cases in which there was evidence of significant otitic barotrauma.

REFERENCES

British Standards Institute BS 6951. *Acoustics; threshold of hearing by air conduction as a function of age and sex for otologically normal persons.* Milton Keynes. 1988.

Coles, R.R.A. & Knight, J.J. *Aural and audiometric survey of qualified divers and submarine escape training tank instructors.* London: Royal Naval Personnel Research Committee, Medical Research Council. 1961

Edmonds, C. & Freeman, P. Hearing loss in Australian divers. *Medical Journal of Australia.* 1985; **143**: 446-448.

Molvaer, O.I. & Lehmann, E.H. Hearing acuity in professional divers. *Undersea Biomed. Res.* 1985; **12**: 333-349.

Molvaer, O.I. & Albrektsen, G. Hearing deterioration in professional divers: an epidemiologic study. *Undersea Biomed. Res.* 1990; **17**: 231-246.

Thomas, G.B., Williams, C.E. & Hoger, N.G. Some non-auditory correlates of the hearing threshold levels of an aviation noise-exposed population. *Aviat., Space and Environ. Med.* 1987; **52**: 531-536.

DISCUSSION

Örnhagen (Chairman): We now need to address the questions: "What are the E.N.T. contraindications to acceptance for diver training? To what extent is existing deafness or previous surgery acceptable?"

McNicoll: Existing deafness is not acceptable because one must start with the highest possible level of hearing. Anyone who has a 20 dB loss when they are starting shows that they already have a problem. The benefit of pre-employment audiometry is identifying those subjects with pre-existing hearing loss. There is no law to prevent an employer from not employing a disabled man if he is diligent enough to have discovered the disability before employing him. One must identify those with pre-existing hearing loss, which might start to manifest as a disability during the new employment for which the current employer is an obvious source for blame and litigation.

So medico-legally at what point can a claim be made? Answer, 10 dB. If I were to do an audiogram on everybody in this room, most will have a hearing loss of around 10 dB. Any notching at 3, 4 or 6 kHz regardless of age which can be attributable to noise, will be. Like Peter, I went through the NPL Acoustic figures (Robinson & Shipton, 1977) which one needs to have for accepting a person around 18 - 20 years. The category H1 (which is the military hearing category of no loss greater than 10 dB) from 256 Hz to 8 kHz for somebody who is wanting to start to dive, that is the figure. At the age of 33, a maximum loss at 8 kHz should be 13.6 dB, at 4 kHz 10.3 dB and at 256 Hz 5.4 dB. That is at the 25th percentile, so if somebody is going to become a diver you must have somebody who has good hearing to start with. We have already talked about the post-surgical contraindications.

Örnhagen: Is there any comment from the floor? *(Pause)* If not, what are the pass/fail criteria in the assessment of Eustachian tube function?

McNicoll: First, one must assess the drum and make sure that it is absolutely normal. Then one would want to see the drum move, the Toynbee manoeuvre is not good for this because one cannot predict in what part of that manoeuvre the drum will move and so one usually will miss it. Therefore you should get the person to do a Valsalva manoeuvre when one should see the drum move briskly. Not opening like a flower: if there is a problem with one side opening briskly and the other one slowly that person will have some future problem, usually alternobaric vertigo.

You also see divers in whom nothing happens while the diver says "I can feel it clear", they have a drum with a low compliance. In this case you can either get them to sink to the bottom of the swimming pool and then look at the drum afterwards. They will either have cleared it or not, so does it look congested? But a far better system is to use an Impedance Meter which basically measures the pressure in one's ear and will draw a graph of how the drum moves. It will demonstrate how the eustachian tube functions. As the patient does a Valsalva so he deflects the stylus and the moment his Eustachian tube opens can be seen easily. No matter how good one's technicians are, this is something one should do oneself. If there is a lag before it goes, then you know he has sluggish movement (McNicoll, 1982). In conventional E.N.T. terms he is absolutely fine. The work that is done in E.N.T. departments on Eustachian tube is done at an equivalent compression rate of 1 metre per minute which, for diving, is absolutely useless. So everybody is normal and "normal Eustachian function" may therefore be a meaningless report. One must note the speed of response.

Örnhagen: Is there any way one can practice this? If one has a candidate coming and he or she has difficulty. Can you give this person practical advice?

McNicoll: I normally get them to try a Valsalva. I therefore say "make sure your eyeballs pop" and do it gently. To do it forcefully also congests the Eustachian tube. The most important advice is that they practice this frequently say 400 times a day.

Örnhagen: The manoeuvre described by Dr. Frenzel is an increase in the intrapharyngeal pressure without a Valsalva manoeuvre and therefore with no increase in intrathoracic pressure. This is a method that you should encourage because if you do not increase thoracic pressure there is no risk of a round window rupture.

McNicoll: Yes, you should just be able to contract your soft palate and do it, but explaining how to do it is very difficult.

Örnhagen: Another question regarding surgery. In earlier days radioactive radium needles were inserted into the tubes to make them open. This is not a technique used today but have you ever come across a diver where some surgery should be used?

McNicoll: If you fiddle around with the Eustachian tube you are asking for trouble. Those people who had the needles, which might have been given for hypertrophic adenoids, may well have developed a carcinoma 30 years on.

My own feeling on Eustachian tube dysfunction is much simpler than everyone makes out. It can be demonstrated with xenon airflow studies and the abolition of dysfunction after surgery to the nose. It is where the vomer and ethmoid unite with the back of the septal cartilage fitting in. If there is a large deformity of the nasal septum there then it's like a rock in a stream, it just flows by. If it's like a small deformity, then its like a stick in the stream and creates turbulence and the air will not flow past easily. I have done now about 5,000 excisions of voma-ethmoid sutures in adults (McNicoll & Scanlan, 1979). If someone cannot clear their ears there is a 95% chance of curing that. However, if there is sluggish mobility then I think about 98% will be cured within 6 weeks. Failures may occur with those who had an over-enthusiastic adenoidectomy.

Turner: I have a lot of patients who have rhinitis, can I have your opinion on the use of inhaled steroids please?

McNicoll: Simple allergic rhinitis is not a contraindication to diving but somebody who has an atopic history, then one finds the mucosa in the nose is grossly oedematous and then the chances are the Eustachian tubes will also be involved. Certainly one can use steroids. Headback, turn to the right, one nostril, two puffs leave it there a while and then sniff it back. The instructions just say sniff it back and, if you do all you get is a throat full of the stuff, useless. If you do not sniff, it tracks over the lining and is effective. Then turn over and do the other side.

Risberg: I sense some difference between today's two sessions. Previously we were saying very cautiously that you had to explain why a person might be unfit and relate this to the consequences with scientific evidence. So I have some difficulty in accepting your very firm, dogmatic, prescriptive approach to these E.N.T. problems. Is there any evidence that some of these contraindications really do place the diver at risk for harm? Though that is really a comment rather than a question.

Örnhagen: Thank you, noted.

LeDez: Many of the applicants going for diving as a second career already have a substantial hearing loss from their previous occupations. It seems unrealistic to fail these persons when everything else is normal.

McNicoll: I take your point. If I can quote the medico-legal view "an abnormal pre-employment audiogram can be detrimental to an employer in that its presence can put the employer on notice that the abnormal susceptibility of the employee. Paradoxically an employee with poor hearing is less likely to suffer the effects of noise than a normal person. The employer must then decide on a course of action after weighing up the risks and benefits. This usually results in turning down the candidate." My own interpretation is that if somebody has a dip at 3, 4, 6 kHz which is probably due to noise then you'll not be doing him a favour by allowing him to work in a noisy environment.

LeDez: At least in Canada if one is doing the examination on behalf of the diver then the results of the individual's tests do not go to the employer, only the certificate that he is fit or not fit to dive.

McNicoll: If you have done an audiogram and you have not informed the employer about this then, when that individual does have a hearing loss, it is to you that the employer will turn because you have not warned them that this person did in fact have the problem. If a person has a hearing loss, you have probably given him the wrong advice.

LeDez: In most of the ones I have seen there has been a marked difference between the two sides. Almost all the saturation divers in the last year or two have almost invariably had marked high figures of hearing loss.

McNicoll: Those are people already diving and what we were talking about was the recruitment of the new candidate. Major industries are doing in-house audiograms in this country.

LeDez: In North America at least, there is no company doing in-house audiograms.

Örnhagen: Peter, do you have any comments on this?

Benton: If a person with unilateral hearing loss starts diving, he is not disadvantaged underwater, but there is a chance that that person may suffer hearing loss in his solitary ear and then become truly disabled. He must at least be aware of the risk in order to make an informed decision on whether or not to dive. The candidate for diving with a unilateral hearing loss should not be accepted. A unilateral hearing loss occurring in an established diver, perhaps due to barotrauma, is not necessarily a contraindication. That is a different decision, ethically.

McNicoll: Five per cent of unilateral hearing loss is due to an acoustic neuroma. So someone with unilateral high tone hearing loss would be a brave man to carry on diving. They grow at 3 - 4 mm per year.

O'Sullivan: You are referring to what is known in legal circles as the "egg-shell skull syndrome". If the individual has some unusual deficit then the employer must take extra steps to protect that individual. The problem that we have with divers is that if they have, for instance, a noise induced hearing loss, the individual must be instructed so that he can protect his own hearing. The diver can be told that if he does have an increased loss at his next examination, it is because he has not been protecting his hearing when in a noisy area.

Örnhagen: How does aural barotrauma affect diving safety and how can this be assessed?

McNicoll: It is either middle ear barotrauma or inner ear barotrauma. Middle ear barotrauma leads to conductive hearing loss which will normally resolve, but an inner ear barotrauma is much more difficult. The perilymph leak or the window rupture will need surgical intervention. There is also an intra-labyrinthine membrane rupture and that presents as a unilateral hearing loss which runs all right to 3 kHz and then suddenly there's a drop. The patient does not usually get vertiginous with it, but may have tinnitus. With an oval window leak, the hearing loss can be anything from 30-40 dB to a totally dead ear. Someone with a better than 40 dB ear should be sedated, repeat the audiogram, if there is no improvement then perform surgery. Explore the ear, if the loss is greater than 40 dB then you have got nothing to lose, go in immediately, the whole operation takes only half an hour. Last April when Fred Pullen from Miami, who was the first person to describe a perilymph leak from a round window barotrauma, was over for the previous Fit to Dive conference, I found that we managed things in the same way. In these cases there tends to be vertigo but its not one that causes vomiting, but they do get tinnitus. They feel as though they have "water in their ears". When there is an oval window leak where the piston and the stapes have gone in, then there will be a roaring tinnitus, very severe vertigo and a total hearing loss. Then it is difficult to get a good result surgically because the foot plate has gone through and hit the sacculus, but one must go in and one must plug the leak.

Örnhagen: Can those divers return to diving?

McNicoll: It is unwise that they do. The hearing will come back in 70 - 80%.

Örnhagen: After a rupture of the tympanic membrane how long should the diver be off diving, I understand it depends on the size of the rupture?

McNicoll: I normally leave him for one month, at that time it really ought to have healed and if it has not then possibly 6 - 8 weeks.

Wendling: Sometimes it is difficult to distinguish between window rupture and the sequelae of decompression illness. Do you propose that anybody with a window rupture should be investigated surgically and have it mended?

McNicoll: Yes.

Örnhagen: The next question, "On what evidence should audiometry standards be defined in relation to hearing loss in divers? At what frequency is audiometry needed in a hearing conservation programme?"

Benton: This depends on what you are looking at. Barotrauma is an acute event and the person needs to be assessed at the time. The annual audiogram will be of no benefit to that person. In other cases the audiometry should be done at a frequency compatible with any other hearing conservation programme. The difficulty with divers is that they are on the whole self-employed, and that they may go to a different doctor each time. The importance of this is that one should look at the audiograms serially on each occasion. There needs to be some sort of follow-up system whereby the diver might bring his own records so that one can look at the previous year's examination. There is also the feeling that diving and low-frequency hearing loss may be associated and so there is a need to look at 250 Hz.

McNicoll: The annual audiogram is appropriate. There is a need to do a second audio at 3 to 6 months after beginning work in a noisy environment to find those who have got potentially tender hearing.

Benton: There is also the need to do one after an episode of barotrauma.

McNicoll: The other thing to do is to find out why he had the barotrauma.

Milne:** No mention was made of the indication for E.N.G. (possibly serially) before return to diving following inner ear barotrauma (including the diver clinically resolved).

Reply from McNicoll: If a diver's hearing returns to the range of normality post-incident, then this usually means that the vestibular system is normal.

Where the audiogram is abnormal post-incident then certainly electronystagmography will give evidence of whether there is canal paresis (i.e. malfunction of the vestibular system or not). There can be varying degrees of canal paresis and an organ of balance may never return to normality. However, if there is total canal paresis so that there is a non-functioning labyrinth, then the diver or any individual may have a problem in environments where there is very poor visibility and in which the eye is unable to focus on a fixed object. In daylight hours or with good visibility under water the individual should not have any great problems carrying out his duties.

Remember also, that inner ear barotrauma can involve rupture of the intralabyrinthine membrane, (i.e. the basilar membrane) and usually, in these cases, there is no diminution of vestibular function.

E.N.G. itself requires to be associated with caloric testing. This is the only way the function of the vestibular system can really be assessed. Straight forward E.N.G. does not incorporate caloric testing.

Örnhagen: "What components of the routine E.N.T. examination may not be necessary annually?"

McNicoll: The only thing that needs to be done is assessment of the ears really, unless there has been some event during the year, like a broken nose which requires a special consideration.

Örnhagen: "To what extent is the examination focused on in-water safety and to what extent on the avoidance of diving-related disorders?"

Benton: One must just avoid barotrauma and noise.

Anderson-Upcott: Could I ask about stress-induced stammer which I have had to fail railway signalmen with?

McNicoll: Have you used delayed speech feedback? This aborts the stutter.

REFERENCES

McNicoll, W.D. Middle ear analysis in the nose/ear distress syndrome. *J. Laryngol.-Otol.* 1982; **96**: 309-323.

McNicoll, W.D. & Scanlan, S.G. Submucous resection: the treatment of choice in the nose/ear distress syndrome. *J. Laryngol.-Otol.* 1979; **93**: 357-367.

Robinson, D.W. & Shipton, M.C. Tables for the estimation of noise-induced hearing loss. *N.P.L. Acoustics Report*; 2nd Edition. 1977.

COMMENTARY

The guidance for ENT (*pages 155*) was considered to be generally appropriate but perhaps insufficiently detailed.

A conclusion that most cases of Eustachian tube dysfunction could be easily rectified by a simple operative intervention led to the observation that only a very small proportion of ENT surgeons have any experience of treating divers, a point further emphasised in relation to the emergency treatment of inner ear barotrauma.

There is evidence that hearing loss in divers may not be so common as has been considered in the past. Only where a risk of noise-induced deafness is identified, is regular audiometry indicated. Audiometry is also indicated, but just once as a clinical measure, after otic barotrauma to assess any associated hearing loss.

VISION

The recommendations from the Guidance Notes on "The Medical Examination of Divers" are:

48. *The corrected vision should be 6/9 or better (binocular). For near vision a standard N5 is necessary which means the ability to read 5 point print from material held at a distance of between 25 and 40 cm.*

49. *The visual field should be normal using the simple confrontation test. Defects in the visual field should be referred for detailed investigation and the opinion of an ophthalmologist. A fundscopic examination of the eye should be made at each medical examination and any significant abnormality referred for a specialist opinion. The assessment of colour vision must be made at the **first professional medical examination** and any deficiency communicated to the diver.*

VISION
Dr. M.R. Cross

My special interest in eyes began when the Moorfield's group came to work with us on retinal degeneration because it was then that I had the opportunity of working very closely with some ophthalmologists. I learnt two things of real importance: if you don't take the trouble to put up the eye chart properly, to illuminate it properly and to cover the unused eye with a blank piece of card, one cannot measure visual acuity accurately. This is a very simple lesson but one which I feel people must appreciate. I had not realised how important that was. The other thing I learned is that most of us waste our time when we stare down the ophthalmoscope. To do this without dilating the eye is, according to the professionals, a waste of time. So as in much of this diving conference, the message is "do it properly". What should one look for in the eye when doing a diving medical? The answer is that what you should be looking for is not going to be visible with ordinary ophthalmoscopy. The retinography of divers needs special equipment and is described below.

Should a diver be able to see? Most divers are likely to work in poor visibility water and need to "see" with their fingertips. What standard is necessary for the examination of divers? The average diver should be able to see reasonably well to accomplish his functions. A person who is capable of passing a standard driving test, i.e. a car number plate at 75 feet, probably has perfectly adequate uncorrected vision for diving tasks. It is also important that one should be able to read diving tables and watches accurately. So, however bad one's vision is uncorrected, it is necessary that corrected vision will be adequate for reading. A real problem which may arise is what sort of correction is appropriate for diving? There is the question of "can divers wear contact lenses?" "What kinds of contact lenses can be worn?" Modern gas permeable lenses are perfectly acceptable in the diving environment. I only have one reservation of wearing contact lenses at depth and that is that when the diver loses a lense, all hell breaks loose. The entire team is sent searching for it. This can also happen during a mask flood and, if the lens comes out, this can be yet one more event in the domino causation of a more serious incident. But I have not yet come across any incident in diving where the loss of a contact lens has caused a real problem.

Colour vision in the diving environment is not essential. On the whole colours don't matter. Only if required for other reasons such as non-destructive testing (NDT) as a specialisation or for other vocational needs, is a colour test required.

RETINAL ANGIOGRAPHY

My interest in retinography in diving arose from the fact that in 1989 I was hard pressed to find a good excuse to visit the Caribbean. I had been impressed with the idea that bone necrosis of divers was very similar to the lesions found in the sickle cell patients. Was there a common mechanism? I became even more interested in this when I discovered the Medical Research Council had a sickle cell unit out in Jamaica. It was there that I met Alan Bird of the Moorfields Hospital making his twice a year visit in order to photograph the retinas of patients with sickle cell disease. As a result, the Moorfields team came down to Plymouth to see if they could find ocular changes in divers. The technique for flourescein angiography and the results of the subsequent study have been described elsewhere (Polkinghorne *et al*, 1988). In summary this was a cross-sectional study of 84 divers with a comparison group of 23 non-divers. The divers were sub-divided into those whose diving experience was less than one year, less than 4 years, or more than 4 years; those whose depth of dive less or greater than 50 m, and those whose last dive had been within the last 3 days, or within the last 30 days to six months, or who had not dived for six months or longer.

TABLE 21 - CAPILLARY DENSITY IN RELATION TO DIVING EXPERIENCE

Groups compared (length of diving experience)	Difference in mean density	95% confidence interval*	p
Non-divers			
Divers (<1 yr)	0.2491	2.0429	NS
Divers (1-4 yr)	2.6360	2.0899	<0.05
Divers (>4 yr)	2.6271	1.8538	<0.05
Divers (<1yr)			
Divers (1-4 yr)	2.3870	2.0676	<0.05
Divers (>4 yr)	2.3780	1.8286	<0.05
Divers (1-4 yr)			
Divers (>4 yr)	0.0090	1.8810	NS

* Multiple-t confidence interval, NS = Not Significant

(Tables 21 & 22 from Polkinghorne *et al* 1988, with permission).

TABLE 22 - FREQUENCY OF PIGMENT EPITHELIAL LESIONS

Duration of diving experience	History of bends	No. of divers	Pigment epithelial lesions
0-1 yr	No	23	5 (22%)
	Yes	0	0
1-4 yr	No	19	8 (42%)
	Yes	2	2
>4 yr	No	24	11 (46%)
	Yes	12	11 (91%)
TOTAL	-	80	37 (46%)

Capillary density seems to drop off with experience (Table 21). We concluded the capillary density diminishes within increased duration of diving and for divers who have been diving deeper. Much more interesting was another finding. These were pigment epithelial lesions (Table 22). The function of the choroid is to act as a heat sink to prevent the retina overheating through the power of the light falling upon it. Normally one cannot see the choroidal circulation because there is the retinal pigment layer in front of it and this does not allow the light through. Where the pigment area is damaged then, through the retina you will see the choroidal circulation shining. A pigment epithelial lesion is not due to obstruction of the retinal capillaries. It is due to obstruction of the choroidal circulation and that is a big circulation.

In those who have been diving for more than 4 years regularly, whether as an amateur or a professional, some 50% of the population have pigment lesions. In those who have had decompression sickness in that time there is a 90% occurrence of such lesions. The Moorfields team have been coming back to Plymouth and now we have around 240 divers and have had no reason to change our relative ratios. There are also bizarre vascular patterns including revascularisation across the macular.

We have often been asked if this will affect the quality of life and I used to think that this condition would not affect visual acuity. We now have 4 divers whose visual acuity may be diminished and this will not be rectified by the use of glasses. We also can see micro aneurysms, non-filling capillaries and occasional dilatation and leakage.

The conclusions of the cross-sectional study was that retinal lesions occur in diver, that retinal pigment epithelial lesions were found in divers with bends and that all lesions could be explained by some form of vascular obstruction. This study is the first evidence of damage to the eye tissue in both amateur and professional divers and it suggests for the first time that a career in diving almost inevitably leads to damage.

There have been some contradictory studies but we believe that our studies are now statistically more valid than originally.

REFERENCE

Polkinghorne, P.J., Sehmi, K., Cross, M.R., Minassian, D. & Bird, A.C. *Lancet* 1988; **ii**: 1381 - 1383.

DISCUSSION

Lewkowicz: Is corneal laser surgery for myopia a problem?

Cross: There has been a computer network discussion on this and the consensus view is that since the orb is incompressible there should be no reason why any surgery on the eye should be a contraindication to diving. But one got the feeling that the American physicians contributing to this discussion each hoped that the first patient with corneal surgery to dive would not be one of their own patients.

Lewkowicz: I have passed one and he has done all right so far.

Cross: I shall send that information back through cyberspace.

Mebane: This is one of our commonest questions at DAN and the consensus view is that there is no reason not to dive.

Francis: It is understandable that we look at the underwater environment but our divers also have other tasks to do, like driving around at night in small boats, and so under these circumstances visual acuity and even colour vision may be essential.

Cross: Those who have special needs must set special standards.

Elliott**: What now is the percentage of retinal lesions in the control population?

Reply from Cross: In our control population it remains at 4%.

Welslau**: Is there any evidence that diving is a contributory factor to acute glaucoma in individuals with a narrow irido-corneal angle?

Dick (F.)**: Is there any evidence of acquired colour vision deficits in the retinography of divers? If so, at what frequency should colour vision screening be undertaken and by which tests?

Reply from Cross: There is no evidence that diving influences glaucoma nor any evidence of acquired colour vision deficits.

ENDOCRINOLOGY

The recommendations from the Guidance Notes on "The Medical Examination of Divers" are:

37. (a) *A proven or suspected endocrine abnormality will require a detailed assessment.*
    (b) *Glycosuria would require investigation.*
    (c) *Diabetes is a case for rejection.*

ENDOCRINE DISORDERS
Dr. J. Seckl

There is no sensible evidence to inform the guidance for endocrine diseases in relation to diving. All that I can present is opinion and give you something to go on as a basis. Most professional divers will not have had endocrine disease, for such persons will have excluded themselves naturally. The first point to raise is the question of those with a stable disease against those with an undiagnosed or the unstable condition because one's approach to each will be different. Then we should consider the various complications of each endocrine disorder that may be relevant to professional diving.

THYROID

Gross thyroid disease is an obvious contraindication to diving but marginal cases may be more difficult to pick up and decide upon.

The commonest endocrine condition one is likely to come across is hypothyroidism. If a person is unwell with this condition then they are also unfit to dive. Thyroxin replacement therapy can cure this condition in which case they are then fit to dive. Missing one or two pills in a week is not going to cause an acute problem. This is no more than hormone replacement therapy and when stable on therapy patients are essentially normal. The half-life of thyroxin is one week, they are unlikely to have any complications but they should be screened annually with a thyroid function test to ensure that the replacement therapy is adequate.

Thyrotoxicosis is also a common condition, the lifetime prevalence is up to 1% in women but very much less in men. It is much more common in Asian societies. Should one screen for thyroid disease? No. Screening might be appropriate for a person who has had thyrotoxicosis if they are coming for assessment of fitness to dive in which case they should have annual thyroid function tests.

A person with active thyrotoxicosis should not dive. If treated, and its usually treated with radioiodine, they will then be hypothyroid and given thyroxin replacement therapy. Thus they are in the same category for fitness to dive as the treated hypothyroid individual. The complications of thyrotoxicosis include thyroid eye disease, with which they should not dive, and the swollen thyroid, goitre, which needs to be assessed as a potential for airflow obstruction if it is of any size. One must be aware that the goitre may be retrosternal. The thyroid eye disease is independent of the course of the thyroid disease itself. The exophthalmos is due to hypertrophic eye muscles within the orbit.

PITUITARY DISEASE

Should patients with pituitary disease be allowed to dive? And should persons who develop pituitary disease be disqualified from further diving? A complication of pituitary tumours is pressure on the optic chiasma with therefore some loss of vision. The nature of the actual visual defect varies from case to case and the classic bitemporal defect occurs in only 50%.

The person with a pituitary problem must be assessed by a specialist. A patient with hypopituitarism on replacement therapy would probably be alright for diving providing they are stable. They can certainly be firemen or policemen but a lot depends on the individual patient and the sort of replacement that they are having. An individual compliant with and well on hormone replacement should be fine, but I draw your attention to persons who are ACTH deficient and require cortisol. If such a patient is injured, stressed to a high degree, just unwell or if they are nauseated and vomiting, they will not absorb their cortisol and may collapse. We advise patients to carry parenteral cortisol, which would appear to be incompatible with diving.

Once a hyperfunctioning pituitary, such as acromegaly, has been treated, the tumour has been removed and the patient is otherwise well, so there is no reason why they should not be able to dive. One needs to assess for the complications of acromegaly, such as cardiac disease and diabetes which may improve with the treatment of acromegaly but should be assessed on their own merits.

Prolactin excess is becoming more frequently recognised. It is treated by tablets (e.g. bromocriptine) rather than surgery and providing patients take the medication then there is no reason why they should not continue to dive.

Active Cushing's disease is a rarity and is a condition not compatible with active occupations unless surgically cured when subjects may dive provided they do not have secondary adrenal insufficiency.

ADRENAL

The problem with Addison's disease is that if the patient becomes unwell, parenteral hydrocortisone is required for survival and that is obviously difficult with a diving career.

A phaeochromocytoma usually arises in the adrenal medulla although it can be outside the adrenal. Clearly these people are not fit to dive while they have the disease (with paroxysmal attacks, including hypertension etc.) but if they have been treated by the removal of the tumour and their excretion of catecholamines become normal, then once again they would be fit to dive like any other person.

GONADS

Hormone replacement therapy is not a contraindication to diving, be it with androgens or oestrogens. Androgens are given by injection 3 to 4 weekly which may or may not interfere with diving practice.

PARATHYROID

The patient with minor hypercalcaemia who is asymptomatic is probably alright to continue diving. On assessment with annual calcium function tests, renal function tests, renal ultrasound and x-rays, if there is no evidence of nephrocalcinosis, then these people are probably fit for diving. I would be much more concerned about hypoparathyroidism because such persons have a risk of tetany. If they are normal on calcaemic treatment there is still a risk of upset to the acid base balance and I believe that for longer duration diving they should be excluded.

DIABETES

If a patient comes with existing diabetes, should they be accepted? Certainly the easiest thing to do is say NO. But there will be shades of opinion on this. For a professional diver to start diving with this condition is inadvisable because of later complications. There is a high rate of retinal disease, of cardiac disease and they should be excluded.

All should be screened by annual urine analysis looking for glycosuria but it is better to ask about symptoms: polyuria, visual blurring, polydipsia, genital infection or irritation etc. The diagnosis is made by use of the glucose tolerance test and anyone with an abnormal result should be referred to a specialist for classification.

Once diabetes is diagnosed they may be managed by diet alone, oral therapy or insulin injections. One's assessment for each of these will be different. If they are already a diver and get insulin dependent diabetes I believe that they should discontinue diving. Those on oral hypoglycaemics can, in fact, be more difficult to deal with because, if they become hypoglycaemic, it could be more prolonged and more difficult to treat than insulin-dependent diabetes.

More difficult to manage is the diver who is controlled by diet. A large number will have self excluded because they are too fat for diving but it is a difficult decision to make. My suggestion is if they are well treated on diet alone then allow them to continue to dive but screen them annually for complications.

The rates of these complications are enormous, of those who have had diabetes for 10 years, 50% have retinal complications and if they have had diabetes for 15 years, more than 90% will have retinal complications. The other complications include: atherosclerosis, cardiomyopathy, peripheral vascular disease, diabetic foot syndrome, nephropathy and neuropathy.

It is important for individuals to be able to regulate their blood pressure and those with autonomic neuropathy cannot baroregulate. One sign is the fixed heart rate which does not vary with Valsalva (the heart rate does not vary between the maximal heart rate during, and the minimum after the release of a Valsalva). The classical ratio of 1.2 or greater, which is normal, is lost. On deep breathing 5-6 per minute a normal person will have a difference in heart rate of 15 heart beats per minute maximum. Those with parasympathetic neuropathy will show less than 10. With an ECG monitor these are relatively easy screening tests. Later on in the disease, a sympathetic neuropathy leads to postural hypotension. Therefore persons should be excluded from diving if any abnormalities are found on screening.

DISCUSSION

LeDez: I have had a few suspicions about the use of anabolic steroids in divers, can you say anything about that?

Seckl: Anabolic steroid abuse leads to people who are hypogonadal. If they are otherwise well, are not hypotensive, have a normal liver function and don't have cardiomyopathy, then, unless there is any other reason to exclude them, they should be able to continue diving. From their health point of view they should be discouraged but there is nothing to stop them.

Griffin: I have been diving with persons who have insulin-dependent diabetes and it seems that there are some who can tolerate it and there are some who, particularly when they are immersed, seem to be entirely disrupted in their metabolism. They may be well controlled in other exercise but when they get underwater they seem to go out of control. Is there any scientific explanation of that?

Seckl: This is an interesting observation and worthy of being investigated fully and written up. There are no data. If a diabetic is stressed then the counter-regulatory hormones may be upsetting diabetic control. Stress causes the release of cortisol, growth hormones, and catecholamines, all of which will antagonise glycaemic control. We do not understand why there are individual differences but there are indeed clear differences. I would be very cautious about somebody who is having insulin continuing as a diver.

MUSCULO-SKELETAL AND HAEMATOLOGY

Chairman : Dr. I.M. Calder

The recommendations from the Guidance Notes on "The Medical Examination of Divers" are:

MUSCULO-SKELETAL AND BONE NECROSIS

39. The diver must have unimpeded mobility and dexterity and must be sufficiently physically robust to meet the demands of the proposed work. In particular, all joints should have a normal range of functional mobility. Divers with a history of back pain should be carefully assessed, bearing in mind the heavy lifting a diver may be required to do when out of the water: recurrent episodes of incapacitating back pain will be a cause for rejection. Successful surgery for spinal lesions may be acceptable if neurological examination is normal and full agility regained.

40. All new entrants should have routine **long-bone radiographs**. These are not thereafter required on a routine basis but the need for such assessment must be reconsidered at each annual examination. Approved doctors should give particular attention in this regard to the following groups:

    (a) those diving regularly more than 30 metres and under pressure for more than 4 hours;
    (b) those who have suffered decompression sickness in the previous 12 months;
    (c) those with clinical symptoms referable to a joint;
    (d) mixed gas divers;
    (e) saturation divers;
    (f) experimental divers;

HSE "Health Notes" : RADIOLOGY AND DIVING

As part of the on-going revision and updating of its guidance on statutory medical examinations, and with the over-riding wish to minimise radiation exposure, HSE has reconsidered the need for long bone radiographs of commercial divers.

The primary reasons for radiography of the hips, knees and shoulders in divers have been the detection of existing bone lesions at the commencement of diving and the early detection of osteonecrotic lesions during a diver's career. It has been acknowledged that such surveillance is particularly appropriate in certain categories of diving.

Various factors have influenced us in the decision to change the guidance. These include:

(i) as mentioned above, a wish to reduce the overall radiation exposure of divers;
(ii) a wish to shift the emphasis of the medical examination from screening towards surveillance in relation to occupational risk and hence to produce information to aid the diver in reaching decisions about his health and work;
(iii) a belief that there should be a balance between the risks of radiation and the benefits to be gained by the diver, and hence that radiography should be the subject of counselling and informed consent;

(iv) our understanding that the incidence of disabling osteonecrotic lesions is very low. Lesions are particularly rare in the air diving range;
(v) whilst the detection of a lesion has no influence on the likelihood of other future lesions the continuance of diving of the same kind may lead to other lesions. The disabling effect of a lesion (if juxta-articular) will naturally be increased by the development of disease in other joints;
(vi) that the removal from diving work of a diver with established osteonecrotic disease does not arrest the progress of that disease, and further that the condition is not amenable to currently available treatment;
(vii) in diving, lesions of the shoulder and hip greatly exceed those in the knees;
(viii) finally, that the finding of a bony lesion at the pre-employment stage would not necessarily, of itself, preclude diving.

We therefore recommend that the practice of <u>routine</u> radiography prior to Part I, Part III or Part IV training should also cease. However, radiography of the hips, shoulders and knees should be carried out before the commencement of Part II training and of the hips and shoulders at intervals thereafter whilst the diver is still engaged in mixed gas or saturation diving.*

Factors in the decision would be those currently advised in MA1 Para. 40 subject to the clinical judgement of the examining doctor in the light of the diver's history and the results of clinical examination. Radiography may be advised on clinical grounds in situations other than those described.

If radiography is not judged necessary on other grounds, it should be repeated at intervals of 5 years during a diver's career.

The decision to radiograph the long bones should be the subject of agreement between the diver and the examining doctor - that is to say the diver should give his informed consent.

Examining doctors would retain the right not to issue a certificate of fitness if they felt that radiography was of crucial importance to their decision on fitness in any particular case and the diver would not agree.

*(Parts I, III and IV refer to different categories of air diving whereas Part II refers to mixed-gas bell and saturation diving).

MUSCULO-SKELETAL
Dr. Ewan Macdonald

I was charmed into coming to talk to this conference because I know a little about backs and knees. Then I discovered it was a conference full of experts on diving and I know very little about diving. However, for ten years I was responsible for the fitness standards of mines-rescue men in the Yorkshire coal fields and the standards of fitness required were very similar, I suspect, to diving. So I'm going to talk about backs and knees and I will start off talking about knees.

You are very familiar with these standards. The diver must:

- have unimpeded mobility and dexterity;
- be sufficiently physically robust;
- have a normal range of functional movements.

Also,

- recurrent incapacitation is a cause for rejection;
- successful surgery is acceptable if neurologically normal and with full agility.

Amazingly detailed and clear, and plenty of scope for different judgements.

KNEES

The prognosis of many knee conditions has improved over the years as the treatment has become more sophisticated and surgeons are less prone to open them up but prefer to use endoscopes. In very active sports people particularly and those undertaking strenuous manual work, but also in the rest of the population, the following may occur:

- Synovitis
- Bursitis
- Strains, avulsions, ruptures
- Patellar subluxation
- Chondromalacia patellae
- Inflammation
- Osteochondritis
- Loose bodies
- Meniscus lesions
- Ligament injury
- Osteoarthritis

What is important in the pre-employment assessment? A history of knee injuries is important as is a history of knee symptoms. Pain if it is mechanical, tends to be local and if it is inflammatory, seems to be diffuse in knee conditions. Stiffness is an important symptom. Swelling, if it is diffuse, is usually above the knee. Locking and unlocking suggests a mechanical problem and "giving way" can be either due to muscular weakness or due to a mechanical instability.

On examination at a pre-employment, pre-placement or pre-diving assessment, I would be interested in normal gait, have they got quadriceps wasting and a normal range of movement or not? I have talked to a few diving colleagues and asked just how thorough and detailed was the examination of the knee and like, I suspect, in many other medicals, the knee joint is not examined in great detail in somebody who is asymptomatic. So I will be looking for this kind of level of examination in somebody who is asymptomatic without problems. The range of flexion and extension are important but that varies and it is important to test that the ligaments are intact.

The range of flexion and extension does vary depending upon the range of activity and you can increase flexion with squatting and I think asking people to squat and crawl is quite a useful test if you are in doubt about fitness.

There are always people who are much more difficult to assess because they have had problems in the past. I always get people to squat and crawl. Look at the quadriceps. One can usually assess the quadriceps size manually and visually. If in doubt, it is important to measure the quadriceps. I take an arbitrary 18 cm above the joint line and a difference of more than 1 or 2 cm accurately measured is a significant loss of muscle mass in smaller thighs. Is there joint warmth? Are there any effusions? Palpate the knee. It is important to do this as it is useful to feel for cysts and remember, round the back as well, for the Baker's cyst.

It is likely that if anyone has any of these positive findings, they have symptoms and the issue always arises, is the individual who is being assessed, motivated to conceal from you musculoskeletal problems or are they motivated to maximise musculoskeletal problems? Are they trying to get into diving or trying to get out of diving? The approach the individual might take in terms of presentation of their symptoms and problems, will vary in that context.

On examining the knee when there is a history of knee problems, it is important to look at the mobility of the patellae, when they are relaxed. The patellae is normally very mobile. You can shove it from side to side and then feel under the edge of it as well. Is it tender underneath, medially and laterally, when you do that? I always check flexion and extension of the knee with my hand over the knee for crepitus. This is very useful to determine the amount of osteoarthritic changes or sub-patella deterioration. The medial and lateral ligaments and the cruciates should be tested. If there is a question of locking, or a suspicion of meniscal damage, it is worthwhile doing the provocation test for menisci: flexion/extension with internal/external rotation of the foot. Of course with knee conditions there are confounders, pain in the knee can be from the hip or pain in the back. There are issues related to unequal leg length which can cause symptoms in their back and knee. Ankle conditions can also affect the knee.

The contraindications to diving which I am proposing are based on experience in examining people with high standards of fitness. I would not recruit someone with Osgood-Schlatters Disease until healed. This is just a traumatic evulsion of the tibial tuberosity associated with retro-patella problems. I am dubious about people with a history of 'locking' or 'giving way'. If they say the knee is locking or giving way because they are wanting out of diving, it becomes a difficult assessment. Then the detailed clinical examination is very important to see if there is any evidence of abnormality. If somebody's got a knee 'locking' or 'giving way', it can be due to a loose body. Chondromalacia patellae, if moderate to severe, will certainly be a contraindication. If it is symptomatic, osteoarthritis it is a possible contraindication. If there's poor musculature and the knees are lax, maybe in someone who's been a footballer with a few knee injuries, I would be dubious about him embarking on a career in diving. A persisting effusion I would regard as a contraindication, but it depends on how tough you need to be. You need to determine how strict the standards need to be.

BACK PAIN

Back pain occurs in 80% of all people. It is a major problem and demands a huge amount of general practitioner time. UK sickness absence is increasing by 25% this year. Why does there seem to be an epidemic of back pain? Probably iatrogenic. An expert group of researchers, gathered by the HSE 2 or 3 weeks ago, came to the consensus opinion in Britain and also North America that the rise of low back pain as a cause of sickness absence, is partly because we all medicalise the problem. In fact, bed rest is the worst thing we can do.

Up to date epidemiology figures suggest that, in a lifetime, 100% of people are going to get back pain. In the last month 25% of people will have had back pain and in the last year 38%. There were 58% of people in a study by Walsh, and Papageorgiou 59%. So divers will also get back pain. Paying attention to the back and being able to assess the back carefully is as important in diving as in any other field.

PATHOLOGY

Obviously, this list of conditions which can apply to the back could apply to any musculo-skeletal problem:-

- Congenital
- Traumatic
- Inflammatory
- Metabolic
- Neoplastic
- Mechanical
- Dysbaric

Facet joint disorders are well recognised as a problem of recurring back pain. Bone spurs can cause impingement of the cord and roots. Pathological studies have shown thickening of the basement membrane of capillaries and thrombosis of blood vessels in the canal. The improved histological studies of cadaveric specimens among low back pain sufferers are showing that the blood supply to the canal and nerves is important. This could be relevant in terms of diving. Fat changes occur around nerves with extra/intra-neural fibrosis and ingrowth of nerves and blood vessels into damaged discs. If you have 10 divers with back pain going to 10 experts, there would be about 80 different diagnoses. The consistency of diagnosing back pain is very poor in clinical medicine. The classical syndromes are at the top of the following list. Prolapsed intervertebral disc, root entrapment syndrome and neurogenic claudication are fairly rare in divers though I saw quite a lot of these conditions in mine workers.

- Prolapsed intervertebral disc
- Root entrapment syndrome
- Neurogenic claudication
- Spondylolisthesis
- Lumbar spondylosis
- Ankylosing spondylitis
- Inflammatory/metabolic/neoplastic/infective

In a US study, of those who get severe back pain, 4 - 10% don't recover. Seventy five per cent will recover in 4 to 6 weeks and most get better within 12 weeks. On autopsy, those who have had chronic low back pain have more double level pathology, more venous dilatation in the spinal canal and more periarticular fibrosis. Those with poor surgical results are possibly due to cotton contaminants from the cotton swabs which are being used in wounds. They also have more calcification.

I think that x-rays really do not have a place. There is a poor correlation with pain, if off work for more than 3 months. In occupational medicine x-rays are not a useful predictor.

Height and weight are relevant. A study looking at a cohort of American GI's showed that those over 182 cm high and those over 82 kg of weight had a 2.6 fold increase in risk of prolapsed and intervertebral disc 20 years later. So height and weight are important in back pain. A more recent study has shown the relative risk of back pain is related to height so the taller you are the higher the risk. Other researchers have suggested that this relationship is not strong enough to be used as a screening test. Weight is important as a predictor of back pain. Risk increases over 82 kg or in the highest fifth quintile.

An old study by Cady confirmed that if you are fit, you have got less risk of back injuries than if you are unfit. I would think that's fairly evident. Chaffin's classic study showed that if your strength greatly exceeds the task requirement, the risk of back injury and of other injury is much less, so strength is very important as a factor in the prevention of back injury.

The individual risk factors include the following:

- age
- height, weight
- fitness, strength
- spinal canal diameter
- past history
- personality
- technique

The best indicator of back pain is a history of previous back pain. Low job satisfaction, somatisation of emotional problems and reduction/pain on straight leg raising: all of these are good predictors of back pain. These are my personal pass/fail criteria proposed for diving. If one needs to be tough at pre-employment, then no history of back pain and a non-smoker. Smokers have a two or threefold increased risk of back pain. Candidates have a normal musculoskeletal system: there's no visible spinal deformity when you look at them and there's a normal range of movement. Straight leg raising is more than 90° in both legs, body mass index is below 25. A dynamic strength test is worthwhile, 50kg seems appropriate because there's a lot of heavy lifting involved. A lot of the issues in relation to back pain are nothing to do with pathology or the precise diagnosis, they are all psychosocial.

The predictors of recovery are:

Individual	-	Physical
	-	Psyche
	-	Lifestyle
	-	History
Social	-	Education
	-	Income
	-	Social support
Occupational	-	Load
	-	Job satisfaction
	-	Work organisation

The pass/fail criteria post spinal surgery are difficult. These are the criteria I would use for high standards of fitness after spinal surgery:

- Troup criteria
- Persisting root pain
- Reduced spinal mobility
- Strength test
- General fitness

Now what are the Troup criteria? Duncan Troup did a very interesting study of those after back injury and looked at the factors which predicted a poor prognosis, a likelihood of recurring back pain.

The prediction of the recurrence of back pain is indicated by:

History	-	Two or more previous attacks
	-	Back pain caused by fall on buttocks or back
	-	Sickness absence over 5 weeks
	-	Residual pain in the leg
Examination	-	Restriction of pain free SLR <45 degrees
	-	Pain or weakness on resisted hip flexion
	-	Inability to sit up from lying flat
	-	Back pain on lumbar extension

These are all quite well validated indicators of a poor prognosis. So I would also suggest that at assessment after a back pain episode the pass/fail criteria would be:

- Recurring back pain
- Troup criteria
- Spinal compression arthralgia

REFERENCES

Apley, A.G. & Solomon, L. (Eds). *Apley's system of orthopaedics and fractures, 7th Edition.* Edinburgh: Butterworth Heinemann. 1993.

Cady, L.D., Bischoff, D.P., O'Connel, E.R. et al. *J. Occup. Med.* 1979; **21**: 269.

Chaffin, D.B. & Anderson, G.B.J. *Occupational Biomechanics.* New York: Wiley & Sons. 1990.

Porter, R.W. *Management of back pain.* Edinburgh: Churchill Livingstone. 1986.

Troup, J.D.G. & Edwards F.C. *Manual handling and lifting.* London: Health & Safety Executive. 1985.

Troup, J.D.G., Martin, J.W. & Lloyd, D.C.E.F. *Spine.* 1981; **6**: 61.

DISCUSSION

Lepawsky: How would you differentiate the back pain of decompression illness from other back pains?

Elliott: This is a diagnostic problem not related to the assessment of fitness to dive. It could be resolved by the history of a dive just before the onset of pain and, if it were the back pain of a decompression illness, would probably be associated with a very rapid onset of paraplegia. It is a totally different issue that needs to be managed as an emergency. Unnecessary recompression of back pain could be wise management.

Bergöö: The contraindications for knee problems seem pretty tough because, if they have joint problems, most divers feel much better when they are in the water.

Macdonald: The stress of heavy manual work that divers have to undergo is likely to be greatest on the surface. In trying to look at this objectively, I developed standards which were similar to mines rescue men who also have to use breathing apparatus and who have to do very strenuous manual work in adverse conditions. For pre-employment the standards are much tougher than those in somebody who has ten years experience and has a good work record. For them the standards become much more pragmatic. I have the view that most people can do far more than doctors think they can, and so I tend to be more pragmatic in the experienced or older worker.

Francis: I was actually going to make the same point, and that is that one is really considering matters above water than below. One has to consider that the diver's equipment is very heavy and has to be carried around. Navy divers operate in small inflatable boats often in foul weather, occasionally at high speed and that back trouble can become a real problem even if at first it seems insignificant.

Bickle: I have always thought the shoulder was the most important joint in diving particularly being able to pull yourself out of the water in a self-rescue situation.

Macdonald: If I had to address the shoulder, I could have taken the whole morning because the musculo-skeletal system is huge and complex.

Blyth[**]: You highlighted the fact that taller and heavier people are more vulnerable to back symptoms. As one with a "tallness gene" I am sure that the explanation is that the designers have made the world too small for us! Work surfaces are too low, tables and chairs too small and cars too cramped. Successive generations get taller and taller so that back problems are bound to increase until such time as ergonomic designers are told to catch up!

Reply from Macdonald: I agree with your observation that with increasing average height, the norms used by designers, based as they are on historical data, will probably become less satisfactory for more individuals. Notwithstanding the above, I believe that there is a relationship between height and weight and back symptoms but that this relationship is weak, and as I said in my presentation I do not think that people can be selected out of employment on the basis of height and weight unless there is going to be an extreme mismatch ergonomically, or there are other risk factors present.

BONE NECROSIS
Professor R.I. McCallum

The knowledge of bone necrosis related to hyperbaric exposure begins before the First World War and was in fact linked with the introduction of diagnostic x-rays. In the diving profession knowledge of bone necrosis surfaced around the 1940's. I would like to go back to a peculiar incident which has not been fully looked into and which happened in 1931. In that year a submarine in the South China Sea, H.M.S. Poseidon, had a collision with a Chinese ship and sank. The collision occurred at 12.12 on the 9th June 1931 and the submarine sank in about 20 fathoms. Six ratings and two Chinese shut themselves in the forward torpedo compartment. The depth guage in the compartment showed just over 100 ft. They then began to flood the compartment to prepare for their escape. This was the first time Davis Submerged Escape Apparatus had been used to save lives. When the hatch was eventually forced open, two men escaped in a rush of air, the hatch slamming shut again. It took a bit longer for the compartment to flood right up and when the water was up to their necks another attempt was made to open the hatch which succeeded the compartment being filled with water. At 14.34 two men appeared on the surface in a burst of air. One man supported the other who was unconscious. Four persons had succeeded in getting out, but two failed to escape although the hatch remained open. All the men who surfaced had decompression sickness. About 12 years later an orthopaedic surgeon in Newcastle published a paper on bone necrosis in three of the men (James, 1945). Thus serious necrosis occurred from a single lifetime exposure to pressure.

Data from the M.R.C. Registry in Newcastle show that a common area for this disease is around the knee joint. It is not true to say, as it does in the HSE Health Note, that the common area is near the shoulder joint, but the important thing is that the lesions round the knee joint do not affect the joint surface itself. In contrast to compressed air workers, a fact about divers is the rarity of lesions in the region of the head of the femur. Most of the lesions will cause no trouble at all and only detectable by x-ray. Illustrations of the lesions, classified in accordance with the M.R.C. diagnostic criteria, are available in McCallum and Harrison (1993). The shoulder is somewhat different. A juxta-articular lesion has the potential for disabling the individual.

So we are looking at something which, most of the time, is not causing disability. There is no reason why somebody with a shaft lesion should not continue to dive.

The Registry work done on compressed air workers led to the classification of radiological lesions which has been of great practical use. However, once one introduces other techniques like scintigraphy or magnetic resonance imaging (MRI) this classification is not applicable. The distinction between juxta-articular lesions and head, neck and shaft lesions are clinically important. How serious is this problem? The following refers to nearly 7,000 divers and at that time there were only 12 who had any form of disability:

	No. of Men (additional suspected lesions in brackets)	
Normal	3355	
Head, neck, shaft lesions	216	(60)
Juxta-articular lesions	77	(37)
Irrelevant changes	3213	
Total	6861	

The factors which are concerned with the onset of bone necrosis are very difficult to disentangle. Estimates of prevalence are dependent upon the choice of population. Men with a lot of diving experience have a high prevalence, but if you dilute the sample with divers having less experience then obviously the figure looks much better. This is why there are conflicting statements about prevalence of this condition.

It is interesting that the earliest description of bone necrosis linked it with decompression sickness. This is intriguing because the Poseidon survivors also suggest that these could be linked. However the data we have indicates that the two conditions are going along in parallel i.e. the same factors which produce the bends are also involved in producing bone necrosis. Bends and bone necrosis are not directly related because a lot of persons who get bone necrosis have not had bends whereas a lot of persons with bends do not get bone necrosis. However there are a few cases which follow the original description of bone necrosis where the onset of pain immediately after an exposure to pressure has continued over some months and in that particular limb the bone necrosis has later appeared. A more recent series of observations by Maurice Cross (1987) has suggested that there is bends pain and there are other "non-bends" pains which together are related to bone damage. This does need going into a little more.

What is the cause of bone necrosis? We have been trying for 30 years to find out but really we don't know. There are many theories raising from fat embolism to oxygen toxicity so we don't know how to prevent it. It is a risk of hyperbaric exposure which therefore has to be accepted.

The questions in the paper which we are asked to address include one about air and mixed-gas diving, "What are the risks of bone necrosis in air and in mixed gas diving? If the lesion does not cause symptoms, what are the criteria for disqualification?" The problem here is that if one is diving with air one is diving relatively shallow whereas with mixed-gas one is going deeper, so here we are really considering the depth factor. I don't know how to answer that question. There is no doubt that one can get bone necrosis from diving on air.

The indications for radiology are less pressing now but it is important to know if the bones are normal in a person who has had an attack of decompression sickness. The pathogenesis of bone necrosis is obscure and the way to prevent it is not entirely clear. It is mostly sub-clinical. There are no symptoms and men can still dive however it would be a mistake to just accept that and do nothing. To produce bone necrosis in an area where it "doesn't matter" is not acceptable.

Finally, the data which I have and which came from the Registry relates to a period between about 1977 and 1984 and therefore to the diving practices of that period. As diving practices have changed there is a likelihood that the picture of necrosis has also changed. Therefore there is still a need to maintain a watch on what is happening to divers, even though as yet it is difficult to prevent.

REFERENCES

Cross, M.R. *Proc. 9th International Symp. Underwater and Hyperbaric Physiology.* Bethesda, MD; UHMS. 1987; Pp 1143-1153.

James, C.C.M. *Lancet*; 1945; **2**: 6-8.

McCallum, R.I. & Harrison, J.A.B. *The Physiology & Medicine of Diving, 4th edition.* London; Saunders. 1993; pp 561-584

DISCUSSION

Calder (Chairman): I agree, but we do not want to crack the problem of bone necrosis too quickly because it is a rich source of higher degrees.

Douglas: Is there any association between bone necrosis and previous trauma to joints? There is the recent case of a 30-year old man with a shoulder dislocation and then 2 years later completed his diver training course with no episodes of decompression sickness. One year later he presented with a crumbling shoulder joint.

McCallum: I don't really know of any similar incident. I would not presume that there is any real connection in that case. One of the problems with the kind of shoulder lesions that I described that they can exist with other shoulder pathology which is totally unrelated. This can be very confusing, particularly medico-legally.

Benton: Do you have any information on the use of MRI for screening?

McCallum: They are being used but there is not the body of knowledge in dysbaric osteonecrosis yet that will enable one evaluate it properly. It may be too sensitive, like scintigraphy which has also been used. The present advantage of conventional radiography is that we know a lot about it. It has the disadvantage of being a late change. In MRI you can find all sorts of changes, but it is not very clear what they mean. Some of these things may disappear; it is a confusing situation.

Elliott:** From your talk is it correct to deduce that you are happy with the recommended intervals for radiography as given in the Guidance Notes e.g. post decompression illness. Personally I find it inappropriate to confine routine radiology to saturation divers when many air divers are making prolonged dives below 30 metres.

Reply from McCallum: Yes, I am happy with the present set of guidelines, particularly as there is at present no Registry nor any similar scheme designed to monitor the overall experience of divers as regards bone damage. However, there should be a policy of central sampling of bone radiographs in order to keep a check on what is happening, particularly if there are changes in diving procedures or types of diving table.

Grönkvist:** Many reports of the frequency of bone necrosis tend to be rather old. Diving tables tend to be more conservative. Is it reasonable to believe that the new tables and more controlled diving will lead to a lower frequency of bone necrosis? When building the Mass Rapid Transit System in Singapore there were more than 180,000 decompressions and not one single case of bone necrosis. The answer is important to decide the frequency of screening.

Reply from McCallum: Bone necrosis is seen more commonly in men who have worked for long shifts (over 4 hours) and at pressures in excess of 25 psig (= 16 metres). The Blackpool decompression tables used in the U.K. have not been found to prevent bone necrosis at higher pressures. In the past there have been a number of problems in assessing the effects of hyperbaric exposures on the bones of compressed air workers. Sometimes only a limited proportion of workers can be radiographed; many of them have been radiographed once only without a further follow-up examination; the time interval between working in compressed air and the discovery of bone changes can be months or even years so that as near complete follow-up as possible over a period of two years or more is necessary before one can say that there has been no bone necrosis. Much of it is symptomless so that unless the follow-up is comprehensive some bone necrosis will be overlooked. At present assessing the effects of changes in decompression procedures takes several years provided the data are available and reliable.

Nome**: What about long bone x-rays prior to start of diving and at subsequent examinations?

Reply from McCallum: Now that much of the natural history of bone necrosis in divers has been mapped out, the relatively innocuous form in which it presents (femoral head lesions are rare for example) and the perceived need to keep to a minimum the amount of ionising radiation to which divers are exposed, there is a much more critical attitude to the frequency at which they are examined radiologically. A reference set of long bone radiographs (skeletal survey) should be carried out at the very start of a diving career. Subsequent radiography should be governed by what happens to the diver, for example if he has decompression illness/sickness, a radiograph should probably be part of his assessment before return to diving.

Nome**: CT and MR examination results do not show the same "final result" of the bone damage as x-rays do, but show the various stages of "repair" taking place in the bone tissue.

Reply from McCallum: I think that this is a reasonable view of the present state of these investigations of bone after hyperbaric exposure. Until the role of CT and MRI in relation to bone changes following hyperbaric exposures is more fully delineated, conventional radiography is the best way to screen for bone changes.

COMMENTARY

The current risk to divers of bone necrosis is probably low but is unknown. There have been potentially significant changes in air and mixed gas diving procedures since the closure of the MRC Decompression Sickness Registry ten years ago which brought the monitoring of necrosis in the populations at risk to an end.

For the prevention of osteonecrosis, there is still a need for epidemiological investigation of the possible causative factors. To achieve this, the central reporting of the x-ray results and the availability of a detailed record of each individual's occupational exposure to pressure remain a high priority.

An X-ray survey of the shoulders, hips and knees, using the MRC procedures, is recommended as a baseline on divers on entry to diving, except only for those entering a category of diving in which the risk of osteonecrosis is negligible. These films must be retained for at least the career lifetime of the diver. Those who dive well within the limits of decompression safety, for example police divers, would appear not to require either a baseline x-ray or periodical surveillance. Those at risk and deserving annual surveillance are those who dive deeper than 30 metres, for longer than 4 hours duration or, even within those thresholds, those who fail to follow accepted safe decompression procedures. The hips and shoulders should also be examined radiologically annually for three years after treatment for decompression illness. X-rays of the knees are required only when shaft lesions are sought for the confirmation of the diagnosis of an otherwise doubtful juxta-articular lesion.

Osteonecrosis of the joints is potentially crippling but at an early stage it will not affect in-water safety. The diagnosis of juxta-articular necrosis should mark the end of a diving career in order to reduce the risk of subsequent joint collapse.

HAEMATOLOGY

The recommendations from the Guidance Notes on "The Medical Examination of Divers" are:

> 50. At the initial medical examination a full blood count, including haemoglobin and haematocrit, sickledex and blood group (unless known), should be performed. Presence of sickle cell trait should be a cause for rejection. Blood group should also be recorded at the **initial medical examination**. Haemoglobin of 12 g.dl^{-1} and haematocrit of 0.4 SI Units are the minimum acceptable levels. Haematology need only be repeated at the Approved Doctor's discretion.

HAEMATOLOGY
Dr. J. Risberg

It is with some pleasure, but with more anxiety, that I present this subject to you. The possibilities of modern medical tests probably excite most of us. Magnificent imaging techniques like CT and MR open a new world of diagnostic and therapeutic possibilities compared with conventional x-ray imaging. Impressive functional testing of pulmonary and cardiac function provide us with tools of still unknown capacity. Within the field of clinical biochemistry, including immunological and endocrinological tests, the menu of tests is ever increasing. We have, however, to be most careful when applying these tests to potential healthy individuals. What are we actually testing for? The Norwegian regulations concerning manned underwater operations in the petroleum activity state that *"he/she, in compliance with regulations issued by the Directorate of Public Health, has been found medically fit for this based on an evaluation of whether the medical condition of the person in question represents a danger to him/herself or to others"*. The document very specifically uses expressions like safety, hazard and danger to differentiate from health effects, the monitoring of medical conditions and so on.

The present Norwegian regulation forces us to be very careful when issuing a certificate of medical fitness/unfitness for an offshore diver. A certificate of medical *un*fitness is a legal document of major economic and social consequences. If the diver raises a law suit, questioning the reason of such a decision, we will have to provide some kind of evidence. We should discuss the subject of blood analysis with this in mind. We may collect a huge amount of biochemistry data from a small blood sample. The question is, of course, do we actually know what conclusions to draw from a positive test result?

Present guidance in the U.K. requires, at the first examination only, a full blood count, haemoglobin, haematocrit, blood typing and sickle cell index. Further haematological investigation is at the discretion of the examining doctor. Norwegian regulations, although rather outdated from 1980, require haemoglobin and sedimentation rate at the annual examination, while haemoglobin-S should be analysed on ethnic indications.

Haemoglobin and sedimentation rate are cheap examinations. Except for anaemia, the specificity of these examinations is poor, and the sensitivity is highly dependent on the extent and development of the disease you are looking for. Without any support from hard facts, I would still recommend these cheap examinations at the annual certification of divers. Haemoglobin >12g/100ml and ESR <20 mm/hr. Anaemia, infections, inflammations and cancer are potentially serious diseases which consequently may be suspected. I see no serious problems with a false positive finding (i.e. a low haemoglobin or high sedimentation rate). A low haemoglobin indicating anaemia should call for a declaration of temporary unfitness for diving, while a high sedimentation rate probably should be followed up without any restrictions if the diver seems otherwise fit. I question the rationale for a full blood count. Bleeding disorders may be detected with the platelet count, but the leucocyte count will hardly provide any useful information as a screening test.

I recommend a reconsideration of blood typing because current practice would not allow a blood transfusion to be based on blood-typing written on some kind of certificate. In case of an emergency blood transfusion, zero-blood would be transfused until laboratory matched blood could be provided. I recommend the practice of blood typing to be abandoned.

The next question is the need for sickle-cell indexing. Let's be very specific when differing the sickle-cell anaemia for sickle-cell trait. Frank sickle cell anaemia is a homozygote Hb-S disorder and is incompatible with diving due to the crises and multiple organ malfunctions in this disease. Sickle cell trait on the other hand is a heterozygote Hb-S disorder, has a prevalence of some 7-8% in the American black population but as high as 40% in some African areas. The sickle-cell trait has a very silent clinical picture, but it has been discussed whether hypoxic regions in the peripheral circulation may induce sickling, increased blood viscosity, vascular stasis and infarction. The proof for such in sickle-cell trait is not convincing. Two recent reports by Gozal *et al* (1992) and Voge *et al* (1991) have reviewed available literature on the field and examined the effects on exercise capacity. The two studies clearly indicate that there is no reason to reject a diver candidate with sickle-cell trait from diving. There is also no scientific reason for putting 40% Hb-S as a cut off level. The U.S. Air Force currently allows pilots with sickle-cell trait without *any* restriction.

Clinically, we should be more concerned with diseases like asthma, ischaemic cardiac disease and potential long term health effects on the lungs, central nervous system and bones, but no good blood tests are available for these. Sudden cardiac death is a major health problem for the age group we are concerned with. It is questionable whether an annual or biannual estimate of cholesterol (Neaton & Wentworth, 1992; Smith *et al*, 1993) would improve diver safety when he is screened already by his personal health statement, an exercise capacity test and an EKG. Nevertheless the cost is small and I would recommend a cholesterol test at first examination and somewhat arbitrarily each fifth year from the age of 40. The frequency of testing should be carefully discussed with qualified internists. A diver candidate with a first examination revealing a hereditary or endogenous hyperlipidaemia should not be accepted, while an acquired hyperlipidaemia should be corrected primarily with diet, or eventually with drugs.

I will remind you that a number of studies have reported changes in liver function (Risberg *et al*, 1992) and even structural hepatic changes associated with diving (Calder & Palmer, 1989). The reports are not systematic and would at this stage probably call for a prospective study, rather than blood testing associated to the annual health examination.

I was specifically asked to mention HIV infection. Personally I would inform a diver with a HIV-carrier state that we do not have the necessary knowledge to tell him how pressure and altered pO_2 will influence further development of the disease. If he is free of symptoms, there is no valid reason to reject him from diving. On the other hand, a diver with manifest AIDS should not be allowed to dive because pulmonary infections and neurological dysfunction are frequently reported as manifestations of the disease, making it incompatible with diving.

I will conclude with recommendations, making no distinction between different classes of divers. For the first examination only, these could be optional items:

> Blood typing: dependent on national practice and equipment for transfusion actually being available *on site,*
> Sickle-cell index: After *informed consent* from the candidate. He should be carefull informed, but not rejected from diving if found to have a sickle-cell trait,
> Cholesterol,

and at annual examination (mandatory):

> Haemoglobin   >12.0 g/100 ml
> Sedimentation rate   <20 mm/hr

REFERENCES *(see page 196)*

DISCUSSION

Rogerson: I want to make a plea to all my fellow examiners that when they undertake the sickle-cell index test and the blood grouping, they enter those results into the log book and then it will not have to be repeated at subsequent examinations. There is no point in doing these investigations unless they are recorded and there is no point in repeating them every year.

McCallum: As far as I know we never found a positive test in all the examinations reported to the Registry.

Mebane: I would like to endorse the business of not disqualifying the diver with a sickle-cell trait. The risk is very slight. A person with sickle-cell disease is too busy trying to stay alive to ever think of becoming a diver, so I really question the validity of the test. If you are not going to disqualify the person with sickle-cell trait, then why do the test? One must also remark about ethnic selection because the last sickle-cell crisis I had to deal with was in a person of Irish-Scots descent.

Risberg: I agree that it should not be mandatory, but it could remain as an option.

Knessl: We don't have sickling in Switzerland but, as we are close to the Mediterranean, what do we do with thalassaemia minor?

Risberg: There may be an individual reason for doing the test, which may be regional or one's own knowledge of the individual. What should be mandatory for all patients? I don't think it is fair to do chromatography on everyone.

Broome: This is a contentious area but would you take this further and do cholesterol testing on persons with known risk factors? Would you then have pass/fail criteria? It really has nothing to do with the diving. Do we actually need it in the medical?

Risberg: You ask what should be the pass/fail criteria for cholesterol. No, once more we have to think of the diving consequences of the disorder we are looking for. A high cholesterol would not incapacitate in any situation. It is diseases that it causes that might do so. It should only be part of some cardiovascular investigation.

Broome: At the initial medical if the person had a very high cholesterol what would you do?

Risberg: If he had a measurement of 9 or 10, I would send him to a specialist for an objective opinion on what would happen in the next 5 - 10 years. But I would probably let him dive.

Griffin: The concept of a hard and fast limit for haemoglobin strikes me, as a woman, as wrong. There should be a recognition of the fact that there is a different range for healthy asymptomatic women from that for men. There is no basis for saying a woman cannot dive because she does not have a haemoglobin in the masculine range.

Risberg: In women the range is from 10.5 g/100 ml and I accept that.

Botheroyd: I expect that the HSE will no longer expect blood grouping to be done for divers. Many haematological departments won't do it except for donors. The second point is the recording of tests in the diver's logbook. It might be OK to record that the tests had been done but not to put results of any kind into the logbook. This might lead to potential discrimination against individual divers.

O'Sullivan: Could the Chairman please give a decision on the way forward on sickle-cell testing in the UK? To test or not to test. It does not seem ethically right to do the test and for the diver to bear the expense of it, if it produces no useful information.

Calder (Chairman): It seems that there is not a problem. Sickle-cell trait has no relevance to diving exposure and so there is no reason to test routinely.

Suprani: I think that it was a good choice to put the haematology session next to the session of bone necrosis in view of the fact that there are haematological disorders which produce bone necrosis and should be a contraindication to diving. So the haemotology test should look for sub-clinical illnesses in relation to the potential for bone necrosis.

McCallum: I agree that there are other conditions that produce bone necrosis and that there may be a big vascular element in the cause, but there is no need for further blood tests.

Bergöö: I would like to go back to HIV testing. Should we put in a provision for this? It is important to know probability for the future development of AIDS and it is also important for the hygiene of those in a saturation chamber.

Calder: This is a problem which is dependent very much upon national attitudes and national legislation. For example, HIV testing in that way would be contrary to the law in this country.

Risberg: The political problem with enforcing a test on a possibly healthy diver is that there is also the problem of latency and the fact that there is no security after the test has been done. It is more important that everybody has the proper hygiene at all times. This is important for Hepatitis B and possibly for Hepatitis C of even greater importance.

Sibley-Calder****:** Why are we considering doing cholesterol tests with a consideration to ban high risk divers when we do not ban heavy smokers? Who must be at greater risk?

Freshwater****:** On the question of cholesterol testing, we should recall that this is only one predictor of cardiovascular disease, and not the most important. Meta-analysis of large trials of cholesterol reduction shows an excess of all-cause mortality in the "treated" groups, much of which is probably precipitated by behavioural changes related to altered lipid biochemistry. Do we want to encourage risk-taking and aggression in divers? Probably not. Thus the question "do we need to know the cholesterol level?" is answered that we positively need to remain in ignorance of it, for fear of increasing mortality iatrogenically.

Nome****:** Testing of cholesterol is irrelevant. Testing of haemoglobin and sedimentation rate are probably also irrelevant if asymptomatic. Liver function testing irrelevant if asymptomatic or, for example, no indications exist of alcohol abuse.

Reply from Risberg: Doctors Sibley-Calder, Freshwater and Nome commented or disagreed on my position in the question of cholesterol testing. Let me first explain my position more precisely.

I believe we should test for cholesterol at the time of entry into diving. Familial hyperlipidaemia may be detected at this stage and the disease is associated with an increased mortality in the young population In general I would not allow a person with familial hypercholesteroleamia to dive unless a consultant considers the specific applicant to have an expected risk of coronary heart disease approximately the same as the reference population.

I would recommend cholesterol testing, somewhat arbitrarily, each 5th year from the age of 40 or 45 to detect an acquired hypercholesterolemia. If an acquired hyperlipidemia is detected I would allow him to dive, but with advice on changes in diet, stopping smoking, increase physical activity etc. I am fully aware that the hypercholesteroleamia is not by itself a problem for diving, it is the contributing factor for CHD which concerns me. We should acknowledge the risk for cardiac death in this age group (men >40-45 years) and appreciate the safety hazard for the diver and his diving companions. High cholesterol is strongly associated with increased cardiac death (Neaton & Wentworth, 1992). I am aware of the study by Smith et al (1993) describing the overall *increased* mortality in groups treated with cholesterol lowering drugs as evaluated by meta-analysis. This conclusion is valid, however, only for the group with initially low risk. Currently I would interpret this study to advise patients with hypercholesterolemia on diet and other clinical advice, and restrict drug treatment to patients with "refractory" high-level hypercholesteroleamia. I believe this is common medical practice in Norway as well. I am not willing to accept this study as an evidence for not screening a *selected* part of the population in which medical fitness is an imperative for the diver himself and his crew for *safety* reasons. I am, however, not confident in advising the exact time and intervals of the tests and am open for any suggestion on this point.

The point on smoking is valid, smoking definitely increases risk of CHD, raises the risk of overall and cardiac death and impairs pulmonary function. I believe that the answer for not rejecting this group is that smoking is a socially accepted abuse, smoking habits are difficult to verify (in contrast with a pulmonary function test or a blood test) and the fact that smoking habits may change from year to year makes a risk assessment even more difficult. In theory, however, we should probably carefully evaluate whether a *heavily* smoking diving candidate, not intending to change his habits, in fact is fit to dive! Such a decision is currently not acceptable, and we will have to wait for the functional impairment of his abuse to appear, to evaluate the consequences for his fitness to dive.

Whether a testing for haemoglobin and sedimentation rate is irrelevant will probably depend on which diseases you are screening for. I have no statistics demonstrating the "overall efficacy" of these tests when screening divers. A low haemoglobin demonstrating anaemia and/or a high ESR would indicate the possibility of inflammatory disease, infection, cancer etc. Although the specificity of the two tests are low, the sensitivity for a number of chronic diseases is good (although usually low at the very early stage of the disease). The cost of the tests are so low that I still believe that the yield of the test is acceptable. Although theoretically the clinical evaluation should be carefully performed for all organ systems, we should acknowledge the fact that a pathological result from a blood sample may increase the sensitivity of your examination somewhat.

Liver function tests were recommended for two reasons. First, there are a number of reports describing liver-function alteration in divers (for a review, see Risberg *et al*, 1992). Secondly, a changed liver function would indicate a *functional* consequent of alcohol abuse, possibly even at a stage when the diver is unwilling to reveal his abuse. To give a valid reply, the *consequences* of doing systematic liver-function surveillance in this work group should be scientifically examined. I do not believe that this is practically possible. Once more, one has to evaluate the price of the examination in relation to the yield of the test and the consequences of a positive finding, when and if it appears. For divers, liver function tests may serve as a test for long-term health effects on the liver (Calder & Palmer, 1989) and to detect alcohol abuse which infers a safety risk for the diver and his crew.

REFERENCES

Calder, I.M. & Palmer, A.C. Histological changes in liver of man and animals subjected to compression and decompression. *Undersea Biomed. Res.* 1989; **16** (Suppl): 88.

Gozal, D., Thiriet, P. Mbala, E., Wouassi, D., Gelas, H., Geyssant, A. & Lacour, J.R. Effect of different modalities of exercise and recovery on exercise performance in subjects with sickle cell trait. *Med. Sci. Sports Exerc.* 1992; **24**: 1325-1331.

Neaton, J.D. & Wentworth, D. Serum cholesterol, blood pressure, cigarette smoking, and death from coronary heart disease. Overall findings and differences by age for 316,099 white men. Multiple Risk Factor Intervention Trial Research Group. *Arch. Intern. Med.* 1992; **152**: 56-64.

Risberg, J., Ulvik, R., Hjelle, J. & Farstad, M. *Sammenligning av tidligere gjennomførte blodanalyser* [Comparison of previous blood tests]. NUTEC Report 31-92. Bergen, NUTEC. 1992.

Smith, G.D., Song, F. & Sheldon, T.A. Cholesterol lowering and mortality: the importance of considering initial level of risk. *BMJ.* 1993; **306**: 1367-1373.

Voge, V.M., Rosado, N.R. & Contiguglia, J.J. Sickle cell anaemia trait in the military aircrew population: A report from the military aviation safety subcommittee of the Aviation Safety Committee, AsMA. *Aviat. Space Environ. Med.* 1991; **62**: 1099-1102.

GASTRO-INTESTINAL, GENITO-URINARY SYSTEMS AND DERMATOLOGY

Chairman : Dr. I.M. Calder

Recommendations about gastro-intestinal and genito-urinary systems from the Guidance Notes on "The Medical Examination of Divers" are:

GASTRO-INTESTINAL

30. Candidates should have a high degree of dental fitness.

31. Any Approved Doctor suspecting dental unfitness may required production of evidence of a professional dental assessment before certifying fitness to dive.

32. Dentures should be removed while diving, but partial dentures can be worn if secured by clasps or attachments to the remaining teeth.

35. (a) Chronic inflammatory intestinal disease would be cause for rejection.

    (b) The presence of an intestinal stoma will be cause for failure except in the case of shallow inshore diving using a dry suit.

    (c) Acute distal colitis or proctitis should be referred for assessment and a decision deferred pending the outcome of investigation and treatment.

    (d) Recurring episodes of abdominal pain should be investigated and the possibility of confusion of diagnosis in diving illness should be borne in mind.

    (e) Dyspepsia will require investigation and the association of reflux oesophagitis with a predisposition of duodenal ulceration should be borne in mind.

    (f) Malabsorptive conditions, because of the likely anaemia or dietary modification required, may render diving impracticable.

    (g) Symptomatic haemorrhoids should lead to referral for surgical treatment and would debar from diving until successfully treated.

    (h) Abdominal wall herniation should be a cause for rejection until repaired.

    (i) Evidence of acute or chronic hepatic disease would render a diver unfit. The presence of gallstones or a history of pancreatitis would also be a bar to diving.

    (j) Symptomatic hiatus hernia and active peptic ulceration (including cases where the condition is under treatment) will debar from diving. The patient should be symptom-free and without treatment for at least one year. A history of peptic ulceration leading to bleeding, perforation or requiring emergency surgical treatment may also debar at the discretion of the Approved Doctor.

GENITO-URINARY

36. *A history of renal disease or of urinary tract investigation will be reason for more detailed questioning and examination. Dipstick urinalysis for glucose, protein and blood should be undertaken routinely. Venereal disease will debar until adequately treated. The presence of kidney stones and other genito-urinary diseases are usually a cause for rejection. (Cases of renal colic may not necessarily be so, but should be judged on an individual basis after specialist investigation).*

DENTAL, GASTRO-INTESTINAL & GENITO-URINARY FITNESS
N.K.I. McIver

DENTAL

There is not very much to say about dental fitness in divers, provided the diver attends his own dentist for regular check-ups. Evidence of a dental certificate of fitness may be required but there have been no Appeal cases relating to dental problems in the U.K.

In a study of 2162 medical evacuations from offshore for all categories of workers, including divers, there were 239 for diseases of the digestive system of which 115 were reported as being for dental problems (Norman et al, 1988).

If a dentist is warned that a patient is a diver he can pay particular attention when performing dental fillings to ensure that the pulp is silent, there is no suggestion of inflammation or the possibility of leakage under a filling. Cases have occurred where gas containing pockets behind a filling have either imploded or exploded (Calder & Ramsey, 1983). Routine 6-monthly dental checks are advised.

No unattached dentures should be worn when diving and at least one diver, who failed to remove them prior to the dive, died by inhaling them (Calder, personal communication).

GASTRO-INTESTINAL SYSTEM

Indigestion

About 30% of the European population is prone to what is termed "indigestion". Four per cent of general practitioner consultations in the U.K. are for the syndrome of "dyspepsia" (Jones & Lydeard, 1989). The broad definition of dyspepsia includes a range of symptoms of upper gastrointestinal disease amongst which may be the following:

- Upper abdominal or retrosternal pain or discomfort, including bloating, distension, early satiety
- Heartburn and regurgitation
- Nausea or vomiting

The main problem is to differentiate between organic dyspepsia with specific lesions (such as peptic ulceration, reflux oesophagitis, cholelithiasis or gastric carcinoma) and non-ulcer or functional dyspepsia. This has been defined as upper abdominal or retrosternal pain, discomfort, heartburn, nausea, vomiting or other symptoms considered to be referrable to the proximal alimentary tract, and lasting for more than 4 weeks, unrelated to exercise and for which no focal lesion or systemic disease can be found responsible (Jones et al, 1988). The same European Working Party reconvened in 1990. They classified functional dyspepsia into the following:

- Gastro-oesophageal reflux-like dyspepsia
- Dysmotility-like dyspepsia
- Aerophagy
- Ulcer-like dyspepsia
- Idiopathic dyspepsia

The first 2 groups account for the majority of patients.

Reflux-like dyspepsia includes retrosternal discomfort especially on stooping after large meals and on laying flat, temporarily relieved by antacids, of cyclical severity and associated with recent weight gain. The dysmotility-like dyspepsia is characterised by abdominal distension, hunger with early satiety, epigastric heaviness or fullness, variable and multiple food intolerances. Pain is diffuse, nausea is prominent and there may be associated features of the irritable bowel syndrome. It tends to be continuous rather than episodic.

The dysmotility-like dyspepsia has a clear overlap with the irritable bowel syndrome whose key symptoms are abdominal distension, more frequent stools with onset of pain, the pain being eased after bowel movements, a sense of incomplete evacuation and looser stools at the onset of pain (Manning et al, 1978).

Acid reflux and dyspepsia are therefore common in the age group of the commercial diver. A diagnosis of functional dyspepsia is more likely with the following if:

- the patient is generally well
- the weight is steady or rising
- the patient tends to be a worrier
- the patient is less than 45 years old

The management of functional dyspepsia includes non-pharmacological measures of explanation, reassurance and lifestyle modification (e.g. cessation of smoking). Physical measures such as weight reduction, posture and food in relation to sleep may also help. Thereafter drug therapy may be commenced. This would entail a 4-8 week trial period with either a gastric motility agent such as Cisapride, an H^2 antagonist, or a Proton pump inhibitor.

Dyspepsia symptoms probably require investigation in the following circumstances:

- in a first episode
- age >45 years
- dysphagia, vomiting or weightloss
- anaemia
- relapse of a previous gastric ulcer

Investigations may include upper GI endoscopy, barium meal, ultrasound, or intra-oesophageal pH monitoring.

Principal causes of organic dyspepsia most of which would require stopping diving until resolved include:

- reflux oesophagitis
- peptic ulceration
- gastric carcinoma
- cholelithiasis

The differential diagnosis of abdominal pain may cause problems during or just after a dive. A recent case encountered in the Southern Sector of the North Sea involved persistent malaise and vomiting coming on 12 hours following a dive and which did not respond to a therapeutic oxygen recompression table. Medical review confirmed acute gastritis which subsequently resolved.

There was also a case of abdominal pain following a dive for which the differential diagnosis could be acute decompression illness. The initial diagnosis had been that of dyspepsia but the diver became a paraplegic.

Other Conditions

Among those divers who were failed and who have come to Appeal, lessons may be learned from the following:

> A 27 year-old commercial diver was diagnosed as having ulcerative colitis and underwent total proctocolectomy with ileo-anal anastomosis. This was converted to a continence ileostomy and 2 years later he presented for his entry medical to commercial diving. He was failed, subsequently appealed and was passed as fit with restriction to air diving range and avoiding saturation.
>
> A diver presented following a dive with abdominal pain and was flown ashore for a surgical opinion. This action was taken once it was discovered the pain had commenced before the dive. He was subsequently found to have a pathological gall-bladder which was removed and he successfully returned to diving. There is no doubt that he would have been treated as a precautionary measure had he been unfortunate enough for the pain to start during or after the dive. It is clearly not possible to screen the diving population for gallstones and a number must have asymptomatic stones. However, once they become symptomatic then definitive treatment should be offered before returning to diving.
>
> A 58 year-old commercial diver (inshore) was found at routine diving medical to have ectopic beats. He was investigated (ECG with treadmill) with negative findings. He did have a hiatus hernia with oesophageal narrowing. He was treated with H^2 antagonists. He had in addition a reduced FEV^1/FVC ratio (below 70%) and he was failed. At his subsequent appeal endoscopy was performed confirming symptomatic oesophagitis and his appeal was turned down.

The contraindications to acceptance for diver training include abdominal hernia until corrected surgically, inflammatory bowel disease with complications such as Crohn's disease, gall-bladder pathology, pancreatitis, haemorrhoids where haemorrhage is a problem, and any form of organic dyspepsia until treated and resolved.

Hepatic Disease

Virus infection (Hepatitis A, B and C) would debar a diver in the acute phase. Once he or she is over the initial illness and has converted from antigen positive to negative for A & B (there is as yet no reliable antigen test for Hepatitis C), is shown to be antibody positive and therefore no longer infectious, then they may return to diving. In the close confines of a saturation diving complex (and at any worksite) bodily secretions, pathology specimens of blood, urine and any open wounds should be treated as if infectious. All divers should be reminded about the need for immaculate personal and environmental hygiene. It is thought unlikely that the AIDS virus would easily be transmitted under normal working conditions (and less likely to do so than the Hepatitis B virus for example) and it is not thought advantageous to screen for HIV. If a diver were suffering from an acute AIDS-related infection then he would by definition be debarred from diving.

GENITO-URINARY SYSTEM

Active genito-urinary infections including herpes will debar until adequately treated and symptom-free. A patient with recurrent herpes infection might be advised against saturation diving. A history of renal disease or of urinary tract investigation will be reason for more detailed questioning and examination. Positive findings on dipstix urinalysis require further investigation. The presence of renal stones and other genito-urinary diseases are usually a cause for rejection. However renal stones may be asymptomatic and some divers have returned to restricted surface orientated diving without problem. A commercial diver in a saturation dive recently was treated for renal colic, was subsequently successfully decompressed and referred for further investigation. A case of renal colic occurring during a saturation dive or just after a dive does cause a diagnostic dilemma. It is suggested that amendments to the fitness guideline in this section are not required at present.

REFERENCES

Calder, I.M. & Ramsey, J.D. *J. of Dentistry* 1983; **11(4):** 318 - 323.

Jones, C.D. et al. Working Party. *Lancet* 1988; **i:** 576 - 9.

Jones, R. & Lydeard, S. *Br. Med. J.* 1989; **298:** 30 - 2.

Manning, A.P. et al. *Br. Med. J.* 1978; **ii:** 653 - 6.

Norman, J.N. et al. *Br. J. Indus. Med.* 1988; **45:** 619 - 623.

DISCUSSION

Calder (Chairman): In the absence of diving data it is interesting to note NATO statistics which suggest that in a recent exercise 60% of the casualties were dental casualties. Perhaps we could now conclude the question of dental fitness:

McIver: There is no real problem with dental fitness providing every diver attends a dentist for a check-up once or twice a year.

Calder: It seems that we are all agreed on that. Now let's turn to the gastro-intestinal fitness and in particular, hernias?

McIver: In the paper by Norman *et al* (1988), the principal causes for evacuation from offshore were haemorrhoids and anal fissure. After that was peptic ulcer (22 cases) and strangulated hernia (10). However I have myself not seen a strangulated hernia in a young person offshore.

Irtun: Hernias should not be allowed to dive. There could be an encapsulation in any hernia. They should not be in saturation and they should not go offshore.

McIver: Do you agree with the criteria for dyspepsia?

Irtun: With dyspepsia but not oesophagitis. It is very difficult to differentiate it from cardiac pain. An individual with pure oesophagitis after endoscopy could go diving.

McIver: Even if he was on continuous cimetidine as a 40 year-old?

Calder: Is there any point in doing occult bloods annually?

McIver and Irtun: *(Indicated that this was not required)*.

Freshwater: I have seen a sports diver with an ileostomy that was continent and well controlled with a bag under a dry suit and a professional diver with a colostomy that was also OK but I restricted him to short duration diving. He had no difficulties.

Ramaswami: Patients who are on antacids or H_2 antagonists may be more prone to gastro-intestinal infections if diving in contaminated water.

Longobardi: Why is a person with Hepatitis type C unfit to dive?

Calder: C is in the same unpleasant category as B.

Lockett****:** The MA1 states presence of gallstones as a reason for rejection. As gallstones are so common and asymptomatic in a high proportion of the normal population, is there any reason to disqualify a diver who is found to have gallstones incidently, if they are causing no problem?

Reply from McIver: If the gallstones are entirely asymptomatic and have been discovered incidentally, then there is probably no reason for disqualification. One might however, ask how these could have been discovered unless his alimentary tract was already being investigated for relevant symptoms.

Broome**: Please address the issue of whether all cases of chronic Hepatitis (B, C, D, E, F, etc.) are disqualified from all professional diving - even if asymptomatic.

Reply from McIver: During an acute hepatic illness the diver would be considered unfit. For Hepatitis B there would have to be evidence of conversions from antigen positive to antigen negative, and to antibody positive before resuming diving. For Hepatitis C & D (Delta antigen, a sub-unit of Hepatitis B with serious clinical manifestations) there are as yet no reliable antigen tests. However it is important to treat all body fluids as potentially infectious. Hepatitis E is endemic in certain parts of Asia, is water-borne and clinically similar to Hepatitis A.

DERMATOLOGY

The recommendations from the Guidance Notes on "The Medical Examination of Divers" are:

23. *The skin is very vulnerable to the repeated and, at times, constant wetness experienced by divers and, particularly, to the high humidity and reduced temperature tolerance experienced in the closed environment of saturation chambers. The main conditions which place fitness in doubt are:*

    (a) *any acute cutaneous infection which must be treated and controlled before diving is allowed;*
    (b) *chronic skin infections, whether fungal, monilial, bacterial, parasitic, or viral (a few warts are an exception);*
    (c) *chronic skin diseases, if severe, such as psoriasis or acne;*
    (d) *most cases of eczema (dermatitis) though mild cases of seborrhoeic eczema may be acceptable;*
    (e) *papulo-squamous eruptions, such as pityriasis and chronic lichen planus if extensive;*
    (f) *the active phase of herpes simplex, or herpes zoster;*
    (g) *any malignant condition of the skin which must be adequately treated;*
    (h) *urticaria which should have resolved before diving is allowed.*

DERMATOLOGY
Dr. R. Aldridge

In reviewing the questions which have been posed I came to an early conclusion that there would be no absolute contraindication to diving for dermatological reasons simply because those who have severe skin disease would be unlikely to consider diving as an occupation. To examine the matter further one must consider the matter in a logical fashion. Firstly, one must consider the occupational risk that diving poses to pre-existing dermatoses and secondly, the nature of the dermatoses that a diver can contract. Central to both of these is the susceptibility of the skin to the increased humidity and to the associated hazards of infection that accompany diving. Conversely one has to exclude the presence of contagious skin disease which might be passed to others. Thermoregulation (Table 23) is another central consideration in diving and one must consider skin conditions which impair thermoregulation.

Table 23 - THERMOREGULATION IN DEEP DIVING

- The high heat capacity of Helium increases respiratory and convective heat loss.

- Narrow thermal comfort zone 32 - 34° C: danger of hypo- or hyperthermia

- At depth there is increased heat production from moderate exercise.

- Normal thermoregulation requires control of cutaneous blood flow and sweating.

A consideration of the structure of skin is important to an understanding of the interaction of skin and water. The epidermis is a remarkably complex structure. The layer which protects the body from the external environment is the stratum corneum. Just below this complex dead layer is the stratum granulosum which is pivotal to its production. The cells of the stratum granulosum contain complex enzymes which produce from the lipids of the cell itself the intracellular cement which glues the dead keratinocytes together within the stratum corneum and produces a surface layer with a buffering capacity at around a pH of 5.7. Within the complex intracellular cement there is a moisture retaining factor which enables the stratum corneum to retain its moisture content at around 2%. This moisture content is central to the extensibility of the skin. If the skin is placed in water it is believed that this moisture retaining factor is responsible for the absorption into the stratum corneum of more water with the eventual effect that has on its structural integrity and eventually the surface pH.

The epidermis is not a sterile environment and Table 24 lists the resident skin bacteria.

TABLE 24 - RESIDENT SKIN BACTERIA

Coagulase negative micrococaceae
Coryneform
24% population carry S. aureus in the nose
Intertriginous areas (e.g. toe webs) also contain:

   gram-negative bacilli
   pseudomonas
   klebsiella
   proteus
   acinetobacter
   coliform-like organisms

The micrococaceae cause no problems nor in general do the coryneform or gram-positive rods. Twenty-four per cent of the population carry staph aureus in the nose but the axillae, groin and toe webs because of the wetness and occlusion harbour a varied population of microscopic life. The factors which control the skin bacterial flora are humidity, skin surface lipids, desquamation, pH, microbial antagonisms, bacterial adherence, toxic products and secretory antibodies. It is the first 4 of these that can be altered in the diving environment. Thus when the skin is wet organisms from the intertriginous spaces spread in these favourable environmental conditions out with their usual confines.

In considering the implications of diving on existing disease I have divided diseases into those in which the integument is compromised (Table 25) and those in which there is some disorder of thermoregulation. Some diseases such as eczema can fall within either category.

**TABLE 25 - SOME COMMON DISEASES
IN WHICH THE INTEGUMENT IS COMPROMISED**

   Dermatitis/Eczema
   Psoriasis
   Pityriasis Rosea
   Lichen Planus
   Acne
   Malignancies

In Table 26 the prevalence of eczema in a mixed industrial and administrative population is listed. Prevalence figures can range from 2% to 15% depending upon the geographical situation and the predominance of industry. About 50% of all eczema is contact dermatitis and 80% of all contact dermatitis is found on the hands (Table 27). Obviously any whole body involvement with eczema is a contra-indication to diving. The problems arise when one is assessing localised eczema and the most difficult local area to assess is the commonest, namely the hands.

TABLE 26
**PREVALENCE OF ECZEMA IN A MIXED INDUSTRIAL
AND ADMINISTRATIVE POPULATION**

Eczema	9%
Contact dermatitis	1.5 - 5.4%
Hand eczema	1.2 - 6.2%

TABLE 27 - PATTERNS OF HAND ECZEMA

Patchy - commonest
Ring
Pulpitis - 10%
Discoid - often atopics
Palmar hyperkeratosis - commoner in male
Pompholyx - 20%

Unfortunately, the patchy pattern is the commonest and each case requires individual assessment. The ring, pulpitis, discoid and palmar hyperkeratotic forms of eczema are usually irritant patterns and not, in my view, contraindications. Whereas an active pompholyx is a contraindication, it is usually intermittent and some account must be taken of the frequency of re-occurrence. Eczema of the ears is another localised area which can be troublesome. It can arise from seborrhoeic eczema, from atopic eczema or contact dermatitis. Clinically it appears very similar to otitis externa and can spread around the ears in an eczematoid fashion. It would clearly be very troublesome to a diver and, if severe, would be a contraindication to diving. Psoriasis is another common condition affecting approximately 2% of the population. Ninety per cent of those affected will have stable plaque-like psoriasis confined to the elbows, sacral areas and knees. This is not a contraindication to diving. Numular psoriasis, if extensive, is a possible contraindication because it is unlikely to clear spontaneously and the same is true of those with widespread plaque psoriasis. On the other hand the so-called guttate psoriasis often clears within 2-3 months and a person may never have another attack, so once it is cleared a history of the condition is not a contraindication.

Pityriasis rosea is often a difficult diagnosis with many differing manifestations. It is an erythematous scaling eruption with rapid onset affecting young adults and is commoner in the spring and autumn. Initially it can often appear urticarial like but if one looks carefully one will see at the edge of a developed plaque, a pityraisiform scale which is diagnostic. One's decision will depend upon the degree of involvement. The more widespread and more active the disease the more rapidly in my view, is the regression, thus sometimes a disease which appears the worst can be gone within the month.

Lichen planus is an intensely itchy condition and in my view sufferers will be unlikely to have any desire to dive. Associated with lichen planus is a loss of sweating which if the disease is extensive could be significant and a contraindication to diving while the disease is active.

Some 10% of acne sufferers will carry gram negative rods in their follicles. These are impossible to distinguish clinically and in general, one would raise no objection to mild cases of acne diving, but anybody with an active cystic component should not dive until they have received dermatological attention.

Effective thermo-regulation is obviously of great importance in diving (Table 23). In considering disorders which can affect thermo-regulation I have divided them up into those in which there is haemodynamic based disturbances (Table 28) and those in which there are disturbances of the sweat apparatus (Table 29).

TABLE 28
DISEASES OF IMPAIRED THERMOREGULATION
BY REASON OF HAEMODYNAMIC DISTURBANCES

Severe Eczema/Psoriasis
Urticaria
Mastocytosis

Eczema has already been considered. Mastocytosis is a contraindication. In the majority of cases, urticaria is a transient condition, but even in those who are troubled regularly providing the condition only affects the skin and never the mucous membranes, it would not appear to be a contraindication. The classic well demarcated red raised plaque of urticaria should cause no difficulties in diagnosis. The more superficial forms of the disease will have a more patchy appearance with central white wheals and a red edge which is often confused with erythema multiform. Occasionally one can see a whiteness at the edge due to blood shunting, the so-called Woronoffs ring. In urticaria the polycyclic nature of the edge and the manner which adjacent lesions merge should enable the condition to be distinguished easily from erythema multiform. Cholinergic urticaria gives rise to small follicular hives which are intensely itchy. Sufferers often require sedative antihistamines which are themselves a contraindication to diving. However, the condition is also associated with odd pulmonary vascular abnormalities so perhaps these should be the determining feature. Pressure urticaria is usually of later onset and more prolonged than the urticarias previously considered and can be extremely disabling if it involves the palms and soles. The disease is always localised and does not itself constitute a contraindication to diving, but obviously involvement of the hands and feet impairing the person's ability to work will comprise a contraindication to diving. Aquagenic urticaria is a real rarity. Small pin-like cholinergic-like urticarial wheals surrounded by redness, this is a reaction to water and must be considered incompatible with diving as an occupation.

TABLE 29 - IMPAIRED SWEATING

Sweat gland dysfunction

Occlusive:
milliaria, rubra, crystalline, profunda eczema, psoriasis, lichen planus

Destruction:
scleroderma, Fabry's

Absence:
congenital ectodermal dysplasia, ichthyosis

Neurological

Hypothalamic disorders
Autonomic neuropathy:-
diabetes, alcoholism, leprosy

Dehydration

Extensive disease within the occlusive sub-category are a contraindication to diving. Scleroderma is an obvious and usually self-limiting contra-indication within this destructive category. In conditions which there is an absence of sweat glands dysfunction, congenital ectodermal dysplasia is extremely small print but an obvious contraindication. Ichthyosis or disorders of cornification are classified into 24 sub-groups. The commonest is the autosomal vulgaris type with a fine white scale which tends to spare the flexors leaving sweating unimpaired in that area. If this form of ichthyosis is not associated, as it often is with eczema, then it is not *per se* of contraindication. The forms of ichthyosis which involve the entire integument may be considered a contraindication to diving.

TABLE 30 - THE SPECTRUM OF BACTERIAL SKIN INFECTION

-	Epidermal:	impetigo
		ecthyma
		infected dermatitis
		pitted keratolysis
-	Dermal:	cellulitis/erysipelas
-	Sub-dermal fasciitis:	necrotising faciitis
-	Follicular:	folliculitis
		furuncles + carbuncles
-	Abscesses unrelated to follicles:	paronychia
		sinus
-	Intertrigninous:	erythrasma
		trichomycosis axillaris

Bacterial skin infections (Table 30) are contraindications and need to be treated before diving can be resumed. In Table 31 I have divided viral infections which may be seen in divers into those in which there is direct skin invasion and those in which were is a secondary rash. The secondary rashes are rarely going to be so extensive as to constitute a contraindication to diving and the consideration will really depend upon the nature of the primary viral infection and the illness that generates. Of the viruses which cause direct skin invasion the assessment problems relate to herpes simplex and warts as herpes zoster is an obvious contraindication to diving. I do not believe that recurrent herpes simplex is a contraindication as it constitutes very little risk to others and no risk to the diver. Orf clearly comprises a contraindication, molluscum contagiosum is unlikely to affect the divers but it is a highly infectious agent and should be treated before the candidate is considered fit to dive. Hand warts would not be a contraindication to diving. Verrucas probably should be but because they are so common it would be inequitable and unjust to prevent a man diving because he has contracted them. I think the diver should be warned of the danger of passing his infection to others and treatment should be initiated. In a diving context I prefer a virocidal hardening agent such as glutaldehyde which limits viral dispersal to the lactic acid/salicylic acid based peeling agents which do give rise to more viral shedding.

TABLE 31 - VIRAL

Direct Skin Invasion (DNA)
Herpes group - simplex - zoster
Papillomavirus group - warts
Pox Viral group - Vaccinia, Molluscum contagiosum
Paravaccinia - Orf

Secondary rash
Mainly RNA groups including Retrovirus

The common dermal fungal infections (Table 32) require consideration. Tinea pedis is perhaps the most important of these because it is the most contagious and least easily treated.

TABLE 32 - FUNGI

Tinea: capitis, corporis, cruris, pedis
Tinea versicolour
Tinea barbae (Cl Sycosis barbae)
Candidiasis

Fungal, bacterial and moulds which may be found in the infected foot (Table 33). If only to prevent the spread of infection to others, tinea rubrum with a moccasin pattern should be cured before the diver returns to diving. The vesicular form of tinea pedis with polycyclic scaling usually spreading from the third toe web is highly contagious and must be settled to prevent spread of the infection to others. "Athletes foot" the common affliction of the third web space is not always fungal. In 75% of cases the infection is primarily bacterial. If fissuring is present it should be treated before the individual returns to diving otherwise the bacteria within the fissure can spread rapidly to other parts of the moist skin.

TABLE 33 - THE INFECTED FOOT

Tinea
Toe Web infection (T. Mentagrophytes)
Chronic scaling of Plantar Surface (T. Rubrum)
Acute Vesicular Tinea Pedis (T. Mentagrophytes)

Bacteria
Pitted Keratolysis (Dermatophilus Congolensis)
Toe Web Pseudomonas

Moulds/Yeasts
Onychomycoses (Scopulariopis Brevicaulis)
Interdigital spaces (Candida albicans)

In the final part of this presentation occupationally acquired skin disease will be considered (Table 34).

TABLE 34 - OCCUPATIONALLY ACQUIRED SKIN DISEASE

Allergic contact dermatitis
Divers' hands
Hypersensitivity reactions

The hypersensitivity reactions include "dogger bank itch" and "swimmer's itch".

Allergic contact dermatitis - the accelerators which are used to vulcanise rubbers are a troublesome contact allergen. Fortunately, they are not used extensively in the manufacture of neoprene which is the isomer of chlorprene commonly found in diving situations and consequently it is moderately safe. However, neoprene does contain antioxidants and the nylon backing is often attached with a glue which can contain allergens so if an individual is apparently reacting to neoprene or other rubberised compound they should be referred to a dermatologist. There are many potential allergens which have to be identified by patch testing before specific advice can be given on alternative products which do not contain the established allergen.

Drilling muds are a complex material and Table 35 lists some of the more common constituents. Drilling fluids do not appear to constitute a major sensitisation problem although I have identified sensitisation to an amine based emulsifier. The alkalis are primary irritants and can give rise to serious skin reaction. The oil-based muds are also irritant. Occasionally reactions to the tannins and chromium have been reported. The problem is, however, potentially complex and anyone who appears to be reacting to drilling muds should be seen by a dermatologist. Those identified by suffering from allergic contact dermatitis must avoid all future contact with that allergen, but the majority of persons will be found to have an irritant dermatitis which should respond in time to rest and thereafter that person can return to diving.

TABLE 35 - COMPONENTS OF DRILLING FLUIDS

Water
Alkaline Earth Metals - density adjustment
Clays - viscosifiers
Organic Polymers - filtration reducers
Synthetic water dispersible polymers - flocculant
Tannins - thinners
Alkalis - lime muds, stabilising, freezing point depression
Surfactants - emulsifiers, foamers, corrosion inhibitors

Table 36 lists the clinical features that are associated with the so-called "divers' hand".

TABLE 36 - DIVERS' HAND

Epidermal Peeling Volar Surface of Hand
Non Inflammatory
Resolves 2/3 weeks
Effects upwards of 80% of Saturation Divers
Probably related to Length & Depth of Diving Experience
Hand often colonised by Gram negative rods

I have seen one case in a naval diver and my own diagnosis was that of keratolysis exfoliativa. This disease commences as a peeling around the sweat glands on the palm of the hands and it seemed to me that it was an extreme form of this disease that was affecting the naval diver. I would be reluctant to consider it a contraindication to diving unless it interfered with manual dexterity.

DISCUSSION

Glanvill**: During a recent diving medical, a saturation diver (whose wife had recently trained as a chiropodist) drew my attention to horizontal ridging of his toe nails. He had no other apparent dermatological disorder. He then commented that other saturation divers he knew had similar ridging of their toe nails. Has this phenomenon been recognised before?

Reply from Aldridge: It is well recognised by divers that ridging can occur in both fingers and toe nails following a saturation dive. The changes are, however, subtle and may well be missed on examination. Ridging occurs because of changes in growth rate. Almost certainly the ridging occurring in divers is associated with changes in the nail growth rate secondary to the profound metabolic changes that take place in saturation diving. When diving ceases the nail would be expected to grow normally.

SPECIAL CONSIDERATIONS OF "THE DIVER'S HAND"
Dr. N. Moe

I wish to present some cases collected over the last 7 years within one particular Norwegian diving company (Table 37). Ahlen *et al* (1991) described a young saturation diver who became medically disqualified by this condition from further diving.

TABLE 37 - CHARACTERISTICS OF THE "DIVER'S HAND"

CLINICAL MANIFESTATIONS:	-	localised peeling
	-	total loss of epidermis
	-	only non pigmented skin of hand and fingers
	-	may affect plantar pedis
ETIOLOGY:	-	bacteriological
	-	toxic
	-	allergic
	-	saturation environment
THERAPY:	-	symptomatic
	-	etiologic

It is only the non-pigmented skin that is affected. The causes may include bacteria in the water in which the divers work and, although it may be toxic or allergic in origin, this condition does occur in divers not associated with drilling muds. There are as many proposals for treatment as there are divers. In some, the condition was ameliorated by the use of otic Domoboro, the buffered ear drops which were then used on the hands. In saturation it may begin during the bottom time and get worse during the subsequent decompression. It persists after surfacing.

In the study by Ahlen *et al*, (1991) some 83% of Norwegian divers have had some problem with their hands. Ninety per cent of the divers also answered that they did not have this condition except when they were diving. There appears to be an association both with length of diving experience and the depth of diving. A pilot study of creams that can be used on the divers' hands is currently underway. Thus divers' hands appears to be an occupational disease, particularly in saturation diving.

REFERENCE

Ahlen, K. et al.   *Proc. XVII EUBS Meeting on Diving and Hyperbaric Medicine,* Crete. Trikilis: Thessaloniki 1991. Pp 493-498.

NEUROLOGY AND MENTAL FITNESS

Chairman : Dr. N.K.I. McIver

Recommendations from the Guidance Notes on "The Medical Examination of Divers" are:

42. *In taking the history, any potentially disabling conditions should be cause for rejection:*

    (a) *claustrophobia;*
    (b) *severe motion sickness*
    (c) *any unprovoked loss of consciousness, recurring fainting episodes or epilepsy other than febrile convulsions occurring up to the age of 5 years;*
    (d) *migraine with visual, speech, motor or sensory disturbance;*
    (e) *any intracranial surgical procedure or depressed skull fracture*

Head Injury

43. *There are inherent dangers in diving if there has been significant brain damage or when there is a risk of post traumatic epilepsy. A history of head injury is acceptable if:*

    (a) *there has been loss of consciousness of less than 10 minutes without focal localising signs;*
    (b) *the period of post traumatic amnesia is less than 1 hour.*

    Minor linear skull fractures are acceptable if the criteria above are met. Depressed skull fractures and penetrating head injuries should disqualify from diving. Other cases of mild to moderate head injury, especially if recurrent, require full neurological and psychometric assessment. Even after apparently uncomplicated head injury with loss of consciousness for less than 10 minutes, the diver should not dive for at least 3 weeks.

44. *Direct enquiry should be made about vision, hearing, balance, co-ordination and sensation including bladder, bowel and sexual function. Any history of neurological disorder should be investigated further.*

45. *The examination of the central nervous system includes both static and dynamic assessment. The patient's manner, attitude, verbal and intellectual response and gait form part of the examination. If in the examining doctor's opinion there is any doubt as to the diver's intellectual or psychological response, further specialist advice should be sought.*

46. *Intellectual and psychomotor performance changes may be the only abnormality in some forms of decompression sickness. A thorough initial assessment is therefore essential. After general assessment, detailed examination should be made of the cranial nerves, motor system, sensation, reflexes and co-ordination. The examination guide is not considered exhaustive in terms of specialist neurological examination but is a screening examination. Any abnormality will require more detailed investigation and may require a specialist neurological opinion.*

47. *Any evidence of past or present psychiatric or psychological disorder (including alcohol or drug abuse) should be cause for rejection unless the examining doctor can be confident that it is of a minor nature and unlikely to recur. Specialised examination may be required to detect suspected latent brain damage. In any case of doubt or uncertainty, specialist assessment must be obtained.*

MENTAL FITNESS TO DIVE
Dr. B. Lunn

Diving is an inherently dangerous activity which, if accidents are to be minimised, requires a candidate to have as few disadvantageous traits as possible and as much training and experience as the task requires. The diving doctor's role obviously encompasses the former including both physical and mental fitness.

This can be looked at in three areas:

1. Psychiatric and psychological disorders unrelated to diving but influencing the safety of the diver in the water.
2. Psychiatric and psychological disorders related to, or occurring as a consequence of diving.
3. Assessing diver fitness and discussing the future needs, in terms of research, areas to be investigated.

DISORDERS UNRELATED TO DIVING

An abstract from current HSE recommendations states:

> "Any evidence of past or present psychiatric or psychological disorder (including both alcohol or drug abuse) should be cause for rejection unless the examining doctor can be confident that it is of a minor nature and unlikely to recur."

The inherent problem with such wording is that for the average dive doctor this is too vague and non-specific to aid much in decision making. Another problem arises when we look at who dives and with particular regard to professional divers, there has been debate as to the "normality" of the population. Biersner and Ryman (1974) compared U.S. Navy divers with a control group of U.S. Navy personnel and quoted a twofold greater incidence of psychiatric disorder in the diving population, but eleven years later Hoiberg and Blood found a result in the opposite direction. It is probably reasonable therefore to assume, not withstanding the doubts about the normality of the U.S. Navy population, that there is little difference in the psychiatric morbidity of the diving population and that of the general population. Indeed in sports diving in particular this has never been more true as over the past decade we have seen an upsurge in the number and range of people entering diving. No longer is diving the preserve of the macho male, nor need the individual experience undue hardship, but the result of this egalitarianism is the likelihood that a broader cross section of mental disorders will be seen.

I would suggest that we look at psychiatric disorders under the following headings:

Psychoses
Depression
Anxiety and panic disorders
Phobias
Recreational drugs
Personality

Psychoses

Psychoses, such as schizophrenia and bipolar affective disorder, should preclude passing a candidate as "Fit to dive". There is a risk that the marine environment and/or other divers may be incorporated into the delusional system of a psychotic individual as has already been discussed in diving medicine textbooks but, more importantly, the disruption of cognition that occurs during a psychotic episode is liable to impair the functioning of the diver and his or her ability to cope with the underwater environment.

Risks are therefore present both for the individual and those diving with them.

Depression

Depression may take several forms ranging from an acute grief reaction to the depressive phase of a bipolar affective disorder, each of these carries with it its own risks and prognosis. Both the medical profession and the lay public use this term to cover everything from minor feelings of unhappiness to the most profound, retarded depressive episode. It is therefore reasonable to make a decision on "fitness" only when it is based on an accurate psychiatric diagnosis and the resultant prognosis.

Suicide is another problem that may manifest itself within a diving population, which after all is just a sub-section of the normal. It is important to remember that this may be unrelated to any psychiatric diagnosis and there may be no warning signs.

Anxiety and Panic Disorders

Diving raises arousal levels in "normals" and, when within certain limits, leads to improved functioning in the diver, however over-arousal leads to rapid deterioration in performance. It is therefore reasonable that a current anxiety disorder should preclude diving as the already high arousal level leaves only a small margin of arousal before the diver is precipitated into a full blown panic attack. It may be, however, that successful treatment of an anxiety disorder may enable future diving.

Phobias

Even minor degrees of claustrophobia may be grossly exaggerated underwater particularly in enclosed environments or poor visibility, both of which are common occurrences in diving. Agoraphobia may only be a problem in certain diving environments, such as wall or open water diving (the "blue orb" syndrome), but entails increased risk for the sufferer. It would therefore appear appropriate to include these phobic conditions in the exclusion criteria for diving. It is also worth noting that simple phobias may also place limitations on diving.

Successful treatment of phobias may allow a monitored exposure to diving for the sports diver, but in the case of the commercial diver this issue is more complicated.

Recreational Drugs

The use of recreational drugs is well established in all societies, the nature of the drug varying with the values of the society itself and, in rapidly changing societies like our own, the pattern of drug using perpetually changes itself.

It is notoriously difficult to screen for drug use when it is in those individuals who are aware of the time periods that drugs are detectable in the body fluids, and even those markers for harmful use have a low specificity and sensitivity. Screening for damage secondary to drug use has its use but it should be realised that it is not a tool which is diagnostic of drug use and is no substitute for a high index of suspicion.

It is well recognised that drug use interferes with the ability of the individual to complete complex motor tasks, impairs concentration and impulse control, and affects judgement. This is clearly evidence in the acutely intoxicated individual but may also be seen as a consequence of chronic use and it is therefore reasonable to consider the drug "misuser" as unfit to dive.

Personality

One description of personality is "The characteristic patterns of behaviour and modes of thinking that determine a person's adjustment to the environment." In itself this is too simple to qualify as an adequate model of personality and various models exist to define personality, including: type, trait, interactionist, psychodynamic, and social learning. None of these give an adequate picture of what in fact personality in the first place. Therefore of course begging the question; what is an abnormal personality?

Assessment of personality is classically by informant interview and personality questionnaires/inventories but these are far from adequate particularly when there is confusion about what they actually measure and assess. We do not know what the "normal" personality of a diver is, how it compares to the general population, nor what aspects of the diver's personality may be either advantageous or deleterious in the water.

Screening of a diver's personality as an assessment tool is therefore unlikely to be an aid to assessment of diver fitness or diver selection.

DISORDERS RELATED TO DIVING

Under the rubric of disorders related to diving the following will be considered:

> Post-traumatic stress disorder
> Panic
> Organic disorders
> Other less common disorders

Post-traumatic Stress Disorder

The ICD 10 definition of post-traumatic stress disorder is: "...a delayed and/or protracted response to a stressful event or situation of an exceptionally threatening or catastrophic nature, which is likely to cause pervasive distress in almost anyone". This will not be covered here but will be by Surgeon Captain O'Connell in a later session.

Panic

Studies have implicated panic as a contributing factor in between 40 - 80% of diving fatalities. It is predisposed to by anxiety and high baseline levels of arousal, both of which have already been covered.

The mechanism of panic can be described as sympathetic over arousal leading to physical sensations which through their misinterpretation result in a "vicious circle". As the diver panics perceptual narrowing occurs leading to increased likelihood of the individual ignoring signs of danger and making errors which because of the environment may prove fatal.

The primary preventative measures are training and a study by Baddeley (1972) looking at selective attention and performance in divers, showed that this was the one protective variable.

Organic Disorders

The diver, because of the alien environment in which he works, is subject to a number of potential insults to the CNS, a far from exhaustive list includes:

- central nervous system DCS
- cerebral arterial gas embolism
- oxygen toxicity
- carbon monoxide poisoning
  inert gas narcosis
- high pressure neurological syndrome

Rather than review these, as they will already by familiar to this audience, I intend to look at two papers, by the same team, which highlight some problems encountered by divers and those who intend to research this area.

In 1987 Williamson *et al* tested 33 South Australian abalone divers and a control group of non-divers. The tests they used included:

Critical Flicker Fusion (CFFT)
Hand Steadiness
Bourdon-Weirsma
Digit Symbol Substitution (DSST)
Motor Reaction Time
Sternberg Paradigm Tasks
Paired Associated Learning (PALT)

These tests had previously been used to assess neurobehavioural impairment in workers exposed to lead and mercury. This is a reasonable approach as they too represent a group of young workers exposed to occupational insults liable to cause subtle cognitive damage.

The results are summarised below:

Test	Difference
CFFT	S
Hand Steadiness	S
Bourdon-Weirsma	(NS between divers)
DSST	S
Reaction Time	NS
Sternberg	"Yes" - S
	"No" - NS
PALT	NS

("S" : significant; "NS" : not significant)

The divers had a faster reaction time on the Sternberg but a greater number of errors, suggesting a sacrifice of accuracy for speed. It was postulated that this reflected greater risk taking behaviour, reflecting the personality of those who work as abalone divers, but another suggestion could be of a greater impulsivity due to frontal lobe dysfunction secondary to the damage incurred in their job.

With the paired associate learning whilst the overall result was not significant on the short term memory subtest, divers took a significantly greater number of trials to reach the criterion of all correct, and fewer actually reached criterion, perhaps a subtle suggestion of impairment too.

In 1989 the same group of investigators tested 80 active abalone divers from three sites; Tasmania (shallowest), New South Wales (longest) and South Australia (deepest). Here they looked at 6 dive variables using the same neuropsychological battery as in their previous study. The dive variables were:

1. Total hours dived
2. Average maximum depth for each dive
3. Incidence of general DCS
4. Incidence of neurological DCS
5. Graded decompression stress/dive risk
6. Use of oxygen

Decompression sickness variables (variables 3-5) were significantly and positively related, and showed a significant positive correlation with maximum depth and oxygen use. Total hours dived was unrelated to other dive variables. This enabled the authors to make a comparison of "Style" versus "Length" of diving. The results are summarised below:

- CFFT was related to incidence of neurological DCS.
- Psychomotor tasks were related to the maximum depth variable in that responses were faster.
- Bourdon-Weirsma test was correlated in the opposite direction with decompression stress tending to place some doubt on the risk taking hypothesis but perhaps giving a bit of credence to a suggestion of frontal dysfunction.
- Sternberg test was poorer where decompression stress was greater for both positive and negative responses.
- PALT was related to incidence of DCS but this correlation was lost when alcohol consumption was included.

NEUROPSYCHOLOGY IN SATURATION DIVERS

As a "taster" the current literature is briefly summarised as a full discussion would required more time than allotted for the whole of this talk.

Psychometry of deep saturation divers in the early-mid 1980's showed little of significance but most used large batteries and summarised results.

Logie *et al* (1985) looked at 16 divers participating in a total of 24 manned dives ranging in depths from 300 - 540 msw using heliox. They showed a decline in cognitive performance on a range of tests ranging from 15 - 20% at 300 msw, to 80% at 540 msw. Whilst at 300 msw results improved over time, there was a continued decline from original levels at deeper depths.

Curley (1988) looked at 25 U.S. Navy deep saturation divers (198 - 335 msw) and noticed transient changes in their psychometry, however these were averaged results, perhaps missing subtle variations in individuals.

Vaernes *et al* (1989) did a prospective study over one year on 82 subjects and showed >10% impairment of some function in 16. Prior to testing these individuals had shown better results than age corrected, non-diving, reference values.

Morris *et al* (1991) looked at neurology and neuropsychology of 282 professional divers in work done for the Department of Energy. Results showed impairment in cognitive function where there had been DCS and also impaired memory/non-verbal reasoning where there had been no DCS but it was suspected that this was age related.

OTHER LESS COMMON DISORDERS

Perceptual Misinterpretations

Here due to a number of factors, both organic and "psychological" the diver may interpret external stimuli falsely as a possible threat, perhaps resulting in errors of judgement, panic etc.

Conversion Disorders

These have been described in the diving population but should only be considered as a diagnosis of last resort when all organic causes have been excluded, and even then be viewed with suspicion.

Munchausen's Syndrome

Individuals presenting with symptoms of diving injuries to serial hyperbaric centres have been reported but this syndrome is thankfully extremely rare.

ASSESSING DIVER FITNESS

Where there is any significant psychiatric disorder, or any doubt, refer to a psychiatrist for advice on diagnosis and prognosis.

Screening for recreational drug use is not reliable in excluding its use, have a high index of suspicion.

Personality questionnaires/inventories have little predictive value.

There is probably significant value in establishing baseline neuropsychological data for all commercial divers, and screening those in whom there has been a dive-related incident at the annual medical.

Refer on to a neuropsychiatrist/neuropsychologist with knowledge of diving-related injuries where any suspicion of an organic brain lesion is uncovered.

FUTURE NEEDS IN DIVING RESEARCH

Research is needed to establish specifically targeted neuropsychological screening batteries for divers.

REFERENCES

Biersner, R.J. & Ryman, D.H. *Mil. Med.* 1987; **139**: 633-635.

Baddeley, A.D. *Br. J. Psychol.* 1972; **63**: 537-546.

Curley, M.D. *Undersea Biomed. Res.* 1988; **15**: 39-50.

Hoiberg, A. & Blood, C. *Undersea Biomed. Res.* 1987; **12**: 191-203.

Logie, R.H. & Baddeley, A.D. *Ergonomics* 1985; **28**: 731-746.

Morris, P.E., Leach, J., King, J. & Rawlins, J.S.P. *Psychological and neurological impairment in professional divers : Final report.* London: Department of Energy 1991.

Vaernes, R.J. Aarli, J.A., Klove, H. & Tønjum, S. *Aviat. Space Environ. Med.* 1987; **38**: 155-165.

Williamson, A.M., Clark, B. & Edmonds, C. *Br. J. Ind. Med.* 1987; **44**: 459-466.

Williamson, A.M., Clark, B. & Edmonds, C. *Environ. Res.* 1989; **50**: 93-102.

DISCUSSION

Dick (D.): Do you think there is a danger of repeated testing producing an improvement in the results? Does the result depend on the interval between the tests?

Lunn: That is very dependent on the test that is being used. There is certainly a learning component. However, there are tests that can be used again and again because one can change the variables. One must be aware of this when designing the test series.

LeDez: Again, I would like to take exception to a great deal of what we have heard in comparison with the criteria we have used for other systems. Is there anything in mental assessment that is related to safety of the diver in the water? We need to apply the same criteria. I know of no evidence that diving aggravates depression. I am not aware if some mental conditions when stable would actually cause a problem during the dive. There is also the disability legislation which is being brought in in the States and which will also shortly emerge in Europe, that one must show evidence that there is a hazard to the individual if one is to disqualify him from a particular job. There should not be arbitrary judgements.

Lunn: I do not totally disagree with you in some of what you are saying. A history of depression in itself should not be something that precludes diving but an active depressive illness should be. Those who have recovered from depression should be judged upon their merits. It would be wise to differentiate between a psychotic depression and an acute grief reaction. Depression must not be a blanket term. One must think about what is wrong with the individual and decide upon that basis. The bottom line is that one must decide not only about the individual's safety but also the safety of those who dive with him. We know that those with depression have altered cognition.

LeDez**: Please give some information about studies or case reports, or from your experience, which demonstrate in working divers the contribution to a serious accident of the following:

(a) previously treated but now resolved depression;
(b) stable bipolar disorder;
(c) recovered psychotic episode.

Reply from Lunn: No absolute evidence exists, but there are anecdotes of injuries and death occurring in sports divers. This raises the question of whether we should be proactive or reactive. Should we try to anticipate problems or should we only respond to something once a tragedy has occurred?

LeDez**: The current wording refers to psychiatric problems of "minor" nature. In other areas of medicine, we accept that hospital admission implies a more "serious" illness. What about the diver (or new trainee) who has a hospital admission for an episode of depression but who is now recovered? Perhaps this section needs to be reworded, instead of "minor" we should consider: "chronic; frequently recurrent" etc.

What about night time hypnotics for sleep? What about the diver on night time low dose amitriptyline but otherwise recovered? Is there <u>any</u> evidence that lithium therapy is hazardous in air diving?

Reply from Lunn: In psychiatry, with the changes in admission policies, community care etc., a division into minor or serious on the basis of hospital admission is invalid.

Decisions on fitness to dive should be based on diagnosis and, most importantly, prognosis. The latter is obviously dependent on an accurate diagnosis. "Minor" psychiatric disorders such as anxiety disorders or claustrophobia may have a major impact on "in-water fitness" and my recommendation would therefore be that active psychiatric disorder should preclude a diver being passed "fit to dive".

When a diver has had a psychiatric disorder that has resolved and the prognosis would suggest little likelihood of recurrence then it may be possible to pass a diver as "fit to dive".

Hypnotics are known to affect motor and cognitive performance, a finding verified in many studies. The use of hypnotics therefore increases the risk for the diver in the water. It could be argued that this is acceptable for a sports diver but I believe that it is not for a professional. Note that insomnia may be a symptom of underlying illness and that long term use of hypnotics is not recommended.

Presumably with amitriptyline what is meant is a diver with a treated depression. If the diver continues to require a tricyclic, or other, antidepressant then they cannot be said to have "recovered" and my reply to the first question still applies.

There have been no studies looking at lithium use in divers, but if an individual is requiring lithium therapy they obviously have been diagnosed as having a recurrent illness and again I would refer the questioner to my first answer. A syndrome of lithium neurotoxicity at normal therapeutic levels has been described (see a review by Bell and Ferrier in "Lithium"; currently in press). This risk is increased where there is any dehydration, a not uncommon occurrence in diving.

Milne**: I would be grateful for your advice on the precise definition of neuropsychological tests appropriate for administration by:

(a) the Approved Doctor
(b) the Diving Supervisor

Reply from Lunn: These are, as yet, unanswered questions which still required to be addressed by research.

NEUROLOGICAL ASSESSMENT
Dr. D.J. Dick

As a neurologist with a special interest in diving I will structure this presentation along the lines of the history and examination of the diver, emphasising those parts of it that are important in the assessment of a diver. Then I will turn to the more specific problems such as head injury, migraine and epilepsy, and finish with some aspects of the clinical neurology of decompression sickness.

NEUROLOGICAL HISTORY

When taking the history, one wants to make enquiries about:

- Mood, Memory, Concentration
- Blackouts
- Senses (sight, taste etc.)
- Speech and swallowing
- Sensation
- Walking
- Dexterity/co-ordination
- Sphincter control

Altered sensibility can take many forms, particularly after an episode of acute decompression illness. It is not just a matter of routine questioning, there are some special sensory syndromes for instance Lhermitte's phenomenon when flexion of the neck precipitates tingling in the extremities. This is characteristic of posterior column disturbance. The sensation of a tight band around the arm or leg is also very suggestive of dysfunction. Sensation is a nebulous phenomenon and often nothing abnormal can be detected. When a patient describes it as being like recovering from a dental anaesthetic, it is usually organic. Do not forget to ask about gait; with pyramidal tract dysfunction the leg may feel heavy and tend to drag. They may catch their toes on raised objects.

One must also ask about:

- Migraine
- Blackouts
- Head injury
- Neurosurgery
- Claustrophobia
- Motion sickness
- Somnolence

Do ask about excessive daytime somnolence. This may be common after lunch but there is a significant percentage of people being increasingly recognised as having a pathological degree of somnolence. A small proportion of these have narcolepsy. The vast majority have another disorder, this may be associated with snoring, periods of apnoea during sleep and headache. These are the symptoms of obstructive sleep apnoea. Their sleep is not deep and therefore they feel sleepy during the day. A question about somnolence should appear in the diving history. Weight reduction and ENT procedures, such as tonsillectomy in some, can cure the condition.

EXAMINATION

Some tips are offered in the following list which is not comprehensive.

Cranial nerve I - This should be done as a baseline for subsequent assessment after a diving incident or other injury. One can use orange peel, coffee, tobacco and there is no need for fancy equipment.

Cranial nerve II - One should test for visual acuity, as already discussed. When doing the visual fields, do not wave your hands around in some mid-position, one must get one's hands right into the temporal fields. Remember that perimetry only looks for disturbances of peripheral vision. If you use a large pin with a coloured glass ball on the end you can look for scotomata. A pin head of 5 mm is just the same size as the blind spot in the eye and, with one metre between the two of you, is a useful part of the procedure. With subtle relative scotomas that are present only with colour, one must use both a red and white pin.

Cranial nerves III, IV & VI - Remember three things when testing eye movements. First do not take the movement into the area of monocular vision. This will induce physiological nystagmus which could be confusing. Secondly, the object should be at least one arm's length from the patient. Thirdly, drugs such as alcohol can induce nystagmus the next day.

Cranial nerve V - The testing of sensation is entirely subjective with the exception of one or two specific tests of which the corneal reflex is one. It is important that one does not approach this test from the front and one should stroke the cornea gently. The other trick, which is objective, is to stick a cotton bud up the nostril which is supplied by the second division of V. The motor division of V must be tested, including the jaw jerk. Do they just have brisk reflexes, or do they have evidence of pyramidal tract dysfunction? A brisk jaw jerk is found in somebody with bilateral upper motor neurone lesions above the level of the motor nuclei of V in the pons.

Cranial nerve VI - Screw up the eyes.

Cranial nerve VIII - Rinné's and Weber's test but which have been superseded by audiometry.

Cranial nerve XI - Trapezius and sterno-cleido-mastoid function. Speaking more generally, when one is testing for power, apparent weakness may be reported if a patient has not given full co-operation. Intermittency of power is bogus. A brief but maximal effort is sufficient to confirm the presence of adequate power. The only exception to this is when there is either discomfort or pain associated with movement.

Cranial nerve XII - A useful test of tongue power is for the individual to push each cheek out with the tongue.

Tone - Test this by pronating and supinating the arm or by moving the wrist passively. In the lower limb assess tone by lifting the knee sharply while the patient is lying supine. In normal tone the heel should remain on the bed and not be lifted off.

Reflexes - The finger jerk is sometimes useful, particularly when compared with the other side. The adductor jerk (L5, S1) may be pathological if the reflexes cross, i.e. tapping on one side produces the reflex on the other. The others are:

-	Supinator, biceps	C5, 6
-	Triceps	C7
-	Finger	C8
-	Knee	L3, 4
-	Ankle	S1
-	Abdominal	T8-10 and T11-12
-	Cremasteric	L1, 2
-	Anal	S4, 5

To elicit the abdominal reflexes draw an orange stick from the outside to the centre. These reflexes may be lost if the person has had surgery, if very fat, or may be lost through age.

For the plantar response pass a sharp stick up the outside of the foot and never do it more medially.

Co-ordination - In the finger to nose test, the subject's arm must stretch to its full extent. Rapid alternating movements are a useful test of cerebellar function; ask the patient to pretend that they are taking a light bulb out. In the leg, run the heel along the opposite shin but first leave the heel on the knee for a while as this may reveal some intention tremor.

Dexterity - This is upset in the disorders of the extra-pyramidal system. Try opposing the thumb to each finger in turn.

Gait - Only by exercising are some features of pyramidal tract impairment revealed.

Joint position sense - Grip very firmly on either side so as not to give any clues about movement.

Vibration sense - It is important to have the patient close their eyes and to do the test with the fork either by vibrating or not vibrating and for the subject to identify which it is.

Discrimination - Two point discrimination, on the lips it is about 2 mm, on the fingers 3-4 mm whereas in the foot it is 3-4 cm.

HEAD INJURY

There is a 1 in 50 incidence of head injury, the commonest group being the 15 - 24 year-old male. Most are minor with only some 4% going for neurosurgery.

One should consider the pathology which will comprise contusion, haematoma and diffuse axonal injury. Most frequent of these is diffuse axonal injury i.e. after a closed head injury there is shearing of the central nervous system axons and subsequent retraction.

The severity of a head injury is measured historically by the length of coma, the clinical state on arrival and the duration of post traumatic amnesia (PTA). The depth of coma can be measured using the standard Glasgow coma scale, which gives a numerical value for the various parameters but the best indicator of the severity of a head injury is post traumatic amnesia (Table 38).

TABLE 38 - PTA FOR PROGNOSIS IN HEAD INJURY

PTA (days)	SEVERE DISABILITY %	RECOVERY %
<7	0	90
8 - 14	0	80
15 - 28	3	60
>28	30	30

PTA is the time from the head injury until the time the patient begins to lay down a <u>continuous memory</u>. Islands of memory <u>do not</u> represent the end of amnesia. PTA does not shrink with the passage of time. This is in contrast to retrograde amnesia, amnesia of incidents leading up to the injury. PTA is always of longer duration than the interval from the injury until when speech starts. PTA may correlate well with the degree of damage shown on magnetic resonance imaging.

Post traumatic epilepsy can follow head injury. In 5% it occurs in the first week. There is an increased risk with depressed skull fracture, intracranial haematoma, prolonged PTA, focal neurological signs and in a young child. Late epilepsy can occur in 5% of this population. There is an increased risk if there is an intracranial haematoma (31%), early epilepsy (25%) or a depressed skull fracture (15%). With none of these, the risk is 1%. Sixty per cent of the first post traumatic fits occur within 1 year, 24% in 1-4 years and 16% after 4 years.

If the severity of the head injury is defined as:

Severe	-	Confusion, haematoma, >24 hours coma, amnesia
Moderate	-	Skull # with 30 mins - 24 hours unconsciousness
Mild	-	<30 mins unconsciousness or amnesia

then, looking at nearly 3000 patients the occurrence of fits is:

	1 yr %	5 yr %
Severe	7.1	11.5
Moderate	0.7	1.6
Mild	0.1	0.6

It is important to note that the incidence in the mild group is no greater than that in the general population. Therefore one can allow unconsciousness or amnesia for up to 30 minutes without any effect upon future diving fitness. Obviously that assessment must include other factors such as neurological impairment and post concussional syndrome which includes headache, dizziness, poor memory, poor concentration and irritability. These are all symptoms similar to those expressed by some divers after decompression illness. Among the problems reported by relatives of head injury victims are slowness, tiredness, depression, anxiety and irritability. Poor memory and personality change are also common in the post concussion syndrome.

I do not therefore disagree with the recommendation given in the Guidance. It is fair that if someone has a minor head injury, they should only be off work for 3 or 4 weeks but you could be more generous about the length of unconsciousness or amnesia for it does look as though the risk of subsequent epilepsy is no greater than in the general population as long as they were not unconscious for longer than 30 minutes.

HEADACHE

As a general rule migraine is improved somewhat by treatment, but with tension headaches nothing works! Migraine headaches have an aura associated with vasoconstriction and then a vasodilation phase which actually creates the headache. Common migraine which comprises 80 - 90% of sufferers have no aura. The classical migraine with aura are in only about 10 - 20% of cases. There are many factors precipitating migraine attacks ranging from stress, worry, menstruation, oral contraceptives, dazzle and glare, physical exertion, fatigue, lack of sleep, hangovers, head trauma and various specific foods and beverages. There are some less common factors in other persons ranging from excessive sleep, high altitude exposures, excess of vitamin A, some particular drugs and refractive errors in reading glasses. It is important to note that this includes change of barometric pressure. This certainly applies to a diver.

Migrainous neuralgia is characterised by paroxysms of severe pain usually peri-orbital or frontal associated with lachrymation of the eye and ptosis. The distinction in the Guidance Note between classical migraine and ordinary migraine is rather difficult, but both conditions can be equally disabling.

BLACKOUTS: WAS IT EPILEPSY?

When taking the story of a blackout one must be very sure of the exact circumstances in which it happened. What warning was there? Was there tongue biting? Incontinence can occur in syncopal events, not just epilepsy. Perception, were there any minor events in which there was just an alteration of sensory perception? I find it useful to ask about any confusion after the event, persons are very rarely confused after syncope but after epilepsy it can go on for quite a while. Aching in the limbs the next day is very common after seizures but will not occur after syncope. Finally a witness account of the attack by an independent observer is absolutely invaluable.

Beware the person who has syncope but is trapped in an upright position so that the patient has a reflex anoxic seizure. It is important that this is not diagnosed as epilepsy.

Any seizure occurring after the age of 5 should prohibit from commercial diving.

DECOMPRESSION ILLNESS

I would like to finish by saying a few words about the neurological manifestations of decompression illness. One may encounter aphasia, field defects, confusion, seizures, monoplegia, hemiplegia or other motor problems, hemisensory loss or other sensory deficits, ataxia, dysarthria, radicular pain or sphincter disorders. This is not an exhaustive list. It depends where the lesions are and the disease is often multi-focal. Spinal cord lesions may give rise to radicular pain. I have often thought that this may be due to bubbles in the dorsal root ganglion, because this is located in a fairly tight bony compartment. The rest are well known. In some 60 cases from the North Sea Medical Centre general fatigue and weakness were the symptoms that occurred most frequently.

Is there any relationship between the latency of onset of decompression sickness and the severity? A rapid onset tends to follow a deep dive, a rapid ascent or a major decompression omission. There is a tendency for slower onset to follow a shallow dive, slow ascents and minor decompression omissions.

There is often reference to "individual susceptibility" but there is conflicting evidence in the literature and many of the cases are anecdotal. Paton and Walder (1954) looked at 376 compressed air workers who had between them some 40,000 exposures with an incidence of decompression sickness of less than 1%, and two thirds of them had an even smaller percentage. In contrast 6% were twice that mean value of 1% "bends", 10% were 5 times the mean and 20% were 18 times the mean.

REFERENCE

Paton, W.D.M. & Walder, D.N. *Compressed Air Illness, Report 281.* Medical Research Council: London 1954.

ACCIDENT INVESTIGATION AND NEUROPATHOLOGY
Dr. I.M. Calder

The advantage of divers is that they are a well contained population and they can be monitored quite accurately. The requirements of an accident investigation are to:

1. establish accurate cause of death;
2. define any pattern which may be of use in future prevention of accidents and
3. to establish any pattern of changes to tissues which may be attributable to the environment.

It is not only the central nervous system that is affected. Morphological changes from the hyperbaric environment have multiple target organs throughout the body.

TABLE 39 - CAUSES OF DEATH IN 117 CASES

	n	%
At work		
Asphyxia	52	44.5
Pulmonary	31	26.4
Hyperthermia	5	4.3
Hypothermia	3	2.6
Medical	4	3.5
Narcosis	5	4.3
Undetermined	6	5.2
Working but not at work		
Murder	2	1.2
Suicide	7	5.9
Myocardial infarction	1	0.8
Cancer	1	0.5

While there may appear to be a lot of suicides but in fact a careful study has shown that the rate among divers is no greater than the rate of a comparable age population of non-divers.

Most people do not realise that while the brain weighs 1,300 grams the cord only weighs 40 grams and that one could get some 4 or so cross-sections of the cord on a single postage stamp. The white matter of the cord itself, the total weight cannot be much more than 25 grams, is a significant target organ.

One of the divers who was killed was a man who had suffered previous acute neurological decompression illness for which he had been treated and from which he had made a good recovery, even though there were some small residua detectable which, had he been a commercial diver, would have prevented him from returning to work. At autopsy the surprising thing was the enormous amount of damage to the cord which in no way reflected the distribution of his original manifestations. His apparent nearly complete recovery was entirely functional. There was an enormous amount of damage on histology (Palmer, Calder, McCallum & Mastaglia, 1981).

After an incident there is oedema which can clear up, and then haemorrhage but the presence of micro-thrombi in the vessels can cause obstruction of very small blood vessels and this produces an infarction in the spinal cord. Interestingly enough the sub-pial layer always seems to be protected against infarction which is related to the vascular arcade.

Under the light microscope it is difficult to detect lesions of 5 microns but in addition it is possible to use specific histochemistry. When axonal death occurs there is myelin sheath degeneration. Normal myelin is a complex liquid but degenerating myelin contains many unsaturated fatty acids and Marchi described an osmium procedure to demonstrate axonal degeneration. Lots of little black dots can be seen particularly in the posterior columns of some divers. Each one is an epitaph to the death of one nerve fibre. In the cases we have so far examined there is no evidence of recent decompression illness and this is evidence of silent damage (Palmer, Calder & Hughes, 1987).

The examination of the brain by HMPAO will be discussed tomorrow but the brain of the only case which has so far come for histopathological examination was unfortunately ruined by a visiting consultant pathologist for medico-legal reasons.

Large lesions in the brain have been comparatively rare. One centimetre diameter lesions have been found in brains of those who have been perfectly healthy as divers. The first indication of possible brain damage was recognised in one unexplained death about 10 years ago in which some of the small blood vessels had inflammatory changes. In general there is a spectrum of microscopic changes in the brain, showing hyalinisation of blood vessels, lacunae, myelin focal damage and focal damage to grey matter. These are interesting evidence to the pathologist in that they do show that damage has occurred. Old pigment may be found outside the vessels showing that they have previously been damaged. Some large spaces around the vessels suggest perhaps that the vessel has expanded in the past and finally one gets tiny areas of dead brain scattered for instance in silent areas of the brain. It does not appear to be a vasculopathy because the vessels hit are fairly random. Perhaps this represents an increased rate of degeneration in the diving population.

The quotation of J. Hughlings Jackson "the study of things caused must precede the study of causes of things" is apposite. In summary "Mortui vivos docet", it is the injured who teach the uninjured.

REFERENCES

Palmer, A.C., Calder, I.M. & Hughes, J.T. *Lancet* 1987; **2**: 1365-1366.

Palmer, A.C., Calder, I.M., McCallum R.I. & Mastaglia, F.L. *Br. Med. J.* 1981; **283**: 888.

PROSPECTIVE EPIDEMIOLOGICAL INVESTIGATION OF POSSIBLE EFFECTS OF DIVING ON DIVERS' HEALTH
Dr. M. Grønning

I will briefly present the plans for a future research project on diving in Bergen, Norway.

The results from the Norwegian research on possible long term effects from diving on the nervous system, LTV-project 1985-1990, were presented at the Godøysund meeting in Norway in June 1993. The results have been controversial, but a consensus was made in this meeting:

> "There is evidence that changes in bone, the central nervous system and lung can be demonstrated in some divers who have not experienced a diving accident or other established environmental hazard. The changes are in most cases minor and do not influence the diver's quality of life. However, the changes are of a nature that may influence the diver's future health".

The Godøysund meeting strongly recommended a prospective long term study which should cover pulmonary function, neurology, neuropsychology and otology, and we have now designed such a study.

The objective is to make a baseline examination at entry of all students into the Norwegian Diving School, and repeat the examination every third year on the same individuals, no matter what their later occupations are. In this way every person will be his own control and the wide variation in the diver exposure which is likely to occur in this population will provide data for evaluating a possible dose-response relationship. We expect that 50% of the students will not proceed to a professional diving career, and these individuals will serve as controls.

The diving exposure will be examined in their "record of dive". Filled in properly, we think this will give an acceptable measure of pressure-time and gas mixture. We will also have a questionnaire asking for other exposures and also for diseases which may be of importance.

The neurological part will be done by two consultant neurologists and one consultant neurophysiologist and includes clinical neurological examination, EEG and evoked potentials.

The earlier LTV cross-sectional study revealed significantly more minor abnormal signs in the divers in the clinical neurologic examination and EEG, but not in the evoked potentials. The longitudinal study also includes evoked potentials; the diver serves as his own control and changes with time will be the important issue. One reason for choosing a limited number of procedures is that most centres have these available and our protocol may be extended to a multi-centre study.

The study will start in April 1994. The follow-up period will be at least 6 years. The statistical analysis will be done after 3 and 6 years.

REFERENCE

Hope, A., Lund, T., Elliott, D.H., Halsey, M.J. & Wigg, H. (Eds). *Long-term health effects of diving: an international consensus conference, Godøysund.* NUTEC: Bergen 1994.

DISCUSSION

McIver (Chairman): The first question which needs addressing is: "what are the psychological contraindications to acceptance for diver training?"

Lunn: As I said in my talk the psychoses are an absolute contraindication to diving due to two reasons:

1. the risk to the diver and
2. the risks to the other people he dives with.

We know that in a psychosis the individual's ability to organise his thoughts and to create logical patterns of behaviour in relation to the stimuli that are presented, is disturbed. Even during the remission of a psychosis there are still abnormalities present. I also believe that where there is an active psychiatric or psychological illness it does influence the individual's ability to cope with stressful circumstances. We have no documented evidence from the diving population obviously but, in an environment where the stresses are frequently unexpected, one cannot predict how individuals will cope and so active psychiatric illness is indeed a contraindication for acceptance for training.

Grønning: I agree.

Francis: How are you going to detect this at a routine diving medical examination?

Lunn: This is a very difficult question. Certainly the most subtle neuropsychiatric damage is very difficult to pick up. We do have to develop tests which are highly sensitive, something that can be administered by the diving doctor to pick up those who might have that kind of impairment. Then they should have an assessment by the specialist.

McIver: Therefore a high index of suspicion is what is needed. In one of HSE's appeal cases a careless facetiousness was all that was needed to alert the diving doctor.

Lunn: Neuropsychiatric disorder is vastly underdiagnosed. If you have a high index of suspicion, you are actually doing better than doctors have done in the past.

Mebane: The Chairman and I have said in print that it is not possible to determine how an individual will respond to stress and so the examining physician does have an impossible task. One of the subjects in simulated saturation diving became psychotic during a 2,000 ft dive in spite of having gone through an enormous battery of testing.

McCallum: One of my present projects is to look at what divers die from. There is apparently an excess of violent deaths compared with the population of England and Wales, there is also an excess of road traffic accidents for instance. So are there personality or psychiatric changes which could have arisen from diving? The problem is to find a suitable comparative population. I looked at a paper on deaths in Icelandic Fishermen and their pattern of mortality has certain parallels of those of divers. They not only get drowned at sea but they also have a lot of accidents on land plus a high rate of suicide. Am I looking at an abnormal population, i.e. the selection process of divers produces such persons, or am I looking at a group with personality changes?

Lunn: There is no easy answer to that. I do not know whether the population is abnormal or whether it is a result of the diving that makes them behaviourally abnormal. There are anecdotal reports of clusters of symptoms in divers which suggests some form of dysfunction comparable to a frontal lobe syndrome. Are we seeing a dysexecutive syndrome in divers? We do know that diving can alter a diver's cognition.

LeDez: As a physician, particularly as an anaesthetist, I am also in a very high risk suicide group. We must be careful not to over-interpret such things. In the respiratory system we gave consideration to the differences between acute, chronic, acute on-chronic, and surely we should do the same with the psychological fitness to dive. We should not have the statement that any psychological condition in a diver's life is a contraindication to diving.

Lunn: That is not the statement that I made, I said any psychotic condition. Also, I do make a distinction between the psychoses and the depressions, whether unipolar or bipolar. An acute grief reaction which is adequately treated, is not a contraindication to diving. So I am making a difference between the chronic and the acute.

McIver: These are certainly the psychiatric contraindications but are there any psychological contraindications?

Mebane: How about the psychotic maintained in remission?

Lunn: Yes, that is a contraindication. They still have active illness, the medication merely suppresses it and one is dependent on the patient continuing to take the medication.

McIver: Can we take the next 3 questions together about the psychological contraindications: "what assessment of psychological fitness has predictive value for safety? What components of the psychological assessment may be needed annually and what is the evidence on the relevance of an 'in-date' psychological fitness examination to the individual's in-water safety during the subsequent twelve months?"

Lunn: The distinction between psychology and psychiatry is blurred. The psychological contraindications are really an extension of the psychiatric anxieties etc. For those who have neuropsychological deficits, they should be excluded as divers. For the assessment of fitness there are no good personality inventories or anything like that which are of any use for the assessment of psychological fitness. This can be done only on a history and then upon a diagnostic investigation. Work is needed on screening people, assessing them adequately and establishing a battery aimed at divers in the same way that it has been done with solvents and other toxic exposures. Commercial divers should have a neuro-psychological examination at the beginning of their training as a baseline and then they can be reviewed should they have troubles in the future. There is no need to test everybody every year. However we should, like the Norwegians are doing, have a longitudinal study.

Then there is the problem of the person concealing illness, it is like the old joke of how many psychiatrists are needed to change the lightbulb? The answer is - one, but the lightbulb must want to be changed. Unless the individual is psychotic or obviously depressed, then the physician is stuck, unless the patient is co-operative. Things like the inappropriate facetiousness that has been spotted by the family doctor shows how important it is for the diving doctor to get to know the diver and see him on successive years. It is then much easier. On the first assessment it is virtually impossible.

Whitehead: Is there any future in applying standardised depressive inventories like Montgomery-Esjberg which, if looked at serially, would enable one to look at the change in depressive features of the divers?

Lunn: The problem with things like that and other inventories, is that they do pick up symptoms but they do not pick up any more than does a psychiatric examination. They are not diagnostic. Others are large and unwieldy and would not be suitable for assessment procedure. The standard history taking is probably more effective.

Elliott: Also that has been extremely successful because there appears to be no evidence of a psychiatric or psychological problem among the diving population. Whatever we are doing now, we are doing it right.

McIver: Now we go on to the neurological questions: "What are the neurological contraindications to acceptance for diver training?

Dick: The neurological examination must be normal. Any abnormality is a contraindication although one must have some common sense and flexibility. For instance a mild degree of wasting of one gastrocnemius muscle because of a long resolved past disc prolapse or someone who had polio with a minor degree of wasting of one calf, would not be a bar to diving provided they were functioning normally. I think that the contraindications in respect of epilepsy should be the same as for a heavy goods vehicle license - free of seizures for 10 years without anticonvulsants.

Grønning: I agree with Dr. Dick. Maybe we should be a little tougher on exclusion for trainees.

McIver: What is the evidence?

Dick: I personally believe that as long as they are functioning normally that is all that is important.

Broome: Could we clarify the word "seizures"? Is everybody allowed one fit? Particularly if there are predisposing factors such as alcohol syncope?

Dick: I meant any seizures after the age of 5, except a syncopal fit. After that I would say that any seizures, even alcohol-related seizures, within the previous 10 years should be a contraindication. The risk of subsequent epilepsy is really quite high in any person who has had a single seizure.

Nome: What about a seizure brought on by flickering of the helicopter rotors?

Dick: Yes, that is a response to a photic stimulus and is classed as a single seizure.

Mavin: I am concerned about your leniency for polio. A successful air diver with just such a problem went into saturation diving and he had quite severe pain. Just minor wasting but he had quite a problem.

Dick: A minor degree of asymmetry from one limb to the other is not in my judgement a contraindication providing he has normal strength. I would suggest the pain in a limb was a coincidence.

Nome: I have examined one diver with a leg many centimetres smaller than the other following polio in childhood. In 1972 there were not many rules around so I passed him fit. For the next 10 years I monitored him and he had no problems.

Foster: If, after a head injury which required the evacuation of a sub-dural haematoma but nothing else, the patient had not had a fit in 4 years, he would be fit to hold an HGV (heavy goods vehicle) license but would he be fit for diving?

Dick: Was he on anticonvulsants?

Foster: No.

Dick: He would be unable to hold a heavy goods vehicle license with that history.

Zachariedes: What about seizures due to oxygen?

Francis: Those who have had a fit due to oxygen toxicity can continue to dive.

Can I ask a supplementary question, if an established diver then has an idiopathic fit, does one have to stop him from diving?

Dick: Yes. The recurrence rate is in the order of 60-70% during the next 5 years.

Lepawsky: Do you screen your divers for oxygen toxicity?

Francis: No, that test is not predictive.

Lepawsky: So you do not stop them if they have an oxygen fit?

Francis: We do not stop them.

Hickish: This is a problem I had the other day, relative to the problem of epilepsy after a head injury in a 30 year-old man who had been a sports diver for 12 years. About 4 years ago he had a compound fracture of his anterior fossa. At no time was he unconscious and at no time did he have a fit. A CSF leak was successfully repaired with fascia lata and he made an uncomplicated recovery, other than some headaches for about 3 months afterwards. Three months later he went to see a doctor for a fitness to dive certificate for recreational diving and he continued to dive. Since then he has made some 400 dives some as deep as 40 m. He now wishes to continue but professionally as a recreational trainer.

Dick: I am surprised that there is no post-traumatic amnesia. In that case there was less than 30 minutes unconsciousness and therefore he is fit to dive.

It is important to realise that single seizures occur in the general population quite frequently. The life-time incidence of a major seizure in the general population is 4% i.e. 1 in 20 persons will have an isolated single attack.

McIver: I would now like to revert to one of the questions that we missed i.e. "Is there any evidence concerning the role of alcohol and drug abuse in the causation of diving accidents? Is there any need for specific screening annually?" Ian, you have some experience in this?

Calder: One of the things one does at autopsy is routinely to screen people for drugs and alcohol. I have come across histological evidence of alcohol but never acute alcohol in diving. What concerns me are the hallucinogenic drugs, they may cause a flashback later. Do these drugs produce a long term effect? Should such a person ever dive again?

Lunn: Triggered memories or flashbacks may be caused by post traumatic distress disorder (PTSD) which will be dealt with by Surgeon Captain O'Connell later. When one has an intense experience which is so emblazoned on one's memory, it takes very little to trigger the memory. It is like the snippet of a tune which brings back particular memories. A minimal stimulus may cause a flashback, it might well interfere with the individual's ability to function at that time, although you cannot predict when flashbacks are going to happen. The only thing one can say is that if they have a history of flashbacks, then they may be at risk, but one is not necessarily going to get a history of flashbacks from the diver when one does the medical.

Do hallucinogenic drugs make a difference to the accidents in divers? There have been no studies of this. There has been a study of the frequency of accidents in oil rig workers with a correlation between the use of drugs on the rigs and the number of accidents that occur. So there is enough evidence in other aspects of society that drug use does affect safety.

Mebane: There were 96 deaths in the DAN series of whom there were 68 forensic autopsies and out of the 68, 4 were over the legal limit for alcohol and driving.

Broome: There are divers found to have abnormal EEG's as a result of experimental diving. Does that affect their diving fitness?

Dick: The abnormalities in EEG's are extremely difficult, there are two problems: first, in someone with established severe epilepsy you can have a perfectly normal EEG. The second is that if you drag a thousand people off the street, a substantial percentage of them will have abnormalities including "epileptic" changes and yet they might all be clinically normal. Thus the diagnosis of epilepsy is clinical and not based on the EEG. In studies of drug withdrawal, the EEG is of not value predicting who will have a relapse. The Civil Aviation Authority are more stringent: a focal abnormality of EEG is a bar to holding a commercial pilot's license.

Bergöö: Should there be screening for drug abuse annually or should it be only after an accident? We made a drug test three years ago on divers in the construction industry. There were about 10% positive for cannabis. This does not solve the problem but it does define it.

Calder: Ten per cent of the rig workers had cannabis and the ones who were taking it were ones who happened to be accident prone. Cannabis was a useful indicator to test for other drugs. About half of these positive cases showed the presence of stimulants and related drugs.

Bergöö: I think cannabis is a major problem on its own, it may hang around for six weeks. You may smoke it in private but it is still with you in working time.

Francis: Do you routinely screen your autopsy subjects?

Calder: I have certainly found cannabis in some offshore workers, but not divers, and a few other drugs as well. It did not necessarily play any immediate part in the accident but it is difficult to work this out.

Masarik: We do routine screening for drugs and we find cannabis but we have a legal problem. What do you do with the results afterwards?

McIver: That is an individual and national problem.

The next question is: "The clinical assessment after an episode of neurological DCI can be related to evidence of individual "bends-susceptibility", length of latency before onset, extent and nature of manifestations, rate of response to recompression, completeness of recovery. What is the evidence that these have a bearing on future fitness to dive?"

Francis: I would like to pass on "bends-susceptibility" because I have no hard evidence. As far as latency is concerned, yes I do have some figures which come from the Institute of Naval Medicine (INM) database, data which are available thanks to the co-operation of the British Hyperbaric Association. There are now some six hundred diving accidents in the database and we have examined those of 1991, 1992 and 1993 who have been given a diagnosis of acute decompression illness, decompression sickness or arterial gas embolism. All had neurological manifestations and they were treated on an oxygen treatment table. We looked at the time to onset of the first manifestation, be it neurological or other. We excluded cases where there was no onset data, where the time of onset was greater than 24 hours, where it had resolved before treatment began or if there was no recording of the outcome. Thus the total number of cases in this particular study is 149.

Cases with motor manifestations and a time to onset of less than 30 minutes, have a 36% complete recovery after the first treatment. This is not yet quite statistically significant but it is approaching a difference of a 5% level from other cases, without motor involvement, who have a time to onset of 30 minutes or greater. Thus it does seem that if one has motor manifestations with rapid onset one is less likely to make a complete recovery than if one has sensory or non-motor manifestations and a longer latency. In the latter category 63% made a complete recovery on the first treatment. If one has a motor manifestation one is likely to have an onset of less than 30 minutes (39 cases out of 55) whereas those without a motor manifestation only 48 out of 94 came on within 30 minutes.

McIver: Is there any evidence from that bearing on future fitness to dive?

Francis: If someone has made a complete recovery from neurological decompression illness, then I am quite happy to let them go back to diving. Where there are residua it is quite clear that there is residual injury and then they should not go back into diving. That is explained to the individual on the grounds that they have reduced their reserve and severely damaged their neurological system.

McIver: If a person has a neurological bend without residua and then has another episode of neurological DCI, which was treated and again without residua?

Francis: One might want to take a look at what this person is doing, whether his dive was provocative. If, however, they were totally innocent divers they may be "bends-susceptible", made a complete recovery after the second insult, they may have some further damage to their nervous system but less obviously than somebody who has not made a recovery. Therefore I would not have any difficulty in sending them back to diving. If they had a third or fourth incident, I would then want to reconsider them.

McIver: If now objectively there is no abnormality but he still has vague symptoms, how would you feel about that?

Francis: Symptoms but no observable abnormality? Does he have a psychological problem with going back to diving? I would not force them to go back to diving.

Elliott: I would like to hear Dr. Dick's experience about this, the two questions are very important. There is a tendency among Approved Diving Doctors that if a person has had two neurological hits he should be made permanently unfit to dive. If those neurological hits have been sensory only, and there was a prompt and complete recovery, then that disqualification seems unjustified. Secondly, there is also the occasional problem that a person after a neurological hit may have feelings of paraesthesia or even a problem equivalent to a post concussion syndrome, i.e. a post decompression syndrome. If those symptoms remain after an otherwise fully recovered neurological hit, is that justification to make the person permanently unfit?

Francis: Subjective symptoms only?

Elliott: Yes.

Francis: If it were real, rather than imagined, I do not think he would be fit to go back to diving.

Dick: This is a terrible question and you know it. If someone has residua after one or more episodes, it is the tip of the neurological iceberg. Would one find the kind of change that Ian has demonstrated at post mortem? If they have got abnormal motor signs they must fail and if they have only got significant sensory loss, they should not go back to diving. But you do see some that have only got a small patch and these people are very difficult. I do not know the answer I am afraid. One is concerned that the small area of sensory deficit on the ankle might hide some more extensive and sub-clinical damage.

Mebane: There was an individual trying to qualify as a scientific diver in the Virgin Islands who had had two episodes of neurological decompression illness for which he was not treated but they resolved spontaneously, so the physician took this diver out diving for a check-up personally! I wonder what the result would have been if the diver had then become permanently paralysed, but then that is the sort of thing people do.

Broome: Is there a role for psychological or psychiatric testing?

Lunn: I feel there is a role. Coming back to the post-concussional syndrome there has been a lot of discussion in the psychological and psychiatric literature about this collection of rag-bag things that are grouped together. To a certain extent it is an excuse for psychiatrists to avoid taking clinical responsibility. If one looks at those with minor head injury who did not need to be admitted for observation there is about 15% of them who developed neuropsychological impairment over the next 6 months. That is very much higher than one expected in an age-matched population. It is consistently the higher executive functions such as concentration, memory etc., that are affected. This dysexecutive syndrome does correspond to damage of the frontal lobe system or associated pathways. It may be that those divers who make a "recovery" but still have symptoms actually have a form of dysexecutive syndrome which has not yet been looked at. We have to take it a lot more seriously.

Elliott: Yes, it is the tip of an iceberg. There may be pathological changes associated with this but everyone has a number of scars from previous injuries. These scars do not necessarily cause a functional deficit. Let us not forget we have the diver's lifetime career ahead. If he is made unfit he is not necessarily going to get any insurance payout, so it is a very serious decision to be made. Although I am inclined in your direction, I do want to be sure that this will not affect his future quality of life or are we absolutely certain that he is now at greater risk for a more serious accident? Those are the two questions which one must answer before making him unfit.

Lunn: There is no hard data but those who have a dysexecutive syndrome are less likely to function adequately under stress. I would be less keen to give a blanket recommendation because there will be a vast range in a variety of individual cases. Each needs to be assessed individually. I think it may also affect the individual's quality of life, but it is a grey area. You must look at the impact that that will have on the individual.

Francis: With respect to the spinal cord there are some who make a very slow recovery over a period of weeks or months and we can be confident that in these individuals there is a substantial injury and this is a functional recovery. This person therefore has a very much less reserve for any future injury. Are we prepared to hazard that individual against a future insult?

Elliott: Or is the diver prepared to?

Francis: Yes. If it is a recovery that is taking some weeks or months, it is obviously a very much more severe injury than somebody who has recovery almost instantaneously.

Risberg: I would not want a diver to go back to diving after two incidents of decompression illness. I have a great problem as this is not compatible with the regulations which suggest that you should be disqualified only if you are a safety hazard to yourself or your buddy. This is a long term health question. There must be some reason why this individual has had two episodes of decompression illness. There are no hard facts but we must protect the diver.

Watt: I wanted to stress the importance of the rate of recovery. I have certainly passed people fit to dive after more than two episodes of neurological decompression illness, but the most important feature is the rate of recovery. A transient visual disturbance which responds completely during compression is a completely different question from somebody who has not recovered until six hours or six weeks after their decompression therapy. My second point is that we have looked at the distribution of decompression illness in divers who have attended for medical examination in Aberdeen. We know that there is a population of divers who seem to get bent more frequently. This does not necessarily mean that they are "bend prone", it may be a factor of the diving procedures.

McIver: I will now proceed with the question of: "What components of the routine neurological examination may be unnecessary annually? Are there components that require less frequent examination, at least until some specified age?" At the end of the 1993 meeting in Stavanger I asked Professor Aarli whether or not the Health & Safety Executive's recommendations for a neurological examination were in fact adequate. His reply was "yes, provided one looks at the lower spinal nerve roots as well". Professor McCallum has suggested that maybe the neurological examination should be taken outside the general practitioners' remit whereas I feel that, providing it is done competently, the examination should be done annually by the Approved Doctor.

Dick: I do not care who does the examination as long as it is done properly. The important thing is that the examiner has enough time to do it and he does enough to maintain expertise. There are elements of the neurological examination that could be left out, for example I very rarely do a cremasteric or anal reflex in general medical practice. However, it does establish a baseline for subsequent examinations.

McIver: Any additional comments or questions?

COMMENTARY

The available guidance (page 213) is not detailed and must be interpreted by the examining doctor on a largely theoretical basis. Several small changes were proposed, for example extending, from 10 to 30 minutes, the duration of loss of consciousness which would be disqualifying after head injury. Such a relaxation is based on studies of head injury data as predictors of subsequent epilepsy. This recommendation provides a useful illustration of where, for the benefit of the diver, evidence can replace an earlier theory which now seems to have been too cautious.

The assessment of fitness to return to diving following decompression illness is continued in the next session but, from this session, it seems that the emphasis will remain upon the skill and experience of the diving specialist to assess each individual acknowledging that much depends upon the attitude of the diver towards a resumption of diving.

Recognition of the psychoses and neuroses is difficult: mental illness is easily concealed by the subject and is widely underdiagnosed. There seems to be a need to develop tests that are highly sensitive, rather than very specific, that can be used to select those who need a detailed psychiatric investigation. However, there is no evidence that the absence of such tests has led to a significant incident in diving which can be related to mental illness.

Similarly, there are no good tests of a candidate's psychological fitness for diving. The present method seems to be by self selection. Developing a set of aptitude tests, to exclude the claustrophobic and others who are psychologically unfit for diving, may not be justifiable. There seems to be no reason to think that such tests would make an important new contribution to diving safety and, because the individual's response to a particular diving stress is impossible to predict, functional assessment might be an impossible target.

Some neuropsychometric evaluation at selected intervals may be of value epidemiologically, but this would be part of the health surveillance of divers for possible long term consequences of diving. This is discussed later.

RETURN TO DIVING AFTER UNFITNESS

Chairman: Dr. T. Nome

The recommendations from the Guidance Notes on "The Medical Examination of Divers" are:

> 46. *Intellectual and psychomotor performance changes may be the only abnormality in some forms of decompression sickness. A thorough initial assessment is therefore essential. After general assessment, detailed examination should be made of the cranial nerves, motor system, sensation, reflexes and co-ordination. The examination guide is not considered exhaustive in terms of specialist neurological examination but is a screening examination. Any abnormality will require more detailed investigation and may require a specialist neurological opinion.*

HSE "Health Notes" : *RETURN TO COMMERCIAL DIVING AFTER EPISODES OF CENTRAL NERVOUS SYSTEM DECOMPRESSION SICKNESS*

Central Nervous System Decompression Sickness (CNS DCS) in commercial divers is now uncommon. In determining fitness to return to commercial diving after an episode of CNS DCS, it would seem appropriate to investigate not only the characteristics of the dive and decompression leading up to the incident, but, where appropriate, factors in the diver which may have acted to increase susceptibility. It will also be important to establish the degree of recovery in CNS function.

Research carried out - mainly on recreational divers, suggests that the presence of a right to left shunt due to Patent Foramen Ovale (PFO) may be one indication of susceptibility to CNS DCS.

Sophisticated investigations of CNS function following CNS bends - again mainly in recreational divers, have indicated more extensive interference in function than might have been anticipated by symptoms or clinical signs.

We therefore advise that commercial divers who have suffered CNS DCS should be referred by approved diving medical examiners for assessment by a diving medical specialist. The diving medical specialist may wish to arrange for the performance of sophisticated tests of CNS function and/or investigation for the presence of intracardiac shunt. Whether or not these investigations were offered to an individual diver would depend on the clinical judgement of the specialist and the consent of investigation following acute illness having implications for cardiac or cerebral function. Whilst Approved Doctors are asked to make referrals for assessment in these cases, the decision on fitness for diving work will remain with the Approved Doctor.

It is believed that PFO exists to some degree in about a quarter of the normal population of the U.K., and hence of divers, without apparent ill effect. Wholesale screening of the diving population does not seem justified in the present state of knowledge.

Similarly, present knowledge of the significance of findings from sophisticated investigations of CNS function does not support their use in screening of apparently fit divers who have not suffered CNS DCS.

RETURN TO DIVING AFTER SURGERY OR ACCIDENTAL INJURY
Professor D.H. Elliott

Fitness to return to diving is something for which there cannot be any prescribed standard. Each case must be assessed on its own merits in relation to a possible resumption of diving. The difficulties of functional assessment by any doctor are related to having sufficient knowledge and experience of that diver's working environment. The doctor must know the tasks which the diver is expected to perform and the hazards which he may have to deal with after his rehabilitation and return to diving. If there is any doubt then the doctor should get the advice from someone who understands that particular type of diving, somebody like a diving supervisor. A limited certificate might then be one of the appropriate options. Too often, it seems, the restriction is made in terms of a maximum depth limit, which is not always a meaningful restriction.

Two cases that can be used to illustrate these principles have already been presented to previous "Fit to Dive" meetings and therefore will be given here only in summary. Each appears at first to be contrary to the advice given in the Guidance Note and illustrates the ability of a diving doctor within the regulations to give a restricted certificate for particular circumstances.

The first was a manager of a single buoy mooring and one of his tasks was to inspect the work being done by the diving contractor. He lost one eye in an unrelated accident at home, but vision in two eyes are required by the Guidance. Monocular vision was deemed sufficient and he subsequently returned to diving with the condition, not unique to diving, that he took out adequate insurance against the loss of his other eye. It was also required that he dived only at that one location with which he was familiar.

The second case is that of a diving scientist who wished to continue diving which was an essential part of his research work, following a road traffic accident in which he became a paraplegic. His pulmonary capacity was not affected and he was given a restricted certificate that required him to have, at all times, a dedicated buddy responsible for his safety in the water. In fact that buddy also had the continuous task of ensuring that the vulnerable lower limbs were protected against abrasions. It should be added that this particular diver was an exceptional individual who subsequently trained war-wounded paraplegics to dive recreationally. His assessment of their fitness to train for this was primarily based upon lung function. He used the simple test of their ability to dive, breath-holding, to the bottom of the deep end of a swimming pool, find their breathing apparatus there and put it on. If they needed to be rescued, they were failed. This pragmatic approach illustrates very well as a functional test. Some years later this individual's regular diving doctor retired and he then experienced some difficulty with his new Approved doctor in retaining his annual HSE certificate of fitness. He remarked to me that he could not understand the problem. "After all", he said "I have less spinal cord to be at risk from bubbles than any other diver". He regained his restricted certificate and now, more than 20 years after his original road traffic accident, he continues to dive worldwide as a diving an active scientist.

These two provide, in contrast to prescriptive standards, reasonable examples of what is meant by individual assessment, particularly for the resumption of diving by experienced professionals.

RETURN TO DIVING AFTER ACCIDENTAL INJURY
Dr. S.J. Watt & Dr. D. Caughey

We have had experience of a number of divers who have suffered significant injuries while diving and who have wished to return to diving thereafter. Many of these are hand or upper limb injuries. One diver's hand was snared in a wire loop resulting, eventually in amputation of the index, middle and ring figures leaving the diver with grossly impaired function in his dominant hand and he abandoned his diving career.

Rather more difficult was a suction injury to the ring and little finger of a right dominant hand. This diver ultimately required partial amputation of these fingers but, despite some loss of function, he maintained normal use of the first three and most important digits and has been able to return satisfactorily to diving. The last comment means he was firstly passed fit by an Approved Doctor and has been reported to have no difficulty in the water by the supervisor who had a particular remit to assess his function.

The last point is crucial - in these situations it is often necessary to have a practical test at the worksite rather than try to make a decision in the surgery. Partly to illustrate this as well as a number of other important issues in management of these patients I wish to present the following case.

> A 40 year old diver working at 150 msw suffered a traumatic amputation of his right arm at the level of mid-shaft of the humerus. His immediate management was remarkably straightforward and following decompression he was admitted to hospital for formal closure of the stump. As a one arm diver he was obviously unfit. It appears easy to make an early assessment that the victim will never dive again. However, we should be considering the rehabilitation of the victim from the moment of injury and carefully managing potential post-traumatic stress.
>
> This man expressed his determination to continue diving and in the overall management of his rehabilitation which progressed at some speed, it seemed inappropriate to terminate his hopes until he had genuinely come to terms with his physical limitations. He apparently accepted that he would not be able to return to saturation diving because of inability to undertake rescues as a standby diver. He started to train as a supervisor.
>
> To do this work he required an offshore fitness certificate. By now he had demonstrated a remarkable ability to undertake a wide range of activities (driving, building work etc.) all before he had access to any prosthesis. As part of an assessment of his fitness to work offshore he attended a survival training course. He did this before he had a prosthetic limb. The basis of this assessment was that if he could achieve a standard as good as the worst of those with 4 limbs who passed the course, it was not reasonable to refuse him a certificate. The trainers were very doubtful about his ability, that they agreed to refund the course fee when he was unsuccessful. The result was an outstanding success and thereafter he went back offshore to work as a life-support technician. By now, unfortunately, it was clear from his general temperament that he was not a suitable candidate for further training as a supervisor and he therefore returned home.
>
> However, he returned after about two months to request a diving medical examination. In the interim he had satisfied himself that he could dive and had undertaken a limited

number of harbour dives abroad working for himself. We agreed to undertake the medical examination, only on the basis that any certificate would have major restrictions. Following examination we undertook discussions with several people for advice. As a result of the consensus view he was offered a certificate with the following restrictions: unfit to act as a standby/bellman diver and limited to dive situations where supervisor agrees he is competent to perform task required. The objective was to allow him to continue to undertake the very limited activities of his own business.

However, he changed his mind and refused a certificate with any restrictions. Perhaps we should have certified him as unfit immediately after his accident, but I think that he ultimately reached the correct decision himself and that coming to terms with his disability was an integral part of his overall rehabilitation.

In conclusion, following injury:

1. Divers require to have the physical ability to undertake the necessary tasks - they do not necessarily need to be able to undertake them in the normal fashion. Physicians may not be the best assessors: other divers or supervisors may be more helpful.

2. We must consider the psychological effects of injury, i.e. the possibility of post traumatic stress, and offer appropriate counselling.

3. A rehabilitation programme should be planned from the start if there is any chance of returning to dive and if the diver wishes to return.

DISCUSSION

Nome (Chairman): The example given by Dr. Watt of the man who had his arm amputated at depth illustrates very well that the most important factor in a return to diving is indeed the personality and determination of the diver himself.

Elliott: A hand injury is important because it may affect the ability the tender to haul on a diver's hose and effect a rescue. It is these aspects of diving that may not be obvious to the examining doctor but which should be revealed if a functional assessment is done together with a diving superintendent.

Another complication of hand injury is alteration to the autonomic regulation proximal to the site of the injury and this may be associated with an intolerance of cold by the diver in the affected part. This can be demonstrated using thermographic techniques following a test exposure to cold. Without the infra-red technique one diver's story might not have been believed. Thus hand injuries are complex and need careful evaluation.

RETURN TO DIVING AFTER IN-WATER LOSS OF CONSCIOUSNESS
Dr. P.B. James

The commonest cause of loss of consciousness in commercial diving has been the supply of the wrong gas, either too little or too much oxygen. This is obviously a problem of mixed gas diving and not air diving. In hypoxia events take place very rapidly. In diving the percentage of oxygen must be reduced as depth increases. Under the circumstances of a 300m dive, as little as 1.9% oxygen will provide a pO_2 of 0.6 bar, three times the mass of oxygen that is breathed at sea level. With such low percentages the boundary between respirable and non-respirable is small and there is a need for meticulous accuracy.

HYPOXIA

The problem in one particular case was generated by the gas supply to the diver which was from a hose supplied by a machine that mixed the gas as it was required. When the machine runs low on oxygen and the limit is reached, an audible alarm should ring. In this case, the system was running so close to the margin, the alarm kept on being triggered and so the topside crew had switched it off. The oxygen supply ran low and the diver, who recognised the onset of hypoxia from his previous experience with mixed gas apparatus in the navy, swam back to the bell but lost consciousness on the way. The standby diver tried to rescue him but breathed the same mixture so there was a period of extreme confusion. However, the standby diver switched over to emergency gas and hauled the first diver back into the bell by his umbilical but there was a delay of about 16 minutes. This particular individual made a successful recovery and returned to diving but this could easily have been a double fatality.

In considering a fitness to return to diving in these circumstances one is really considering fitness after cerebral oedema. The problem in making an assessment after an incident like this is, how long does the local injury in the brain persist? The assessment of brain function is difficult.

A second case with a similar outcome occurred when the diver became asphyxiated by a rope which became wrapped very tightly around his chest. After recovery to the bell, he was in coma with fixed dilated pupils. The oxygen level was then kept high and about 20 hours later the eyelids moved. He had some pulmonary oedema but over the next six hours he appeared to make an almost full recovery. How is the effect of hypoxia to be assessed? The neurological assessment of decompression sickness and gas embolism by Curley *et al* (1988), is a relevant paper. Though these changes may be different from simple hypoxia, the common denominator is that of cerebral damage. The U.S. Navy quote this paper as the basis for their policy of further hyperbaric oxygen treatments in any person who after a decompression accident has any evidence of a focal abnormality or perhaps a change of personality. This paper evaluated 4 cases by the use of psychometric tests and they may be appropriate for the assessment of those who have suffered hypoxia.

OXYGEN TOXICITY

An extreme example of exposure to oxygen occurred in 1976 when a diver was given pure oxygen to breathe at 78 m. On the tape recording of the incident it is possible to hear the change of gas as the oxygen creates greater resistance within the demand valve of the breathing apparatus than did the oxy-helium, which was the mixture he was initially breathing. After about 30 seconds the diver tries to communicate to the surface but the helium voice unscrambler was adjusted for helium and so the pitch of the voice was lowered greatly. The time to his actual convulsion was just over 6 minutes and occurred after he had been recovered into the bell. In fact the convulsion occurred about 20 to 30 seconds after his helmet had been removed: the so-called oxygen-off effect.

An oxygen fit in the bell is reasonably secure because there need be no change of pressure and the diver can breathe from the atmosphere of the bell. In contrast, an oxygen fit in the water is potentially dangerous because the diver may lose his breathing apparatus and if ascent occurs when the glottis is closed, there is the additional risk of pulmonary barotrauma. There appear to be no long term sequelae of oxygen convulsions.

LOSS OF CONSCIOUSNESS DUE TO TRAUMA

A saturation diver, whose face-plate was blown in by an underwater explosion, had the presence of mind to open his bypass for plenty of gas before he lost consciousness which prevented drowning. This individual therefore suffered from a blast injury with a pneumothorax, and near-drowning due to the inhalation of water. He was kept at his storage depth for about 10 days breathing intermittently high levels of oxygen. He made a good recovery and decompressed successfully. He made a complete recovery and returned to diving.

CARBON DIOXIDE

Unintentional rebreathing can lead to carbon dioxide retention. This has occurred with gas reclaim systems. When the diver is recovered to the bell or returns to a normal breathing pattern, his recovery is very rapid.

The factors which increase carbon dioxide retention in diving are:

- increased respiratory dead-space
- increased respiratory work load
- increased thoracic blood volume
- increased inspired pO_2
- exercise
- hydrostatic pressure
- cold

Carbon dioxide retention was first investigated by Haldane in 1905 because of episodes of loss of consciousness in hard hat diving. He recommended a free-flow rate into the old-fashioned standard helmet very much greater than had been used previously. CO_2 build up can also occur in rebreathers that have a soda-lime scrubber but with demand breathing apparatus carbon dioxide is not possible.

CONCLUSION

I think there is a place for neuropsychological assessment after in-water loss of consciousness, more so than for neurological assessment which cannot reveal subtle changes in intellectual function.

REFERENCE

Curley, M.D., Schwartz, M.J.C. & Zwingelberg, K.M. *Undersea Biomed. Res.*, 1988; **15:** 223-236.

DISCUSSION

Elliott: The cases presented by you were predominantly of mixed-gas divers. Would you please also consider deep air divers and comment on the so-called "carbon dioxide retainers" and the possible association of that with "deep-water blackout"? A number of open circuit compressed air divers swimming hard at depth in excess of 50 m have passed into unconsciousness. The factors of CO_2 retention, oxygen toxicity and nitrogen narcosis are considered to be synergistic.

James: The basic evidence for CO_2 retainers is controversial. I don't see how one can distinguish between the other contributory factors. I agree that these incidents are not easy to resolve but I agree it is important to point out that loss of consciousness can occur on open-circuit compressed air.

Welslau: Are CO_2 retainers generally unfit to dive? Are they unfit after a blackout in-water? Are they unfit when reporting frequent hour-long headaches as the only symptoms? Would you see a difference between professional and recreational divers regarding fitness to dive?

James: There appears to be little evidence to support the concept of carbon dioxide retention in diving (see Donald, 1992). Clearly the response to carbon dioxide will vary slightly from person to person but only within close limits. The use of breathing apparatus will tend to increase carbon dioxide levels which will have an effect on diving with enriched oxygen mixtures and may also be relevant to nitrogen narcosis. The increase in the liability to oxygen convulsions with increased levels of exercise is well known. Loss of consciousness due to nitrogen narcosis has occurred in dives to 30 m. Clearly someone who is susceptible to this effect should be limited in depth.

REFERENCE

Donald, K.W. *Oxygen and the diver*. Hanley Swan, Worcs: SPA. 1992.

POST-TRAUMATIC STRESS DISORDER
Dr. M.R. O'Connell

Before we begin to talk about the particular disorder on the agenda, it is necessary to state that the military psychiatrist is more concerned than are his colleagues in hospital psychiatry with occupational psychiatry: keeping persons at work and, where necessary, restoring them to full duty. The military psychiatrist is not involved in the selection of individuals for particular jobs, with which this conference is primarily concerned, but with those who are subject to trauma, and as soon and as close as possible to that incident in order to get them back to duty. The majority of people who I see therefore are those who are not able to cope with such stress. I was pleased to hear in the previous presentations about the diver who was hoping to cope even though he had lost his arm. That sort of individual does not need a psychiatrist. So the first question to ask is how does the average person cope with the stress of trauma.

A post-traumatic stress disorder (PTSD) is a result of:

- a realistic traumatic event
- the perception of potential danger to life or limb
- an intense activation of the autonomic nervous system

these last two may occur before, during or after the event.

It is important to realise that what we are dealing with is not a true illness but a mis-management of perfectly naturally feelings. Many lessons have been learned from civilian disasters. After the tragedy of the Herald of Free Enterprise a study of coping strategies among the divers was proposed. This was to include divers of the Belgium, Dutch and British Navies but none of the divers were prepared to volunteer because they felt their future livelihood might be at risk.

In a collage produced by a Piper Alpha survivor, a diver, he uses the words "grief, guilt, anger, confusion, depression and despair". Another Piper Alpha diver said "am I going crazy down here?" We used this collage therapy in the fourth week of a post-traumatic stress (PTS) management programme to allow them, perhaps for the first time, to bring out many of the issues that they had previously avoided. They then have to describe what they have put into their collages to their colleagues and we video-record this. At this stage they learn that their recovery will continue perhaps for the rest of their lives.

A significant proportion of those with post-traumatic stress enter a period of depression which is perhaps the most common diagnosis after a multiple disaster. This kind of depression, though possibly reactive, needs active intervention and counselling alone is not sufficient. In, for example, a fireball situation the individual senses may be suddenly overloaded. Subsequently the memories of what was heard, seen, smelt and felt may return to the individual, recurringly.

The emotional needs of rescuers include the need to express:

- guilt over not rescuing more
- anxiety over being survivors themselves
- anger over weather or hostile forces
- resentment over lack of praise from survivors

It must not be forgotten that the media who cover such events are also at hazard.

The emotional needs of survivors include the need to express:

- relief at escape
- anxiety over the future
- fear of further trauma
- anger
- loss of companions - grief
- guilt over survival

From my experience of the very few commercial divers that I have seen, I understand that they do not work in significant teams but nevertheless have developed relationships in their work. Anger is probably the most difficult emotion to deal with. This is compounded if the anger is directed towards one's boss.

The basic philosophy of military psychiatry revolves around a statement by Dr. Salmon in 1917 that "the closer to the front line and the sooner you identify your psychological casualties, the sooner you can expect that the majority of them are going to return to duty, and the lower is the incidence of long-term psychiatric illness". This is the basis for the theme "PIE" (Proximity, Immediacy, Expectancy). In the diving industry therefore I would recommend a similar principle: "SPRINT" (Special Psychological Rapid Intervention). SPRINT is the military response to disaster, a team who can go rapidly to the site of an incident.

Following the earlier discussions this morning I was interested in the concept that if one's morale is maintained, then there is a very much better chance of returning to what is a potentially threatening environment. Morale is the "general sense of well-being felt by the group with confidence in their ability to survive environmental stress, faith in their leader, and an overall sense of cohesiveness amongst their number". As far as I am concerned the most important word is "leader".

DISCUSSION

Elliott: This is the first time in our "Fit to Dive" meetings that we have considered PTSD in relation to diving accidents. My concern is that you have presented a very simplistic scale from coping to not coping. When one is seeing a diver after he has had a severe incident himself or he may have seen a buddy killed, and he <u>appears</u> to be coping, how do you assess very quickly that he has not got it all bottled up and it will all collapse the next time he goes into the water?

O'Connell: I do not know, but I will tell you what I do. I make sure that I see his partner. As more often than not he or she is more likely to give you the whole picture, including the picture that the subject may be concealing. I put up that definition of 'Morale' because my understanding of divers, and I liken them to the special services in the military, is that to get to their degree of expertise one must have a tremendous belief in oneself and that implies a very high morale. If morale is impaired for any reason, and in our example we return to duty successfully about one third of our uniformed personnel whereas the rate of recovery of those who are not in the services is very much less because there is a less perfect system. The system in which they operate may have less confidence than that within the services. Among the divers who we saw from the Piper Alpha, they are being referred to us again as a tertiary referral, their morale and their belief in their backup had been significantly impaired by their experience to the point that they believed themselves to be unfit to dive. We have to accept that divers are professionals who, at the end of the day, must make the professional decision as to whether or not they are themselves fit to dive. There is no test but if you have not interviewed a significant "other" you have not completed your assessment.

Douglas: How does one prevent PTSD in relation to mere drowning and also perhaps prevent inappropriate litigation after the treatment of a decompression disorder?

I will illustrate that with a case from a commercial diver who had a near-drowning episode and was rescued. He had no physical residua and there was a lot of pressure from the diving school to put him back into the water. He then completed his diving course successfully and, after two years of commercial diving, he was then diagnosed as having PTSD with flashbacks and alleged that he was unable to continue his diving career. There was an out of court settlement with a very substantial sum. I have often wondered whether my decision to allow him back to diving so soon was correct.

The second illustration is that of the treatment of severe neurological decompression illness, a near-wheelchair experience. During the acute phase I often see an acute grief reaction with denial, guilt, anger etc. Sometimes when these people are sent to a specialist centre for further investigation where the grief reactions are not properly managed and that is when the sniff of litigation comes into the air. I would like some practical advice please, on the prevention of PTSD in such cases.

O'Connell: The more I see of PTSD the less sure I know what it is. The more I see people with this condition the less certain I am that they are going to recover completely. Certainly we are now beginning to see relapses in people about whom we had made some very confident statements. I would advocate getting people back into the water similar to the old adage that you must get back up on the horse after a fall. I saw a pilot about two years ago who was awarded a bravery award for his time in the South Atlantic. He presented again when he took up a position similar to that that he had occupied previously, except at a more senior level. Within 36 hours he had a panic anxiety state with all the hallmarks of PTSD. By the time he got back to see me he had worked out what the problem was. In 1982 he was single but in 1989 he was married with one and a half children, and the pressures applying to him were significantly different to those that occurred previously. The difference with coping and non-coping may therefore be a very small addition to circumstances.

I would like to know therefore what might have transpired in the diver who had his relapse two years after the original incident. It may have only been a very small trigger. I would certainly encourage though that you get a diver back into the water as soon as possible after an incident associated with the water.

IMAGING TECHNIQUES
Dr. F.W. Smith

It is my purpose to tell you about the newer imaging techniques in the demonstration of brain and their potential for showing function. Based upon the imaging methods used in the dementing disorders, one may use x-ray, particularly computerised tomography (CT scan) which is a good screening procedure, relatively inexpensive and widely available, but non-specific. Magnetic resonance imaging (MRI) is relatively expensive and of limited availability. Its specificity is not proven, but it is superior to CT for showing morphology and metabolism. Single photon emission computed tomography (SPECT) is inexpensive, widely available, can demonstrate metabolism but its specificity is not proven.

The cost of MRI has now come down and the cost of examination is about the same as a CT scan. MRI specificity is not proven, particularly when we use different pulse sequences. The new and more modern applications of MRI e.g. echo-planar imaging may allow us to learn something about the images of the brain made in about 30 milliseconds and allow us to learn something about cerebral perfusion. This may begin to give us a handle on metabolism because of changes that can be seen between eyes open and eyes closed and when a loud noise is made.

X-RAY C.T.

X-ray C.T. is good for demonstrating:

- Ventricular size
- Cerebral atrophy
- Space occupying lesions
- Infarction
- Ischaemic changes

MAGNETIC RESONANCE IMAGING

Magnetic resonance imaging quality is superb. Depending on the pulse sequences that one chooses one is able to highlight grey matter, white matter or the ventricular system. One can see blood vessels as flow voids or one can use a system that enhances a signal from the flowing blood and suppresses that from the brain and displays the arterial and venous system within the skull. However it is a sensitive technique and one can see abnormalities without knowing their cause, which may be for example an old virus infection. An MRI picture shows how sensitive the technique is, the brain slice may be 4 mm and the pixel-size is small and there are 250 pixels per square cm so very small lesions and demyelinisation can be seen.

Thus if MRI is to be used for specific diagnostic criteria, the conditions must be standardised. At the present time the resolution is not good enough to see small lesions within the spinal cord.

REGIONAL CEREBRAL BLOOD-FLOW

The assessment of regional cerebral blood-flow has developed over the last 9 or so years. It may be performed by the following methods:

- ^{133}Xenon,
- Xenon enhanced x-ray C.T.,

- Positron emission tomography (P.E.T.) and
- Single photon emission tomography (S.P.E.C.T.)

^{133}Xenon is the most accurate method of measuring cerebral blood-flow but does not produce an image. Xenon enhanced C.T. had a short period of popularity but is difficult, a bit expensive and is not readily available. Positron Emission Tomography has been the way forward where one can use short life isotopes such as oxygen, hydrogen, fluorine as labelled water or as fluorinated de-oxy glucose to study regional cerebral blood-flow. This is at present limited to 3 facilities in the U.K. and is expensive.

Single Photon Emission Tomography (S.P.E.C.T.)

This gives reasonable morphological information and a display of regional cerebral blood flow distribution. The commonly used radio pharmaceuticals are ^{123}I-Iodoamphetamine and $^{99}Tc^m$-Hexamethyl Propylene Amine Oxime (HMPAO).

^{123}I-Iodoamphetamine is not readily available whereas $^{99}Tc^m$-HMPAO is available in every nuclear medicine department in the country. HMPAO is administered by injection and is taken up by the cerebral grey matter and basal ganglia on the first pass. The data is collected by a gamma camera for 3 dimensional reconstruction. One can use the technique to section the brain in each of the 3 main planes using relatively crude images on a colour display and from that to surmise what the cerebral regional blood-flow is. It is not possible to quantify this uptake.

The majority of people working with HMPAO will display their images on a colour scale.

CEREBROVASCULAR DISEASE

Each centre using HMPAO in the United Kingdom is probably doing it with a different combination of gamma camera and data processing unit. Very few centres will produce images which are comparable to images made in other centres. The work that has been performed on patients with stroke has demonstrated that HMPAO is useless at differentiating occlusive disease from haemorrhage or tumour. It has indicated that we can show areas of no-flow but that can be deduced from the clinical picture.

DEMENTIA

From P.E.T. studies using unfluorinated de-oxy glucose it has been shown that there are different uptake patterns by cerebral grey matter between those patients that had a true Alzheimer's disease and those that had a vascular based multi-infarct type of dementia. So there is a place in psychiatry for using this technique in order to separate these two types of dementia.

DIVING ILLNESS

A large number of divers have been studied using HMPAO. Some of the findings have been quite abnormal and worrying since, clinically, many of the divers appeared to be normal. For example:

> **MR. G.M.:** 19 year-old male diver from Scapa Flow who treated himself for the bends during a weekend diving there and came in complaining of dizziness, some vertigo and feeling sick, had numbness in the right foot, tingling in the right hand. The HMPAO scan appeared identical to the Alzheimer picture. He improved over the next week or so, and psychological testing later was normal.

Now finally, some scans of divers have been studied, comparing HMPAO appearances with their diving history, their alcohol history, tobacco and drug use and with any other appropriate parameter. No correlation was found between those that appear normal and those that do not. In some individuals there are areas of decreased flow in the fronto-parietal region which were considered to be abnormal. However, the patient may have no neurological deficit and no psychological upset. So is one to stop him diving?

Another individual was psychologically normal and had no neurological deficit but he had had a bend. In the motor region there was good uptake but in the parieto-temporal area there was patchy uptake, and then it became normal again. There are a certain number of divers who will give this appearance, there is no correlation between this and their physical findings, social history or even their diving history. This one observation is not sufficient to stop a person from diving.

There was one diver who had suffered decompression sickness, his original brain scan was very patchy, more abnormal than the previous individual, and was followed up six months later when he was feeling a lot better, physically fit and well. One can still see the apparent perfusion deficits. The scan is no better, but the patient is.

The next case with a similar story, is fit and well and has a patchy appearance on HMPAO through the parieto-temporal region while the motor cortex is essentially normal. In contrast an 87 year old following a transient loss of power in her right arm and scanned 4 days later has an essentially normal HMPAO for somebody 87 years old. It is certainly a lot better than the previous 4 divers. I do not know what that means. Until we are able to follow these men and, when they have a fatal accident, be sure that we can compare HMPAO results with autopsy results, we will not know.

We are not in a position that we should stop somebody from diving merely on the grounds of an abnormal HMPAO study. It is a non-specific study which gives very elegant pictures, pictures we can draw inferences from, but its findings are not proven.

REFERENCES

Evans, S.A., Thomson, L.F., Smith, F.W. & Shields, T.G. $^{99}Tc^m$-HMPAO-SPECT imaging in divers. Pp 175-185 in: *Proceedings of the XVIIth Annual Meeting of the European Underwater Biomed. Soc.* EUBS: Heraklion. 1991.

Evans, S.A., Ell, P.J., Smith, F.W. & Shields, T.G. ^{99}Tc-HMPAO-SPECT in diving illness. *Long Term Health Effects of Diving; an international consensus conference, Godøysund.* NUTEC: Bergen. 1994. Pp 65-73.

EVOKED POTENTIALS
Dr. D.J. Dick

I had intended to confine my comments to evoked potential studies but in view of yesterday's interest in the EEG I would like to start by saying a few words about the electroencephalogram. The E.E.G. shows the following rhythms:

>   Alpha   8 Hz
>   Theta   4 - 5 Hz
>   Delta   is even slower

There is also a fast rhythm which is occasionally seen called Beta which is usually connected with drug use such as benzodiazepines. Abnormal EEG's are either abnormal in rhythm or activity. The interpretation of EEG is subjective and should be left to experts. There are three major reasons for these difficulties:

1. individual variation
2. natural changes according to age
3. variation with the time of day and according to recent meals, hangovers etc.

There is also a considerable overlap between normal and abnormal. Epileptic abnormalities may be found in perfectly normal persons who have never had a seizure. The EEG is not useful as a screen after decompression to look for epileptiform complications or evidence of central complications.

SOMATO SENSORY EVOKED POTENTIALS

In clinical practice evoked potentials are usually used for the diagnosis of multiple sclerosis. They include the visual evoked potential, the brain stem evoked potential (auditory), the somatosensory evoked potential and the P300 which is a useful research tool. Today we will deal with somato sensory evoked potentials which are generated by stimulating a peripheral mixed nerve in the upper limb, median or ulnar, and in the lower limb usually the posterior tibial. To record the signal there is a spinal electrode and a cortical array of electrodes. The stimulus is repeated many times and averaged to give a trace and from this can be derived the central sensory conduction time.

>   EP's change at depth
>   SSEP's change at extreme depth
>   SSEP's: - abnormal in DCS
>   - latency increased
>   - amplitude decreased

From the diving literature one can conclude that the evoked potentials can change at depth particularly in the visual and brain stem but these are reversible and are normal on return to atmosphere. The somato sensory evoked potentials may be abnormal in decompression sickness and James Francis has used both latency and amplitude to study this in dogs.

Of the 9 divers with abnormal SEP's described by Yiannikes (1988), 6 were neurologically normal on examination and so they suggested that the SEP was sensitive enough to pick up subclinical damage. However Overlock (1989) in a separate study, found the only abnormalities were in 4 divers confined to wheelchairs while 9 of those with abnormal signs had normal SEP's. It is difficult to reconcile these two extremes but there is a certain degree of variability between laboratories. They need to be standardised for height which was not done in all these studies. One must also remember that the SEP's measure the sensory tracts and many of the disabilities are motor. So far the evidence is rather mixed and further investigation with standardised techniques is required.

MAGNETIC CORTICAL STIMULATION

The cortical stimulation is a technique for stimulating the motor pathways. A coil is placed over the head and a DC current discharged through it. Due to the sudden discharge a magnetic field is generated and a small current will be induced and cause neurones to be activated. It is not a comfortable technique for the subject. Electrodes are then put on to peripheral muscles such as the thenar eminence and then evoked potentials can be used to measure central motor conduction time.

I have looked at a few divers who have had abnormal motor signs after an episode of neurological decompression illness and the findings are not terribly convincing. Technically it is quite difficult to do the study on the lower limb.

REFERENCES

Overlock, R. et al. *Undersea Biomed. Res.* 1989; **16** (Suppl.): 89.

Yiannikas, C. & Bevan, N.A. *Clin. Exp. Neurol.* 1988; **25**: 91-96.

DISCUSSION

Boonstra**: Is it possible to predict if an O_2 fit is imminent if we have an EEG running on a patient breathing 100% oxygen at increased pressures? Are there any data/studies available on alterations of EEG's in situations of hypoxia and hyperoxia? Do EEG changes occur before the patients get unconscious or get an O_2 fit? If these changes have been reported, what are they and do they have predictive value as to the occurrence of an O_2 fit/loss of consciousness?

Reply from Dick: The EEG will certainly have become abnormal prior to an oxygen toxicity fit. However, it may only show abnormalities in the 20 or 30 seconds prior to the seizure. If there was a longer prodrome of confusion prior to the seizure then it would be correspondingly abnormal for a longer period of time.

COGNITIVE FUNCTION TESTING FOLLOWING A DIVE INJURY
Dr. B. Lunn

When do you assess a diver for return to diving? I would argue that you should start at the time of recovery of the diver from the water. There is some suggestion that complex cognitive function testing should not be given to the diver by someone without experience. I do not disagree but I would say that basic cognitive function testing is not difficult. In audio tapes presented by Dr. James, but not reproduced in the proceedings, we listened to people with degrees of cerebral damage and we were all making crude cognitive assessments. Cognitive assessments include the most simple assessments such as: is the patient conscious or not, is he oriented, has he got gross memory deficits? This level of assessment can be done by lay individuals, as long as they are adequately trained. It is quite possible that the technicians, bell superintendents and other divers can be trained to do cognitive testing as soon as the diver is out of the water, as soon as he is beginning to recover. What is difficult is interpretation. As long as the data is properly recorded it can be interpreted by somebody else later.

There are pen and paper tests that can be done without a great degree of understanding their theoretical basis. The difficulty comes when you get fairly subtle deficits. I would argue however, that it is not important at this stage of treatment. If any disorder is discovered it does not matter if the memory disorder is due to frontal lobe dysfunction, a pure memory loss or aphasia, it demonstrates that there is something that needs to be treated.

The next stage in assessing the diver is immediately following the initial recompression, when you think treatment is complete. Curley *et al* (1988) examined five subjects. Three of them were U.S. Navy sailors, two experienced divers, one a trainee, one was a male Coastguard who had made a chamber dive, and the fifth was a female U.S. Army technician who had been exposed by sudden decompression to an altitude of nearly 8,000 m. All developed manifestations of decompression sickness or gas embolism and all were treated in a recompression chamber. They were discharged from the recompression chamber and it was not until afterwards that it was realised that these people had residual problems. One for example could not write his own name and could not remember the names of his friends. It is amazing to me that these simple tests could not have been done before. It does not take complex neuropsychological tests to pick up such gross deficits. We must always look for neuropsychological deficits when divers are being treated.

The third stage of assessing fitness to return to diving is, perhaps, the most technical. This one should not be left to people who do not have a great deal of experience. There are two ways in which people may present which can be problematic. They may say "I want to go back to diving" and if you test them and find an abnormality you can be fairly sure that it is genuine, but you have to persuade them they cannot go back. The person, however, who claims to be disabled and has no demonstrable deficits is much more complicated. A criticism of one of the papers quoted yesterday is that the workers had been looking at divers who were involved in litigation.

I would like to tell you a story about a man who had gone through a lot of traumatic events:

> He is not a diver, however he does live in a village called Lockerbie. On the night that the aeroplane fell from the sky he and his wife, who is a nurse, went out to do whatever they could to help. His wife coped very well with it, but although he, as a lorry driver, had seen many accidents, he had never been so intimately involved. Following these events he was treated locally for post-traumatic stress disorder with some success.

Unfortunately a couple of years later he was driving his lorry down the A74 when he was hit from behind. His lorry rolled several times but he sustained no significant injuries. Again post-traumatic stress disorder was diagnosed but this time there was also an associated depressive disorder. Initially he seemed to be responding well to treatment but began to complain of memory loss and "blackouts". He was referred to Newcastle for assessment and his "blackouts" were diagnosed as migraine; however a clear cause for his memory problems was not forthcoming. The memory deficits did not follow a typical pattern and in the initial assessment were thought to be factitious. There was however, evidence on testing of a mild aphasia leading to a possible difficulty in disentangling poor performance due to an amnesic syndrome or aphasia, or indeed due to a functional disorder.

The point of this is that there are now tests available that will aid in the differentiation of organic and functional memory problems. In one of these tests the subject is shown a four digit number on a card then, following either a five or twenty second interval, a card with the original number and another card with a previously unseen number. The subject is then asked to identify the previously revealed number. In a subject with no recall or recognition memory there is a 50% probability that they would get the answer right (i.e. by chance) regardless of the time interval. The majority of the population believe that memory deteriorates over time but, when no element of interference is introduced and within the time limit used in this test, there is no deterioration.

The patient from Lockerbie got 40% right when there was a five second interval between the cards, perhaps indicative of an organic memory problem, but only got 10% right following a twenty second interval. So this man had recalled the numbers and had, consciously or unconsciously, selected the wrong responses. In other words his memory disorder was functional.

It is much more difficult to assess loss of concentration or mood swings. The main problem here is that the best way to elucidate such a history is to use an informant. The informant however may stand to gain from the subject being considered either fit or unfit to work.

In summary therefore we should, in the first instance, start performing neuropsychological assessments at the time of recovery of divers from the water. This will require adequate training of those personnel involved in this process. Secondly, we need to do a formal neuropsychological assessment when the individual completes recompression. This stage will require an experienced neuropsychologist or neuropsychiatrist to become involved. Finally the diver should be comprehensively assessed by an experienced and competent neuropsychiatrist prior to any return to diving.

REFERENCE

Curley, M.D., Scwartz, M.J.C. & Zwingelberg, K.M. *Undersea Biomed. Res.* 1988; **15**: 223-236.

DISCUSSION

Head**: There is proof of asymptomatic gliosis in brain/cord and of some psychometric changes with time related to depth exposure. Even in the diver with a full recovery from a decompression illness, surely they have a "residua" which is at the moment unquantifiable and immeasurable, but does that mean we can advise them to return to the water? Is this an acceptable occupational hazard that we can allow to continue until an overt clinical result appears?

Reply from Lunn: This is a difficult question. At the present level of knowledge I believe we are unable to do anything other than respond to overt signs of cognitive impairment. This "goal post" may well shift as our neuropsychology improves and becomes more focused. Our primary need is to delineate the long term consequences of diving, and only then will we have a rational basis for issuing recommendations.

PROBLEMS IN DIVING PATHOLOGY
Dr. I.M. Calder

The problem for pathologists is that we are very limited in the material we can acquire. We will begin with an accident in which a section of lung showed a lot of mucopus in the terminal airway. A trivial condition in a person who felt just "one degree under". This led to air trapping and he had a number of emphysematous blebs of quite long standing over the surface of the lung. These would have been of no consequence until there was a differential pressure, and the result was rupture of the blebs with arterial gas embolism. Trivial disease causing a major disaster.

The organs of special sense have received scant attention and are summarised by the quotation:

> "Of all the organs assigned to the use of animals, we have least knowledge of those of the senses ...."
>
> Du Verney: Traite de l'Organe de l'Quie (1683)

So far, from examination of the eyes of both men and experimental animals, little has been found. However the inner ear is a useful example. Some early electron microscopy studies showed changes to the hair cells of the inner ear. Further work using experimental animals showed the loss of hair cells suggesting that there is *prima facie* evidence of pathological change within the inner ear, due in fact more to compression than to decompression profiles. Human autopsy material does not lend itself to satisfactory electron microscopy.

From the histopathological aspect in the CNS, there are some firm elements of mechanism in the formation of damage. Minute gas bubbles within the small blood vessels show development of platelet aggregates on the intima. These can lead to mural thrombi and the ischaemia of tissues supplied by the vessel. In addition, the damage to the intima with loss of physiological integrity can allow the transudation of blood break-down elements in the perivascular tissues. The local changes of ischaemia range from oedema, through infarction to gliosis. With treatment it is possible to limit the damage, but the time zone for this is small. It has to be considered that recovery is due to re-education rather than regeneration of tissues.

The long-term effects of CNS damage may be reflected by the volume of tissues exposed. The brain with a weight of 1300 gm has the possibility of greater redundancy when compared with the spinal cord of 40 gm. This is further confounded by the fact that the white matter in the cord is the target organ, and this is approximately 25 gm. It is therefore not surprising that with a tissue weight ratio between brain and cord of 35.5 to 1 that injury manifests itself with greater effects in the cord.

There is *prima facie* evidence of small areas of infarction in the brains of divers of 0.2 cm with no observable functional or psychological effects. Much of the material available is rare and has to be treated with state of the art technology. In the single case of a well-documented case of decompression injury with HMPAO and followed by suicide, much of the value was lost by unsatisfactory autopsy techniques.

REFERENCE

Palmer, A.C., Calder, I.M. & Yates, P.O. *Neuropathol. Appl. Neurobiol* 1992; **18**: 113-124.

CRITERIA FOR RETURN AFTER DECOMPRESSION ILLNESS
Dr. T.J.R. Francis

The present revision for the multinational Diving Medical Advisory Committee (DMAC) of their Guidance was undertaken to put the old guidelines into the more modern terminology of decompression illness. It is not possible to lay down guidelines for every case because each one is different and so minimum lay-off periods have been produced relating to the different types of illness. There are also suggestions about recovery which were made this morning and these must be borne in mind. We are looking at minimum lay-off periods recommended after completion of successful treatment i.e. there are no residual manifestations as tested, as we have heard this morning. If we take category A, which might traditionally be called the less severe forms of decompression illness with uncomplicated recovery: minimum lay-off times are 24 hours before going back to diving. If however the treatment is not uneventful, there may be a recurrence or relapse requiring further recompression, then that time should be extended to a minimum of 7 days. In category B, the neurological or pulmonary manifestations (the old Type II decompression sickness), on the whole return to diving should only ever be after consultation with the company's diving medical adviser. The neurological category can be divided into cases with altered sensation only, where one can go back after at least 14 days, and the more serious neurological manifestations with a minimum lay-off period of 28 days.

TABLE 40 - FITNESS TO RETURN TO DIVING AFTER DECOMPRESSION ILLNESS

1. The following minimum lay-off periods are recommended after completion of successful treatment (there are no residual manifestations).

    A. Limb pain, cutaneous (skin rash with severe itching), lymphatic (swelling of tissues) or non-specific (persistent headache, excessive fatigue, loss of appetite, nausea), manifestations only.

i	With uncomplicated recovery	24 hours
ii	With recurrence or relapse requiring further recompression	7 days

    B. Neurological or pulmonary manifestations:

    (Return to diving only after review by the contractor's diving medical adviser)

i	Altered sensation involving the limbs, only	7 days
ii	Other neurological manifestations (including audiovestibular) or pulmonary manifestations	28 days

    C. After an incident of pulmonary barotrauma resulting in a pneumothorax or mediastinal/subcutaneous emphysema, the diver should be assessed by the contractor's medical adviser. Return to diving may be permitted, but not normally until at least 28 days following complete recovery.

2. In cases where there are residual manifestations, even after repeated treatment, the diver should be considered unfit to dive. Return to diving should only be permitted if sanctioned by the contractor's medical adviser.

DISCUSSION

Nome (Chairman): I would like to compare the new recommendations with the old. It is interesting to compare the changes made from the ones prepared about ten years ago:

Manifestations not needing treatment:

12 hours lay-off (but less if into deeper saturation)

"Type 1" full recovery:

24 hours (but less if into saturation); (after recurrence or relapse: 7 days)

"Type 2" full recovery:

>7 days (and review by an Approved Doctor);

Residua: NOT FIT

Pulmonary barotrauma: 3 months after a full recovery and assessment by an Approved Doctor

These guidelines are an example of prescriptive recommendations and they are currently under review by the Diving Medical Advisory Committee. I have given them as the basis for our revision, where we are coming from, and as James Francis has indicated there is definitely room for much improvement.

Elliott: Can James Francis please put his overhead (Table 40) up again. It has got there "treatment (there are no residual manifestations)". To me this means <u>clinical</u> manifestations but then you went on to say "as tested this morning" which implies therefore those special investigations, some of which are dubious at best. Could you please clarify whether or not by "residual manifestations" you meant primarily the purely clinical assessment of the individual at the end of treatment?

Francis: This morning we heard about different ways of assessing people and, in these circumstances, some may be indicated and some may not.

In the past we have looked at HMPAO but this proved to be unable to discriminate between normal and abnormal. We now no longer use it at all. At the moment we do not use any sophisticated tests but limit assessment to a clinical examination. MRI and other investigations are not specific for the decompression illnesses. If the individual is sound physically on examination then that should be sufficient.

Nome: What is the basis for temporary disqualification before a return to diving after recovery from decompression illness? James, could you deal first please with simple limb-bends.

Francis: The problem is that we don't know what is the mechanism of limb-bends. Does it include involvement of the nervous system? We know from the work of Ian Calder that people who have not had a decompression insult may have some abnormalities in the cord. This makes us very much more cautious in our recommendations for any return to diving. The element of caution is not based on scientific knowledge but a sense that, because we do not understand the condition, we should be more cautious than in the past.

Nome: In this session we have had some very good presentations on the use of advanced techniques and have learned perhaps, the reasons why they do not work. We have sound advice on what to do but, perhaps, not enough on when to do it? We need to be more aware of the possibility of long term damage and therefore we should perhaps send more divers for specialist investigation. This would have the additional advantage of giving the specialists a broader experience which is important for the maintenance of high quality training.

Wendling: Is it correct that we have agreed that one can examine for a PFO after neurological decompression illness, but this is not essential?

Francis: The PFO studies are difficult because they are not conclusive. They have shown that a diver with a bend has a greater chance of having a PFO than a diver who has not had a neurological bend, but one cannot turn that around to say that those with a PFO have got a greater chance of having a bend. To do that, one needs to perform a longitudinal study. We know that there are plenty of divers who do have a PFO who have dived successfully with no episodes of acute decompression illness. Thus to eliminate all divers who have a PFO would not make a lot of sense. Just because a person has had neurological decompression illness, I do not feel that should automatically demand an investigation for a PFO. If you find one what are you going to do?

Grönkvist[**]: A question for the Panel please. The discussion about fitness after a pulmonary barotrauma (PBT) with AGE dealt only with possible neurological sequelae. Is there an elevated risk for another episode of PBT after the first one? Does that risk differ if the mechanism is a properly performed ascent, a "spontaneous" PBT, or follows an emergency ascent where the performance is unclear? How do we deal with the pulmonary aspect of fitness after a PBT without clinical sequelae?

Reply from Elliott: The proposed DMAC advice is for a minimum period of 28 days of diving, whereas the existing advice ("pulmonary barotrauma") is for a 3-month rest period.

There is no hard evidence for either figure but certainly the intent is that this period without exposure to pressure changes should be sufficient to heal the lung. There is little or no evidence about the risk of a further episode but case histories suggest that if there is a recurrence then the manifestations are more severe. Hopefully, the collection of medical data in a central registry will provide us with hard data in due course.

It is generally thought that an undeserved pulmonary incident, i.e. one following a normal ascent, deserves a more cautious evaluation than one in an individual in whom the incident followed a buoyant ascent. A similar provocation would be the rare example of a shallow diver subjected underwater to the effects of significant wave action.

COMMENTARY

Much attention at Edinburgh was rightly given to the meticulous assessment of the candidate for initial diving training, and this review has extended throughout the various organ-systems.

An important additional feature of this meeting was that it also tackled the problems of the experienced diver and, in particular, the resumption of diving after a diving-related incident or period of unfitness. In relation to a return to diving, many general medical and surgical conditions have been reviewed in the earlier sessions but, to resume diving after trauma or a diving-related incident, was not covered. This assessment can rarely be made on the basis of pre-determined standards. The decision in each case should reflect those aspects of impairment which could affect future safety. To do this competently requires doctors who are knowledgeable about professional diving. The central collection of such cases for analysis and review would do much to resolve present uncertainties.

Post-Traumatic Stress Disorder

Problems arising after a stressful incident of any kind may be reported by the subject, friends or relatives, in which case the diagnosis of post-traumatic stress disorder (PTSD) should be considered and appropriate action taken. There is no requirement after each diving incident for routine psychological assessment of the specific potential for a PTSD. In most cases an early return to diving would be beneficial.

Return after Trauma

Because of the wide variety of possible residua from injury, a thorough knowledge of the diving tasks that may need to be undertaken by the individual is necessary for the medical assessment. In the assessment of, for example, hand injuries, thermography may be needed to determine the thermal sequelae in the region of the injury. Also for hand injuries, an example of a functional test is that of the ability of the diver to haul in a tended diver by hose or lifeline. The assessment may lead to the issue of a restricted certificate if appropriate. In specified circumstances divers with significant injury can be assessed positively: a paraplegic diver and a monocular diver have been returned to restricted diving work.

The effectiveness of appropriate decisions depends upon the breadth of knowledge and experience of the diving doctor in the relevant category of diving.

Return after Impaired Consciousness

Safe resumption of diving largely depends on the identification of the cause of the unconsciousness. Medical causes should be assessed on their own merits. If hypoxia was present, a return of full mental function must be assessed, including possible neuropsychological testing.

If oxygen toxicity can be identified as the cause of loss of consciousness, then there should be no reason to discontinue diving, but within the safe limits of oxygen neurotoxicity. Although CO_2 retainers can be identified among those who lose consciousness when working hard and breathing dense gases, tests of ventilatory response to inspired CO_2 are insufficiently discriminating to provide a practical pass/fail test.

Return after Decompression Illness

Clinical assessments of cognitive function are needed during and after a recompression. Testing cognitive function again is appropriate before a return to diving. These are usually simple clinical measures but could be enhanced by the development of a more specific protocol. A neuropsychometric evaluation should preferably be in reference to appropriate baseline of data for that individual.

The period of temporary unfitness to dive following a full recovery from a decompression illness depends on the nature of the manifestations and also on the rate of a complete recovery.

Those divers who have had two or more episodes of neurological decompression illness and who have made a full recovery can return to diving, though consideration may be given to the possibility of a PFO as a contributory factor. It is suggested that peripheral motor manifestations should regarded as more sinister in making a prognosis than purely sensory symptoms. Transient sensory disturbances are not a barrier to the resumption of diving.

An immediate clinical recovery before or during the recompression treatment would seem to support a favourable prognosis and a return to diving. If, however, the divers have some residual symptoms, such as parasthesiae, but no observable residua then, unless the diver is determined to continue diving, the consensus is that he should not be given a certificate of fitness.

The specificity of MRI examination, though better than x-ray CT, is not yet proven and its role in the follow-up of decompression illness has not yet been defined. HMPAO scanning in normal divers has shown no correlation between its results and any aspect of the decompression history or episode of decompression illness. Similar scans can be found in other conditions including drug abuse. Thus, in the absence of other clinical findings, there is no justification for disqualifying a diver only because of some "abnormality" in an HMPAO scan.

When neurological recovery takes weeks or even months, functional recovery may be due in a large part to a re-learning effect in the presence of persistent lesions. In these persons, who seem functionally fit to return to diving, the potential for serious sequelae from a subsequent incident should lead to consideration of the long-term health of the individual and the strong advice that person should give up diving. It needs to be recognised that this would not be a disqualification on the grounds of a lack of in-water safety. Where there is no evidence that a return to diving would be hazardous to the safety of that individual but only perhaps to his future health, the final decision should also take into account the views of that person on the effects of disqualification upon his or her quality of life and future earning capacity.

Cautious recommendations have been made on a theoretical basis by the Diving Medical Advisory Committee. These suggest specific minimum intervals but the emphasis will remain on the full and careful assessment of each individual case by suitably experienced diving physicians.

THE FUTURE HEALTH OF DIVERS

Chairman : Professor H. Örnhagen

TRAINING DOCTORS TO EXAMINE FOR FITNESS OF DIVERS
Dr. B. Minsaas

The goals in examining the physical fitness of divers are several and these will come in contradiction with each other because they are done for different reasons. In the current atmosphere of a new Europe with deregulation, it is time to take a closer look and may be even re-think the whole approach to the medical examination of divers. Do these examinations achieve anything useful? Do they improve the in-water safety of the diver? Do they provide increased knowledge of the long-term health factors of a diver? How do we train doctors to meet these concepts? There are many questions and this paper will try to answer some of them.

GENERAL LEGAL ASPECTS

Current legislation in the U.K. and Norway clearly states the need for a qualified MD to examine a working diver and evaluate whether he is, at the time of the examination, fit to dive.

U.K. Guidance, 7: *Approved Doctors must keep abreast of the developments in diving generally (including important changes in the legal and regulatory positions) as well as those in diving medicine.*

Norway, Diving Regulations, 83: *Personnel engaged in diving operations shall have a valid certificate from a medical practitioner confirming that he/she, in compliance with regulations issued by the Directorate of Health, has been found medically fit for this, based on an evaluation of whether the medical condition of the person in question represents a danger to himself or others.*

These regulations have been referred to throughout this meeting. I placed the emphasis on the overall goal of the medical examination : "in-water safety" has been employed and should be thought of as the "under-increased-ambient-pressure safety". We employed it extensively during our first sessions and then it disappeared into the more general terminology like "fit for work". It is time to bring it back.

"In-water safety" is based on a "statistical" probability of surviving and living under pressure without serious or debilitating illness resulting from increased ambient exposure. The concept of "fit for work" is more the individual's ability to perform a defined work task under these conditions.

This is underlined by the I.L.O. principle of adapting work to man and man to work. Norwegian legislation is based on the safety concept which is strong in the legislation of many countries. The need is strengthened by a total confusion on what is considered to be safe in the regulations for seamen world-wide.

The legal power of a physician only goes as far as the law allows. In the papers presented throughout this conference, the concepts seem to vary. We have been presented with a broad overview of the regulatory status on different types of diving in Europe. Unfortunately a simplification is not easily possible in the regulatory area.

The issues in question can be covered by Acts, seemingly far removed from our main issues. Norway has an Act for physicians governing most of what they shall do and what they cannot do within the legal framework. Currently other countries are introducing similar Acts. Most European countries have Acts on the work environment and these vary a lot as they were passed from just after the war until the late 1970's. These Acts place tasks on physicians which may be difficult to follow. The EU has since placed a lot of effort on the health and safety at work directives.

The Act for physicians in Norway is far more powerful than most other legislation and may completely override any diving regulations and guidelines. The most important aspect, in this observation, is that the absence of regulations and guidelines is not acceptable. On the other hand, the existence of such regulations does not remove them from the hierarchy of the law, whether it is the English case-based law or the more common Napoleonic European legal system.

The regulations should exist and they should be understood in a context where the life, health and personal integrity of the diver remains intact. The power or authority of a physician in any country to do something about a certificate of fitness for a diver is based on a net of Acts and Regulations. This brings us to the first and paramount need in the training of physicians: such a legal jungle requires to provide continuing guidance on the training and role of physicians in the evaluation of a diver's fitness to dive.

Outside the actual power granted by the legal system, the medical practitioner can only do what he is trained to do: advise! The medical practitioner based on some ethical principle, cannot place himself over the law except in very rare cases. Normally he would be placing himself outside the law: wide open to litigation.

The examining physician has three foundations to operate from:

- qualities as a general physician;
- knowledge about diving and diving medicine;
- knowledge of the regulatory basis for the actions that the medical practitioner can and must take.

In a European atmosphere of deregulation as well as harmonisation of regulations it is important to grasp the self-regulatory, goal-setting, functional requirements of regulations which are appearing. The well known "cook-book" prescriptive pass/fail approach is disappearing and is being replaced by what is the consensus of the medical community.

Current Norwegian regulations covering the offshore scene with regard to fitness to participate in offshore operations are dated November 12th, 1990. Other regulations cover the inshore diving activities in Norway undertaken for pay. Only "pure" sports diving activities are beyond any official regulatory governance. Sports diving is only subject to voluntary acceptance of internal rules and regulations without any formal status. Even the sports diving community, however, recommend the formal training of physicians to examine divers and it is mandatory in the U.K. and Norwegian Regulations that the doctor shall be qualified in some way to examine working divers.

THE TASKS OF THE PHYSICIAN

If the first point of training is the medical examiner's understanding of his legal position, his second task is to be a good clinician. The basis of a good clinical review is:

- the medical history (the anamnesis)
- the physical examination
- the supportive examinations (laboratory, x-ray)
- any referral for a second opinion

Based on these principles, and within the framework of the changes in the legal system in any country, the goal of any examination of a diver is to state if the health of the diver is in conformance (compliance) with "in-water safety". This is called "fit to dive", and not "fit to work".

The major tool is the medical history. In sick patients the medical history has been found alone to account for more than 50% of the accurate diagnoses made. The physical examination is, to a large extent, governed by what is found during the taking of the medical history. The improvement in diagnostic accuracy is then raised from 50 to only 60%. Finally, the laboratory examinations gain at best only another 10%. So the medical practitioner, at the end of a rather comprehensive and complete medical review, is reasonably certain in 70% of the cases. "Blind" laboratory testing, or so-called screening, is not common in this context and is difficult to handle. In diving we still discuss the value of long bone x-rays and urine testing, and we have discovered during this meeting, once more, how easy it is to debate the value of measuring the blood pressure.

After more than 20 years of research and experience, we know little about divers and we should not and cannot exempt them from their livelihood based on what I called the "probability of a possibility". If we do not know positively that we must bar a diver from diving, then we cannot do so, but we have an obligation to advise on the best of our knowledge. Being a medical practitioner is to help - not to be a barrier. The task of performing a "barrier" function can be imposed only by regulatory means.

The task is thus to find what makes the diver an in-water risk and then to remedy the problem as much as possible. When this is beyond the capabilities of the medical practitioner, he moves into his third state as a medical practitioner in diving medicine, the referral.

Referral and Advisory Services

Section 15 of the Norwegian Regulations on medical requirements offshore covers this aspect:

> *"... duty of the medical practitioner to ensure adequate clarification of the case".*

The medical practitioner has without any doubt a duty to collect all relevant information before making a decision concerning a certificate of medical fitness to dive. In addition, the same chapter, section III states:

> *"If during the examination the medical practitioner discovers anything to indicate that a certificate of medical fitness should not be issued, the medical practitioner in cases of doubt should consult a specialist before making a decision as to whether a statement of non-compliance with medical requirements or of a certificate of medical fitness can be issued".*

This third section has its counterpart in the Norwegian Act for Physicians. Once more, acts, regulations and guidelines tell how a medical practitioner should act on his professional findings. Above all, the regulatory system indicates the limits of liberty at the disposal of the medical practitioner. For 20 years the driving force of regulation has been to limit the qualitative judgement required by a medical practitioner in most of his cases. The effect is to turn the medical practitioner into a person trying to comply with legal requirements that, far too often, are opposite to his medical training and thinking. The net effect is to produce very confused doctors.

This demonstrates so well why continuous, or revision, training is so important. It has three aspects:

- basic understanding of the problem;
- basic understanding of limits to knowledge and the answers;
- application of knowledge (or lack) in a regulatory context.

This four day meeting demonstrates why regular gatherings are so important at a national and at an international level. There are few medical practitioners who deal with divers. Too often they can be up against problems about which they have never heard or read. The network approach of referral and counselling is far more important in this area than in most areas of medical practice.

COMPREHENSIVE HEALTH CARE

Throughout this meeting we have been exposed to a wealth of information and an unbelievable breadth of knowledge about diving medicine. It demonstrates eloquently that diving medicine can be the apex of medical knowledge and confusion.

This seeming contradiction may elicit two responses:

- stricter requirements in the Regulations;
- more stringent emphasis on the training and knowledge of the medical practitioner.

The second requirement already exists in most countries and cannot be replaced by regulatory polishing.

Norway went a step further in 1985 by forming, in their Regulations, a complete and comprehensive health care service for divers as was feasible at that time. It is time to renew the whole concept of health care offshore as well as for divers, but that is far beyond the scope of this paper. There is still a lot to be done.

TRAINING REQUIREMENTS

The major concern in training physicians to handle people who have to survive, work and maybe live at increased ambient pressure, should be to train them in just what this means. The medical practitioner already has a sound basis for medical thinking. The problem is that of adapting it to an environment which he never has to consider in the rest of his daily work.

In my initial paper I referred to the risks of the unforgiving underwater environment, where man cannot live without an envelope of man-made protective systems. To survive, the man exposed must face the problems of increased ambient pressure and its many implications.

Thus the trained medical examiner must understand:

- the hyperbaric environment;

- the risks of such an environment on health and safety;
- the problems of certain diseases in this environment.

A medical practitioner has to do what he always should do, make: "a qualified judgement on his client, in this case a person exposed to the in-water risk".

INITIAL AND PERIODICAL MEDICAL CONSULTATIONS

During these four days we have approached a more dynamic concept of the assessment of the diver or a person exposed to increased and varying pressure. There should be an extensive initial examination where the goal is to avoid launching people into a career where there is a greater probability than in other careers of losing their livelihood for medical reasons. A competent initial examination would also provide a good baseline for long-term follow-up studies on the diver's health.

The diver then needs to pass a periodical medical examination which is to detect the pathological deviation from normal health. This can possibly be done in a more simple version of what is common today. Every 3 to 5 years the same stringent considerations applied in the initial examination can be applied again. These extended medical examinations will establish a better longitudinal basis for the evaluation of the health of the diving population.

It is critical to distinguish between the medical examinations for a continued safe career and those made to study long term health effects on the diving population. In most countries these two can be in conflict. On one hand we perform a public licensing and on the other hand we perform the surveillance of a population that has a health risk. The most stringent adherence to who does what in these circumstances is paramount, otherwise the results can be used for unintended and undesired goals.

CONCLUSION

Those involved in the assessment of the health of the diving population need to understand the hyperbaric environment, the legal aspects as well as medical matters. This is mandatory in order to be able to assess the in-water risks of a diver both in the short term and the long term surveillance system.

In my presentations I have not touched on the relative and absolute contraindications. One of the reasons is that any such system should be based on a full understanding of the meaning of the diagnostic terms employed. If such lists are to be a standard for the medical community, any diagnostic criteria must be supported by scientific proof that a condition should bar the person from work. Otherwise it is easy to fall into the trap of having a list tending to the ridiculous, like "enough teeth to have understandable speech" and how many teeth is that?

What the medical community should do in diving is what they do for the rest of society: provide a health service. They should also stop the practice of barring divers from their work based on flimsy or contradictory medical evidence. The medical practitioner should have sufficient training in the area of the hyperbaric environment to provide him with qualitative judgement for the assessment of in-water safety of the diver.

During these four days many things have changed and I believe we are now on our way to creating an appropriate medical community perspective, but there is a lot left to be done.

DISCUSSION

Örnhagen: The best way to know the environment is also to be in it, do you know of any offshore diver who is also a doctor?

Minsaas: No, but many of the doctors present here are sports divers and a number of us have been through training programmes which have included professional equipment. A few have been trained to professional standards of diving.

PROPOSAL FOR A DIVER HEALTH SERVICE IN NORWAY
Dr. M. Kromberg

We have been hoping to establish a medical register for divers for about 15 years. The purpose was to be the long term follow-up of health effects of diving. The method was supposed to be the compilation in one large database of data from the annual exams. It has not yet come to realisation. The first problem was legal. Although employers were made responsible in regulations for facilitating the collection of such data, there is no automatic provision in Norwegian law for their storage. So far the divers have refused to agree to the proposed systems for such data storage. The second issue which has delayed implementation has been the problem of relevance. Will an annual fitness checkup designed to screen for risks to safety be appropriate to provide the data that we need for long term follow-up?

In this connection we also have to consider some related questions. Who should pay for the examinations to collect the relevant data and for maintaining a register? Who would be the owner of the information in such a register, and for which purposes could such information legitimately be used?

A third problem was the structural problem of the diving industry. Increasing competition and the tendency towards even briefer contracts which, as we have heard, may be for only 3 weeks, has now made it impossible to ask that divers competing for jobs should provide their entire medical record and lay it before their prospective employer. Also, to ask the industry to take the responsibility for follow-up of each person over the next 50 years each time that they employ an individual for maybe only 3 weeks, is perceived to be unreasonable. We have therefore come up with an alternative proposal.

We propose a national or public health service for divers. We cannot and should not alter the responsibility of the employers for the safety of diving operations, and we will retain that part of our regulations which makes it mandatory for diving operations to use the services of an occupational health service. Such an occupational health service should retain the present 3 main functions:

- advice of medical doctors with defined competence in planning of diving operations and in the preparation of the statutory Safety Case;

- continuous supervision of the working environment and its risks, aided by pre- and post-dive examinations as advised by the competent doctor;

- duties and responsibilities in an emergency as defined by the emergency preparedness plans.

We now wish to introduce a new health service for all divers, preferably both offshore and inshore divers, with areas of responsibility which will be different from those required by employers. This new service might be responsible for the first medical selection before training. We think the service should offer periodic medical examinations which are relevant to detecting the long term effects of diving. The health service should also offer medical rehabilitation guidance for the purpose of insurance and also help provide the medical certificates necessary for insurance purposes. With the diver's consent the medical data from this health service should go into a medical register with the dual purpose of recording the individual diver's health status and being available for research purposes.

It must be an offer of a health service which the divers can be free to refuse, and the divers will have to agree to be registered. It will also be necessary to find ways of linking health data to exposure data. Although some data may be available from offshore records, for some types of diving the only exposure data available will be that from the diver himself. We hope the divers will then be prepared to make truthful information available to the registry. A proposal has been sent out for discussion and we do not yet know whether it will be accepted.

In summary, these are the questions which have to be answered before a new health service can be established:

- Are annual health fitness checks based on safety considerations appropriate for long term follow-up?

- Which parameters are needed for long term follow-up?

- How often should they be carried out?

- Who should do them?

- Who should pay?

DISCUSSION

Örnhagen (Chairman): Is this to be arranged through your Board and how many doctors do you expect will be involved?

Kromberg: Such a service would be the joint responsibility of government and industry and we will have to negotiate an appropriate share between them. For self-employed divers it would be tax-deductible but the details have not yet been worked out.

THE NEED FOR SPECIALIST CENTRES
Professor D.H. Elliott

I will use the need for a specialist centre as the focus for a number of other aspects of the provision of medical support for divers because this is not a simple subject but one with many intertwining threads. One could summarise the whole week in this context but we need the opinion of all present on all aspects of this, so please take part in the subsequent discussion or submit supplementary comments.

The need for specialist centres exists because there are some aspects of the diver's periodic examination which require the use of specialised techniques which are not readily available in the normal practice. There is also the occasional need for a review by persons of consultant status. The techniques of occupational health and safety have become more sophisticated than they were when the Navy first required divers to have an annual physical. There is now a need for a number of special investigations for the health and safety of each diver to be conducted at various points during his or her career and we seem to have achieved the consensus view that, for these, he or she should be reviewed at a specialist centre.

The turning point in this meeting came near the start of the clinical sessions when, you will remember, we tried to be precise about the numeric value for blood pressure that would be disqualifying for a diver: should it not exceed a systolic pressure of 140 and a diastolic pressure of 80? The response to that and several other issues was "do not make rules because it all depends ...". That marked the moment, which has been a long time coming, when we had to abandon the original title of this meeting "MEDICAL STANDARDS FOR FITNESS TO DIVE". At the end of these four days we have adopted the phrase "MEDICAL ASSESSMENT FOR FITNESS TO DIVE".

Standards can be prescriptive; assessment requires special knowledge.

When it comes to the need for examinations in a specialist centre, what precisely do we need? What does such a centre do? How often does it need to do this? In fact, does it need to do the same thing every year? We have already agreed that for some examinations these need not begin until the age of 30 or perhaps 40.

From this debate emerges a way ahead. Definitions were made by the European Diving Technology Committee in 1978 for each of the following:

- The Medical Examiner of Divers
- The Diving Emergency Medical Doctor
- The Diving Medical Consultant

The consultants are of two types. Like the many who have joined us so helpfully during the week, there is the hospital consultant who, as an individual, knows a lot about diving. The other is the diving consultant, the doctor who not only knows about diving medicine but also about diving physiology and operational diving. This includes the structure and selection of decompression tables, the physiological criteria for the acceptance of breathing apparatus, and other topics. This knowledge often comes from having worked with an operational or experimental diving team.

Dr. Botheroyd in his "Health Notes" refers to the *"Diving Medical Specialist"* and, in his presentation,

Surgeon Commander Francis refers to the "contractor's Medical Adviser" as a person who should have a more detailed knowledge and considerable experience. Thus to define a specialist centre is to formalise what we already have.

The specialist centre should be defined by the qualifications and experience of those who are in it. These doctors should be "Diving Medical Specialists" for whom diving medicine is a significant portion of their professional life. This will thus formalise the concept which we have discussed of a "2-tier system" and which, in an informal way, already exists.

The first time that such a specialist centre should be visited is for the initial examination before acceptance for training. Then at set intervals which have yet to be defined, there will be occasions when the diver should be reviewed again at a specialist centre. The Approved or Appointed Diving Doctor, who will still be the backbone of the annual medical examination system, will then form a closer relationship with the Diving Medical Specialist who, in the intervening years, can advise on any difficulties that may arise for the individual diver.

Thus a specialist centre will have one or probably more specialist medical consultants in diving. It will have special equipment, for example for the investigation of the long-term health effects. It will also be a focal point for the specialist hospital consultants who know about diving and the system will favour those consultants who are geographically close to such diving medical centres.

I think we can safely conclude from this meeting that no longer can we have a simple pass/fail set of criteria for diver fitness. Individual assessment is required and it must be done against a thorough knowledge of what the diver's tasks are and what are the occupational hazards which he has to confront. Not only will the specialist centre become a key component of the referral network but also, by the careful collection of medical data, it will provide a feed-back loop having audited the effectiveness of the decisions that we now made. It will be able to advise on the future "standards" or guidance that we should consider when making subsequent assessments. There is also the important opportunity, to be discussed later, for epidemiology and for the links with dive-data storage banks that, in theory at least, will enable links to be made between the nature of the occupational illnesses of divers and the possible causative factors within a diving career.

DISCUSSION

Burges: I am strongly in favour of the suggestion that you should set up centres of excellence around this country. This would harmonise and standardise a lot of the work that we are doing. We already refer our divers to one of the local private hospitals and find that we have no discussion, such as we had here on Wednesday, about what type of exercise testing should be done. That decision is made by the clinical consultant. These centres should be manned by consultants with experience of diving and would be the focal point for decisions on return to diving after decompression illness. Those are my very strong views.

Örnhagen (Chairman): Is there to be some sort of quality assurance for these centres?

Elliott: In my original notes I wrote in large letters the word "AUDIT". This is an essential part of modern medical practice.

It is worth mentioning that there are, of course, a few doctors of diving medical consultant status, who do not need to come to the revision courses. There are also a significant number of examining doctors like yourselves, who come to these courses regularly. Our concern must be about those Approved Doctors who, since their one week of basic introduction, have never come for any refresher training (though there are a few who have sent their apologies as to why they were unable to come to Edinburgh). Thus, if we had a two-tier system with specialist medical centres, then audit would be a natural part of the process of continuous improvement.

Lewkowicz: What you were saying about accreditation can be compared with what, in general practice, we have with child health surveillance doctors. There are special training courses spread over several years controlled by the Royal College of Physicians. It is a specialist field with continual updating, and diving should be exactly the same.

Elliott: I agree with that. I fear that a number of doctors do not understand the complexity of the environment in which the diver works. I believe that suitable training should include not only medicine but also diving.

LeDez: I want to endorse strongly what you said about looking at the diver as a whole. That should be our emphasis, not looking at some particular standard or whether he passes it.

Freshwater[**]:** Outside the world of the North Sea diver working for the oil industry, or those working for government agencies such as the police, there exists a large number of divers who earn precarious livings doing such work as clearing salmon cages, scallop diving, cutting ropes from propellers, etc. Many of them, perhaps most of them, live and work in areas of relative remoteness, often diving part-time between other marginal occupations.

Already, the complexity of regulations mean that some diving is being done which is not strictly in compliance with the law, or is frankly illegal, because the cost of compliance is greater than the money to be earned. Where there is enough work, divers try to work legally, but costs remain tight and diving medicals for a team of divers remain a significant operational cost.

If we increase the complexity and thus the costs, of the medical examination, we shall reduce the number of divers attending for examination; however, this is unlikely to be matched by a reduction in the number of people actually diving. Similarly, travelling to a specialist centre may easily double the cost of a medical, with the same result.

Centralisation of diver examinations will have advantages of making standards more consistent, and will help to improve the data available for research. However, knowledge of diving medicine is already thinly spread in the profession, and there may be disadvantages to restricting it further.

The divers pay for the medical examination, not any regulatory body. That being the case, we need to be sure that we are meeting their needs, not ours.

They need to have the benefit of health surveillance which protects them from unacceptable risk (and this does not mean no risk). They need to be given acceptable, realistic and justifiable reasons if disqualified. They need to be offered standards that are relevant to the work they do and the environment in which it is done. Finally, if they are obliged to finance the examination, they need an examination they can afford.

We can meet these needs by refining the present system of examination. Greater consistency might be addressed by increasing the data supplied on the forms (MS-80) returned to the government agency (HSE); collation of this would supply much useful information for research.

Let us make sure that changes are made for the benefit of our patients, not merely to show that we can organise our work differently.

Reply from Elliott: That is an important consideration but we must not forget that we agreed at the beginning of this meeting. There should be no difference between the different categories of diving in the requirements for fitness which relate to in-water safety. This implies that there can be differences in the special investigations needed for long-term health effects and these should be at the examining doctor's discretion.

In accordance with the law, it is the employer of divers who should pay for the medical examination, though I do appreciate that most of the divers to whom you refer are self-employed. In spite of that, the principle must be maintained and any omission of medical or safety procedures, including insurance and equipment, gives the "cowboy" an unfair financial advantage over the truly professional. The offshore industry is now relatively safe: no fatalities in the last ten years and with no neurological decompression illness last year from compressed-air dives. The inshore divers still have many problems and must be encouraged to set progressive targets for improvement.

Blyth**: (1) "New entry diver failed by one Approved Doctor and subsequently made fit by another". We can only audit our work if we have feedback. An Approved Doctor whose decision is overruled should be given a full written explanation.

(2) "Special centres" - can they meet the demands of the customer for an instant medical prior to urgent deployment overseas? Will they be evenly spread over the U.K. as the Approved Doctors are, or will Alverstoke, Plymouth, Great Yarmouth and Aberdeen be the only choices?

(3) What figures are available to show that Approved Doctors are inefficient and if the opinion is that Approved Doctors are competent, why not limit the special centres to carrying out the more advanced investigations over and above the current requirements.

Reply from Elliott: I agree with your concerns and am sure that these will be addressed. We were asked by the Health & Safety Executive to aim for consensus conclusions and this we have done. We have to leave the consideration of such concerns and the implementation of our recommendations to them.

Saliba**: I support the idea of specialist centres. These should serve also for postgraduate education. In this way doctors with an interest in Diving and Hyperbaric Medicine can follow Diploma or Degree courses which will then be recognised as a postgraduate course in its own right.

Grönkvist**: Harmonisation of fitness standards within Europe is of course extremely important. The discussion was very occupied with limits and personal dispensations. I want to point out the importance of an overall clinical evaluation of each case. The decision to pass or fail must be based on this evaluation and not on prescribed figures of what is considered acceptable and what is not.

APPEALS
Dr. E.M. Botheroyd

In the last few days we have been bombarded with a large amount of information which will take some time to assimilate, but nevertheless it is important to draw some rapid conclusions before the general feelings of this consensus may be forgotten. One of my jobs is to run the Appeals system, or diver review system, as it is more formally known, in the U.K. I am also responsible for approving the Approved Doctors and for pruning from the list those who do not conduct enough medical examinations to keep themselves in touch.

In the review, I am often called upon to make a Judgement of Paris and one value of this week has been to better define the uncertainties.

There are 300 Approved examiners of whom 200 are in the U.K. and 100 are from overseas. They average 17 medicals per year : few do very many and many do very few. The Tables (41 and 42) below show the steadily increasing number of medicals each year.

TABLE 41 - MEDICAL EXAMINATIONS CONDUCTED

YEAR	U.K.	O/SEAS	TOTAL
1990	2971	972	3943
1991	3401	1345	4746
1992	3525	1224	4749
1993	3695	1359	5054

TABLE 42 - THE FINDINGS OF THE MEDICALS

YEAR	TOTAL	UNFIT	REVIEW
1990	3943	29	7
1991	4746	33	6
1992	4749	61	6
1993	5054	43	5

I suspect the numbers found unfit are too low but, of course, some divers just quit without going for a final medical. Very few come to review. The reasons for applying for a review, it had been thought, was a desperate desire to get back in to the water but another reason is that a number are seeking confirmation of their unfitness in order to pursue civil litigation.

TABLE 43 - OUTCOMES 1990-93 OF 24 APPEALS

SYSTEM	NUMBER	UNFIT	FIT	FIT WITH RESTRICTION
C.N.S.	6	3	2	1
RESP.	5	3	1	1
C.V.S.	5	1		4
E.N.T.	3	2	1	
M/S	2	2		
G.I.T.	2	1		1
PSYCH.	1	1		
G.U.S.	0			

The fact that a number are found fit with some restriction upon their diving activity (Table 43) gives us a clue to the assessment that is needed for divers in relation to their particular work, instead of adherence to "Standards". The following were confirmed unfit:

TABLE 44 - UNFIT UPON APPEAL

SYSTEM	NUMBER	REASON	STATUS E = Experienced T = Trainee
C.N.S.	3	History of Polio & DCI	E
		Episodic loss of consciousness	T
		Disabling migraine	T
RESP.	3	Pneumonia with residua	E
		B/P, aspergillosis	E
		Chronic bronchitis	T
C.V.S.	1	Cardiomyopathy	E
E.N.T.	2	Stapedectomy	E
		Bilateral inner ear damage	E
M/S	2	Complex ankle injury	E
		Complex pelvic injury	E
G.I.T.	1	Chronic active hepatitis	E
PSYCH.	1	Paranoid illness	T

At present, a medical conducted before training begins is not a statutory examination and strictly should not be included in this report. But we did realise some years ago that at the point of entry to diving we do need an *exclusive* standard. It is worth noting that the second case listed under the respiratory system is unique.

The stapedectomy case in this list was a policeman who had been diving for 14 years having had his stapedectomy while still in the Armed Forces. After some years he changed medical examiners to one who realised that this had been a contraindication to diving and considered that, in spite of so many years of safe activity, he was nevertheless unfit. After much discussion between many experts, this decision was upheld. He subsequently retired from the police on the grounds of deafness.

The following were found fit:

TABLE 45 - FIT UPON APPEAL

SYSTEM	NUMBER	REASON	STATUS E = Experienced T = Trainee
C.N.S.	2	Recurring headache	T
		C.N.S. DCI without residua	E
RESP.	1	Reduced FEV_1/FVC ratio	E
E.N.T.	1	Grommet scars eardrums	T

This is not a procedure of reversing an Approved Doctor's decision so much as collecting additional information and opinion for an advanced review. This is not an adversarial review.

A certificate of restricted fitness was given to the following:

TABLE 46 - RESTRICTED FITNESS UPON APPEAL

SYSTEM	NUMBER	REASON	STATUS E = Experienced T = Trainee
C.N.S.	1	C.N.S., DCI, HMPAO anomaly, PFO	E
RESP.	1	Pneumothorax following infection	E
C.V.S.	4	Systolic hypertension	E
		Labile hypertension	E
		Myocardial ischaemia	E
G.I.T.	1	Colectomy with continence stoma	T

The first case showed some HMPAO changes and also had a confirmed PFO but we felt able to permit a return to diving in very closely controlled circumstances. The same applies to the others on this list and shows that we can limit the diver's exposure to hazard and can assess him fit for that particular environment. This means that their safety is not compromised but there may still be risks for their future health which they themselves must accept.

The review system is difficult to operate because it needs to be fair. One has to consider not only the diver but the people he dives with, the implications upon those who trained him and for his future employer and insurers. One needs to be fair to the industry as a whole and also to the original medical examiner. Finally, of course, one must be fair to the taxpayer who has to foot the bill and therefore we must keep control over unjustifiable expense.

The advantages of the current system are its impartiality, it is usually fairly quick and it is fairly cheap. The disadvantages are that there is much nagging and lobbying and I would accept that there is deficient feedback on outcomes to other medical practitioners. This only happens at meetings such as this and we do not publicise the outcome of the Appeals. The Appeal system also has doubtful relevance to those divers who may be made unfit when they are overseas. In these circumstances the review must be conducted within the U.K.

I would like to include the translucency of this process. We ought to be better at getting information back to the Approved Diving Doctor network. The information gained is used as a feedback to our medical guidance on fitness. In fact, at the present time we are engaged on a complete review of this guidance. It has been suggested that we should have a panel of referees rather than different consultants for different cases. This idea has some logistical difficulties such as travelling expenses and similarly whether to provide some kind of tribunal decision, but this would be a formal review procedure with tripartite representation (trades union, industry and government). This might become rather unwieldy and difficult.

I was asked how we might extend a review system internationally. That would depend on there being uniform criteria within Europe and the identification of referees with a decision-making process. A secretariat would need to be established to run this, at the present moment this is done on a part-time basis by one secretary in Aberdeen. This could indeed take much longer to reach a decision and possibly cost more money and for this the obvious question would be "who pays"?

We should keep a sense of proportion about these things. If we examine 5000 people each year roughly 50 are found unfit, 6 apply for a review and, of those 6, only 3 are confirmed unfit. Two are confirmed fit but with restricted employment, and only 1 of the 6 who had applied for review, is confirmed fit without restriction.

DISCUSSION

Sibley-Calder**: The number of divers certified as unfit may be artificially small because: (1) unfit divers do not present for re-examination and (2) the first two examinations sometimes decide whether or not to proceed, therefore forms are not sent back.

Reply from Botheroyd: I am grateful for your thoughts on the reasons why the figures may suggest an unexpectedly low rate of finding of unfitness to dive. As you say there are all sorts of possibilities, the difficulty is that we simply do not know about divers for whom we do not receive examination returns and it would be good if we could know why divers do not return for medicals and/or decide to abandon diving as a career.

Hawson**: If during the course of a commercial diver's medical an exclusion finding is detected, for example a major joint problem, should the examination be terminated at that point and a FAIL certificate issued declaring only that single finding, or should the examination be completed in entirety including tests and ECG etc. so that the FAIL certificate can properly state whether that was indeed the only abnormality, or whether there were other excluding findings?

Reply from Botheroyd: I think if you come upon a major FAIL point during the course of the examination, it would be a matter for agreement between you and the diver whether you terminated his examination at that point and returned his fee. Some doctors do that. It creates problems for us in conducting a review if one becomes necessary because, as you will appreciate, the review can only deal with identified FAIL criteria.

Sometimes we get round this by adjudicating only on that particular FAIL criterion and returning the individual to the Approved Doctor who found him unfit in the first place, but naturally some of the divers are reluctant to return there particularly if we appear to have overruled the doctor's judgement. It is all a matter of human relations I guess and explaining the problem to the diver at the time.

Doig** The slide showing 5000 medicals - 50 fails, 6 appeals with 3 succeeding. This implies that we Approved Doctors are producing perhaps around 25 false negatives i.e. failures, where the subjects are fit. Should the Health & Safety Executive not be collating the notes of all failures to review the reasons and contacting those who may actually be fit?

Reply from Botheroyd: It would be a nice idea for a benevolent government agency to try to identify false failures of divers! We prefer however, to leave these things to the judgement of the Approved Doctor and the diver. In other words if a diver feels that he has been unnecessarily found unfit he has access to us as appellant. Sometimes, of course, divers are ready to agree with the finding and do not wish to question it.

On the whole I think it would seem odd for a governmental body to interfere in something which was the outcome of agreement between an individual and his, for the time being, medical adviser.

Douglas**: Please can the initial medical require a report from the diver's own general practitioner for 2 reasons: (1) it stops past medical history e.g. of epilepsy being hidden and (2) is a permanent record kept in the diver's own doctor's records to state that the patient had a career in diving and, if the patient dies or suffers from certain illnesses e.g. pre-senile dementia,

psychiatric problems or Parkinson's disease, that contact is made with a central point, perhaps the HSE, for post-mortem or clinical follow-up.
This should be necessary for <u>all</u> prospective divers, to make the system universal and fair.

Reply from Botheroyd: We do intend to introduce a statutory requirement for a pre-training assessment of fitness to dive. This would mean that a certificate of fitness could be obtained "at leisure" before commencement of diver training. This in turn would allow for the time delay we might envisage in obtaining general practitioner reports, if sought. I do not think, however, that we can insist that general practitioner reports are made available or that they are required.

It is also our intention to make available to divers a copy of the findings of their examinations. Quite how this will be done is yet to be decided, but clearly if the diver wanted that information to be held by his own doctor it would be an option for him.

RECORDING THE OCCUPATIONAL EXPOSURES
Professor D.H. Elliott

Several Norwegian speakers have already referred to the Godøysund Conference in 1993 from which one conclusion was that, in order to prevent adverse long term health effects, the need is to have for the epidemiological studies a continuous record of occupational exposure to hazard.

In a study of posterior tibial somatosensory evoked potentials (PTSEP), which has now been reported to the Health & Safety Executive, its sponsors, it has been shown that there are a greater number of persons in diving with an increased latency than there are in a control population. To achieve accuracy, it is important that each PTSEP measurement is controlled for height. The conclusion was that in healthy and experienced divers who have never had any recompression for decompression illness, there is, in contrast to non-diving control subjects, a proportion of individuals who have significantly delayed responses. However, it is important to emphasise that, although these results are statistically significant, the consequences to that individual are not necessarily of clinical significance.

More important for us and for the diver is the known long term health effect, dysbaric osteonecrosis. As discussed by Professor McCallum, there has been little research in this subject since the closure of the MRC Decompression Sickness Registry some ten years ago. If one is to assess the prevalence, time course and causative factors of long term health effects, whether they be neurological, bone or other tissue pathology, it is necessary to know the nature and degree of exposure to hazard of the individuals affected, and of unaffected persons. In order to do this in diving it should be possible, within the next year or so, to benefit from the introduction in the U.K. by the government, the oil industry and the diving industry (HSE, UKOOA and AODC) of a dive data recording system.

Depth, breathing mixture and other parameters are to be recorded continuously on-line from each air-range dive. The results will be recorded centrally and be available for analysis. Dive data recording should:

- encourage compliance with decompression schedules;
- provide accurate records of the actual dive profile;
- allow cumulative analysis of decompression safety;
- provide evidence of company and individual, responsibility.

The cumulative analysis would be one which, by looking at the occasional cases of decompression illness, should be able in due course to analyse any particular causative factors and thereby provide evidence for the subsequent improvement of decompression tables. However the primary justification for the cost of introducing depth-time recording together with a host of other relevant operational data, is that it displays an on-line image of the diver's depth over time. With this technique it is possible to monitor divers, perhaps as their compression is temporarily halted with ear problems or as their depth varies around their bottom depth. One can measure the maximum depth exposure with accuracy and then watch their decompression not only in the water but also if they transfer to a compression chamber.

The value of such a record is illustrated in Fig. 18. which shows the final minutes of a 120 ft x 50 minute dive in which the diver had been breathing nitrox with 32% oxygen. During his ascent from depth he heard an "engine" in his head and realised that he might be losing consciousness. He wedged himself into an anode on the structure but subsequently fell from that towards the seabed.

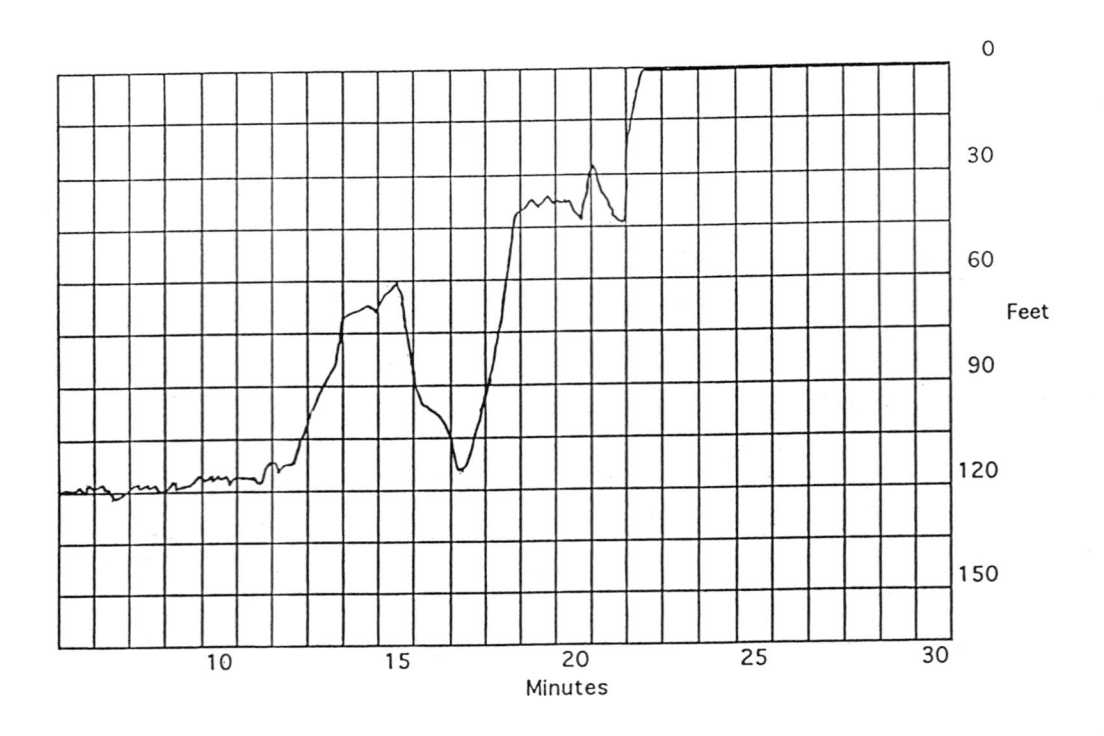

Fig. 18. - Example of an on-line dive record

These events are shown dramatically on the on-line display. Another diver, whose depth-time data is not displayed on this graph, was sent down to the appropriate depth to rescue him and, as you can see, having brought him up to a shallower depth spent a little time getting him into the basket for a return to the surface. The evidence from a helmet-mounted television camera confirmed the occurrence of a convulsion but the diver, who required recompression only for omitted stops, suffered no lasting ill-effects. The purpose of this example is to demonstrate the on-line value of dive-data recording which one hopes will soon become universal and to make a plea for the central storage and analysis of dive records in order to provide accurate information for epidemiology.

From such records, which for an individual air-range diver need to be collected from all his diving activities both home and abroad, an accurate work history can become routine.

REFERENCE

Elliott, D.H., Pearson, R.R. & Sedgwick, E.M. *Neurological and cerebrovascular abnormalities in divers.* Final HSE Report, MATSU/8565/3073; 1994.

DISCUSSION

Robertson: Should the conference recommend the instigation of a system so that the information from a diver's previous medical is instantly available for the doctor conducting the next one?

Botheroyd: First, I agree that this is a difficulty and at the present moment all the clinical records are retained by the examining doctor and not forwarded to a central point, such as the HSE. Instant availability is therefore not feasible but we can provide the name and address of the previous doctor upon request, from whom these records should be available. It would not be appropriate to put any confidential information into the diver's logbook.

Anderson-Upcott: When a diver's fitness has been subject to an appeal, who signs the certificate?

Botheroyd: Strictly speaking the decision is that of the Director of Medical Services, but in fact it is usually mine.

Douglas: From the point of view of a medical officer of a commercial diving school, very often the initial diving medical is such that I have to bale-out people who should never have been allowed to come. Other doctors have passed them as fit with poor eustachian function, poor respiratory function, obesity etc. The consequences in cost for all concerned are considerable and the hassle devolves upon us at the training school. We need clear limits for the initial examination before the potential diver comes for training. There is also a percentage of wastage of divers who, after training, find that diving is not for them and go and seek employment elsewhere. These would make an ideal control group because we would have a good baseline on them. Thirdly, there is the opportunity for the medical officer at the school to assess the future potential for a diver while under training, in relation to the functional tasks which he may be required to perform in different branches of diving in the future. It must be remembered that our thoughts on long term health effects must also be applied to the inshore diver.

Charters: Specialist centres would be convenient for doctors but not so user-friendly for the divers and this is a service that we provide for them.

Elliott: That is so but the overriding priority is for the quality of the medical examination which they need. It may require some travelling for occasional medicals but in general the diver would continue to see the Approved Doctor of his choice.

Hawson: You have suggested that specialist medical centres should be approved but my feeling is it should be the doctors who should be approved.

Elliott: I agree, I said that it is the doctors, and this includes the consultants, who need to be "approved". The specialist centre should be defined by the persons in it.

Hawson: I would like to remind people of the importance of the telephone, perhaps the most important diagnostic tool available.

Elliott: I agree, particularly in the treatment of diving emergencies, but the telephone is no substitute for the special investigations which are proposed at such specialist centre.

Minsaas: In Norway we already have 3 categories of diving physicians but we have never "approved" a centre.

Knessl: Dr. Botheroyd, you mentioned a case in which the diver was made partially fit because of myocardial ischaemia. Was this a clinical diagnosis or by ECG?

Botheroyd: It was an ECG finding. This individual, incidentally, works in a ship model testing tank which is immediately opposite a major general hospital. The risks were not so great for safety even though, of course, he might suffer an ischaemic attack in the water.

Minsaas: We have an appeal system in Norway also and we have 20 divers who have lost their medical certificates since 1980. But not a single one of these Norwegian divers appealed.

Elliott: This is slightly relevant to Appeals, but maybe more relevant to the conclusions which we might draw from the overall view of diver fitness. I am concerned by a number of cases among those divers whose documents come to me for review from the loss adjustors for employers' liability insurance. I am aware that a number of divers are made unfit to dive for reasons which, in my view, were not valid. However, unless those individuals then appeal, the inappropriate decision by their Approved Diving Doctor legally stands. That is a gap over which of course the HSE has no control. It is also important to remind divers when they are made unfit that they do have the opportunity for an Appeal.

Botheroyd: This is also a concern for us, we do not want to have more appeals but yes, I do agree that the majority of those made unfit to not appeal and we just have no way of assessing these.

Farrell: If I make a diver unfit and send the appropriate form off to you in Aberdeen, is there a safety net that ensures that he must not go round the corner to get a fitness certificate from somebody else?

Botheroyd: This gets picked up at the time that the entry is made into our computer when it will be found that there has been more than one medical within the year. These are then compared. So there is a mechanism, but it is not foolproof.

Örnhagen: An additional advantage of a specialist medical centre is that, given that there is a limited number of divers, the work and therefore the experience will be focused on a few such centres and the quality of assessment would be enhanced.

LONG-TERM HEALTH SURVEILLANCE: NATIONAL/CENTRAL REGISTRIES FOR OCCUPATIONAL EXPOSURE HISTORIES
Professor R.I. McCallum

The general impression I have gained from this conference is that there is an important interest in registries. A registry is the old terminology for what is now known as a databank. The former Medical Research Council Decompression Sickness Central Registry in the University of Newcastle upon Tyne was started by Professor Dennis Walder somewhere in the 1960's, initially to collect information about decompression sickness and to relate it to compressed air exposure. It began with compressed air workers from caissons and tunnels but during the 1960's divers were included. The particular interest of the Registry then was in bone necrosis. The Registry had a unique collection of data on bone necrosis, both the exposure records of the worker and the medical examinations reported annually including in many cases the bone x-rays. This enabled us to analyse the data to make certain observations of a practical nature. It was funded first by the Medical Research Council and later by the Health & Safety Executive.

I have selected 5 activities of the Registry which were concerned with divers. The first was investigation into bone necrosis based upon the records of nearly 5000 divers (MRC Decompression Sickness Registry, 1981). The second investigation was into the age of retirement and this was at the request of the insurance industry. It was based on 2,665 divers (Trowbridge et al, 1982). In 1984 a study of the relationship of ventilatory capacity to hyperbaric exposure in divers was published, based upon 858 divers (Davey et al, 1984). In 1984 we also looked at the weights of more than 1500 divers (McCallum & Petrie, 1984). Finally, there started a study, that is still continuing, into diver mortality. A group of 2000 divers has been identified and in due course their death certificates will be provided for review. This project will continue for some years but some results from the earlier deaths are already available (McCallum, 1993).

All the information upon which these studies have been based was collected from the details on the form returned by the examining doctor who conducted the annual fitness examination. From this it can be concluded that a great deal of information can be obtained from even the simplest collection of data; information that was not collected especially for research but which otherwise would have remained in the files of the examining doctors. Of course, a lot of the information with which we were provided was not very good. For example the study of ventilatory capacity drew some very rude comments about the poor quality of data provided but, in spite of that, a good paper was produced and published.

One of the things that worried us in assessing the information was, for example, that when a blood pressure was recorded, there was not information on how it had been obtained. Similarly when our study of obesity of divers' weight was recorded it was not very clear as to how it had been measured. It turns out that most doctors use ordinary bathroom scales which are not very accurate.

The criteria against which height and weight are judged were the Metropolitan Life Assurance figures which were at that time related to middle-aged American males. It appeared that at any age the mean weight of divers in the North Sea was greater than the Life Assurance criteria which might mean that some divers would be excluded from diving on the basis of an inappropriate standard. Audiometry provides another example of where quality of data can be poor.

The question which has not been addressed so far is one which I would like to emphasise. Are we going to do anything about a Registry or a similar databank now? If there is a general feeling that this should be the case, what is to be done? In an informal discussion between Dr. Kromberg and myself over lunch there was a large measure of agreement about what was needed and how it could be done. The solution must be grasped at the national level. Although it could be done internationally, this might be difficult.

The mortality study mentioned earlier has encountered a problem due to the mobility of divers during their working life and subsequent retirement. Once they leave the country and therefore the social security numbering system, they are lost to our tracing. The difficulty in our mortality study is indeed to define "the diver". The solution which I have adopted is that each of the 2000 people we have selected have got 2 medical examinations in the Registry in which they were certified as fit to dive. There is often a range of occupations given on the diver's death certificate that have nothing to do with diving.

I hope that, as a result of this meeting, there will be a move to set up a Registry of medical data but the question that must be addressed outside this meeting is, who should fund it?

REFERENCES

Davey, I.S., Cotes, J.E. & Reed, J.W.   *J. Appl. Physiol.* 1984; **56**: 1655-1658.

McCallum, R.I. & Petrie, A.   *Brit. J. Industr. Med.* 1984; **41**: 275-278.

McCallum, R.I.   *Long-term health effects of diving: an international consensus conference, Godøysund.* Hope, A., Lund, T., Elliott, D.H., Halsey, M.J. & Wigg, H. (Eds). NUTEC: Bergen. 1994. Pp 179-186.

MRC Decompression Sickness Registry. *Lancet* 1981; **2**: 384-388.

Trowbridge, W.P., Walder, D.N. & McCallum, R.I.   *Undersea Biomed. Res.* 1982; **9**(i)Suppl: 11.

DISCUSSION

Simpson: A comment would be welcomed on combining a register of diving history with a databank of dive data. Is there any value in setting up a registry that excludes either the medical or the diving component of the information?

McCallum: Both the medical and the environmental data must be together. This was so in Newcastle and there is no problem about it. The diver entered his own diving experience on the form and later it was possible to check using the diver's logbook. As described by David Elliott, a method of collecting such data from operational records would now seem to be feasible. It is important to emphasise that the essential feature of a registry is its long term potential. If it is not set up for a long time it is not worth doing.

Douglas: I wish to make a plea that the general practitioner records in some way get linked into the diving medical records and long term health results. For example in providing a "tick box" summary of a potential trainee diver's past medical history, there could be some flagging within the individual's notes about his occupation which would enable a future general practitioner to follow-up with the registry should some condition such as senile dementia or bone necrosis emerge in later years.

Whitehead: Going back to the comments by David Elliott, one of the advantages of the Approved Diving Doctor system is that we are indeed general practitioners. As such we are fully computerised and, with modems, putting information into a central registry could be routine.

McCallum: That is a very useful contribution as input of data would be both simple and cheap.

Elliott**:** Could you please comment a bit more on the appropriate standards for height/weight (obesity) criteria?

Reply from McCallum: The problem with standards lies in the assessment of data derived from many different observers carrying out examinations in different parts of the country but untrained in a uniform way. Where skinfold callipers have been used in this sort of way, uniformity of standards has not been achieved and the data are suspect. Reliable measurements of weight and height should be more easily attainable but only if accurate scales (not cheap bathroom scales) are used. This would mean that the Quetelet Index (wt/ht^2) could be used with more confidence in assessing obesity. It should also be standard practice to weigh people in minimum underclothing and to record height in socks or barefoot. With regard to reference standards the Newcastle Registry data could probably provide a normal range of weights or height for divers.

Bickle: I like the idea of the diver having a contact point for the time between his medicals, preferably a general practitioner who is an Approved Diving Doctor, since there are so many general practitioners who know nothing about diving.

Örnhagen (Chairman): I recognise that we have been focusing on the specific visit of the diver to a doctor to meet the fitness requirements, but I would like to make a plea for a doctor to be available to evaluate whatever happens in the months or even years between these periodic examinations. I would favour a system where the divers are expected to visit a specialised diving centre every 5 years and that, in between these times, the diver has a selected diving doctor who can see him as required. This idea of a nominated doctor is essentially what I was proposing.

Lewkowicz: We run the system that anybody who visits us for an annual diving medical can come back and see us at any time during the following year with a diving related problem at no extra charge.

McCallum: Could we come back to the problem of who takes the initiative for a registry?

Elliott: This is happening and it must happen. The Godøysund Conference said that the top priority is surveillance for long term health effects and this cannot be done without having a registry.

In closing this meeting I have no intention of re-iterating everything that has been said already. This meeting has been a milestone. We started off with the title of "Standards" and, at the very first clinical session, demolished the concept of pass/fail criteria in favour of the need for greater emphasis upon individual assessment.

In the middle we acknowledged the need to match the assessment to the changes of ageing.

In conclusion we are thinking of continuity and Ian McCallum has just led us into that with the importance of setting up a new registry for the study of long-term effects.

At this meeting it has been a great joy to see so many doctors from so many different countries agreeing on the way ahead. Some 23 different nations and more than 200 participants, and all seem to be in reasonable agreement. I would like to thank not only the speakers from the podium and from the floor but also those who provided the special award at the Banquet to the doctor who had asked the most questions. I also thank my colleagues, Eric Botheroyd and Nick McIver on the Programme Committee; the HSE and Astra Pharmaceuticals who supported much of the expense; the various Chairmen and the consultants who came in to help us; the University who have provided us with these superb facilities and Karen Reeves who organised it all. I thank you all.

This meeting has worldwide implications and I look forward to reports of progress when we next meet.

COMMENTARY

Training

The Edinburgh and Luxembourg meetings have concluded that the training objectives, necessary experience and the need for periodic refresher training for the medical examiners of divers, are of vital importance and need to be adequately defined.

The new emphasis has been on the necessity for each medical examination for fitness to dive to be much more than just an application of pre-determined guidance. If each examination is to be a careful assessment of the individual diver in relation to the requirements and hazards of his particular working environment, it means that the doctor must have a good knowledge of the tasks and the risks of the job. The course content for examining doctors needs to include the physiological aspects of diving, work procedures, types of equipment, and emergency procedures. Periodical refresher training is required. Assessment of knowledge and audit of performance are essential.

Traditionally the diving medical specialist has been trained as a diver, often in a navy, and gained experience with an operational diving team, but this route is becoming rare. Another way must be found to provide adequate experience in air, mixed gas and deep diving procedures.

Specialist Centres

While there was agreement on the continuing role of an approved doctor or "medical examiner" in the annual assessment of diver fitness, there was also consensus that there are certain important aspects of the medical examination of divers which need more resources than are available to the majority of examining doctors. The concept of a "two tier" examination scheme for diver fitness achieved acceptance by consensus. Regular surveillance is to be conducted by a trained medical examiner. Before beginning training and at critical points in the diver's career, it is important that the diver is reviewed by a diving medical specialist.

It was agreed that the "Specialist Diving Medical Centre" would need to be defined by the training and experience of its diving doctors, and not by its location, buildings or medical gadgets. It was recognised that for special investigations it would need to have additional equipment not normally available to the diving medical examiners. The centres would also conduct some of the longitudinal health surveillance which also requires special equipment. The likelihood is that the Specialist Centre will be a medical centre which is also on call for the management of diving medical emergencies.

Review System : Appeals

Important precedents can be set by the cases that appeal for review. There was support for a Panel to review appeals and other difficult cases in order to function as a national professional memory bank and so enhance consistency. A number of divers each year fail to seek re-examination and the reasons for this, medical or otherwise, remain unknown. It is also probable that some divers are disqualified for reasons that, had they wished to appeal for review, would not have been upheld.

Recording Occupational Exposure

For the study of the occupational effects of diving, the history of each individual's exposure to diving hazards at work, in particular pressure, breathing gas and duration, needs to be available. The current introduction of on-line dive data display and recording for offshore air divers is primarily related to diver safety but could also fulfil this function. It could lead also to the retrospective analysis of actual decompressions and in time to the safe enhancement of air diving decompression tables.

Epidemiology of Long-Term Sequelae

The annual examination for safety is not a suitable opportunity for longitudinal surveillance, other than requesting bone x-rays when appropriate. Health surveillance requires a different set of investigations from those related to diving fitness, and they may be needed at a different periodicity.

Each procedure should be directed towards a specific occupational illness, the diagnosis of which would lead to effective preventative or therapeutic measures. Each investigation should use a standardised and validated technique, be relatively safe and inexpensive, have an internationally agreed diagnostic classification, provide reproducible results with good specificity and be associated with a statistically valid population of matched control subjects.

Radiology for bone necrosis is a good example of surveillance which meets these principles. Possible long term effects on pulmonary function are being assessed and future surveillance would need to be done at a specialist centre though not necessarily every year. Prevention of diving sequelae would be enhanced by the introduction of a central registry of divers' medical data linked to a record of their dive exposures and decompressions. Studies are needed also to review the health of divers beyond retirement into old age in order to assess the significance of alleged health effects.

CONCLUSIONS

David Elliott

The Edinburgh meeting and the medical section of the European Diving Technology Committee meeting in Luxembourg a few weeks later were together attended by more than 250 persons representing some 20 nations. Many participants in Edinburgh submitted, as requested, supplementary comments or questions in writing which means that one can be reasonably confident that all opinions have been considered. It would be presumptuous to suggest that conclusions can be drawn which represent the views of all but, from the lively discussions on the podium and from the floor, much experience was presented together with some innovative ideas that need to be more widely recognised.

The conclusions that follow are intended to be unbiased and to reflect those of the two meetings as a whole but the words are the responsibility of only the Editor. Any misinterpretations or omissions are entirely unintended. Some associated recommendations are offered and represent a more personal view, but each has a firm foundation and should be acceptable to those who participated in the discussions. Some of these need further debate and refinement. They are given here so that the contributions made by those who attended the meetings will not be lost but can be used as a foundation for the further enhancement of diver health and safety.

FITNESS ASSESSMENTS

It was concluded that medical fitness examinations are essential for diving safety. They can reveal medical conditions which are not only incompatible with the individual's safety in the water but which also could put the safety of companions at risk. This is true for both the recreational diver and the diver at work.

Though reviewed at the same time, those aspects of the medical examination which assess the effects of diving upon the health of the diver, but not upon in-water safety, should be considered as a distinct and optional activity.

Applicability of Fitness Assessments

Those aspects of the fitness assessment which relate to in-water safety should be the same for all categories of diver. Those aspects which relate to safety in other circumstances, e.g. night-time eyesight standards for handlers of diving boats, do not need to be applied universally.

Though consensus was not achieved, there was a widely held view that the professional instructor of amateur divers must have, for the safety of the novices, the same standard of fitness as any other working diver. For individual recreational divers, exceptions to otherwise essential aspects of mental, medical and physical safety can be made for diving in particular circumstances but only with the informed consent of all concerned. For the diver, such as a scientist who has suffered a traumatic paraplegia, there is the solution of a fitness certificate with specific safety conditions.

Initial Assessment on Entry to Training

There is a need for the medical history and examination of a candidate to take place <u>before</u> entry into training for a career as a working diver. This examination should be especially stringent because, at this stage, the consequences of rejection are relatively straightforward whereas medical disqualification during or after training implies avoidable financial penalties for the individual.

The guidance for this examination should reflect both diving safety and potential long term fitness for the job. This examination should be comprehensive and must be conducted by a doctor who is trained and experienced in diving medicine. The special investigations should include AP chest x-ray (inspiratory and expiratory), audiometry (preferably by an audiometrist) and rigorous pulmonary function testing including FV-loops.

Fitness for the particular vocational aspects of the diver's future employment (e.g. police, navy) may be performed at the same time but the need for these standards is related not to the diving *per se* but to the nature of their particular duties. These will vary within each category of diving and such standards should be determined by the employer.

Baseline Data

About the time that a professional diving certificate is awarded, a number of baseline investiations should be made for future clinical reference. These are not necessary for assessing in-water safety but are related to the future assessment of health particularly in relation to occupational illness. For instance, baseline bone radiology is considered essential for all divers who may be expected to be at risk by working for durations greater than 4 hours or at depths below 30 metres. These x-rays must not be discarded after a few years (in accordance with hospital practice) but retained, perhaps in a diving medical centre, for at least 3 years longer than the individual's diving career.

Subject to the validation of current research, the initial examination may in the future also include pulmonary diffusion capacity (TLCO) and somato-sensory evoked potentials (SSEP's). Another baseline which needs to be developed for all exposed to the risk of decompression illness is that of a test of neuropsychometric function to be used during treatment to assess recovery. At present several of these investigations would be for epidemiological purposes and, as such, should be funded as research projects.

Re-Assessments

The existing, almost universal, convention of a standardised examination repeated annually, could be improved. After a comprehensive initial examination and assessment, a young fit diver should have an annual fitness review but for some years this can be quite brief. As the diver becomes older, a selectively more detailed assessment will be needed of chosen aspects of fitness. Some additional investigations may be introduced in the ageing diver to ensure an appropriate assessment of continuing fitness.

Annual Fitness Review: In the interests of diving safety it is recommended that there contnues to be an annual review of fitness for each diver by any doctor who is trained as a diving medical examiner. This review can be relatively simple, particularly if done by the same medical examiner on each occasion. The routine examination should be capable of being conducted without the need for special investigations. It should include, as a minimum, a full medical and diving history of the past year, examination of the tympanic membranes, a cardio-pulmonary and neurological examination and a simple test of physical fitness. Such fitness tests are purely functional and the results should be considered qualitatively, without precise pass/fail criteria. Should there be any uncertainty concerning fitness, the diver should be referred to a diving medical specialist.

Periodical Detailed Assessment: At selected times in the diver's career, which should probably be defined by age, a more stringent examination than that of the annual review is recommended. This examination will require the use of special equipment which may be expensive and is not necessarily available to a family practitioner. This assessment must be conducted by a diving medical specialist (a consultant whose competencies are reviewed later). It should focus upon the possible effects of ageing upon continuing fitness, and health surveillance for the known occupational consequences of diving, such as bone necrosis. This detailed assessment should be repeated at pre-determined intervals during the diver's career, with the more simple annual fitness review by a diving medical examiner in the years between.

Physical Fitness: A general test of physical fitness is needed each year. A suitable annual test, such as the extended step test or the time taken to swim 1 kilometre, has yet to be agreed. It should be supplemented periodically by the direct measurement of maximum oxygen uptake.

Continuity of Assessment: It must be possible for the records of all the previous fitness examinations to be available to the examiner at each re-examination. This will enable the medical examiner to look for any trends in that individual at an early stage. A national repository of the medical records would facilitate the maintenance of comprehensive records spanning each diver's previous medical reviews.

MEDICAL FITNESS STANDARDS

For fitness assessments, the concept of a "pass/fail checklist" was rejected in principle. Certainly there are a few absolute medical contraindications to diving for which prescriptive rules can be made. However, there are very many more relative contraindications to diving where fitness can be decided only by individual assessment. Guidance is helpful but needs to be interpreted by a doctor who is fully aware of the hazards of the underwater environment, who understands the functional implications of the work and who appreciates the constant need of the diver to be able to respond to some unexpected emergency.

Current guidance for the medical fitness of divers is largely based upon years of cumulative experience and there is little scientific evidence available to confirm its validity. To acquire scientific backing for much of the opinion expressed would demand experimentation that is not likely to be approved by an ethical committee.

Advice is usually qualitative and can be subject to varied interpretations. Current guidance appears to be effective, but this may be because it is over cautious, eliminating not only those at risk but also, unnecessarily, many individuals who would have been fit. Some relaxation of existing guidance seems possible without compromising safety and the central collection of medical data could provide retrospective evidence in support of further such action.

The details of the recommended guidelines have been reviewed on a systematic basis and largely agreed. Some modifications have been proposed and some uncertainties remain. This guidance is a helpful basis for assessment but needs to be interpreted by a doctor who is aware of the hazards of the underwater environment and who understands the functional implications of the work. A few diving medical standards relate to bell and surface safety and not only to those in the water. A study is required of the functional requirements of each category of diving and these could be used to enhance the future medical assessments of the individual diver.

RESUMPTION OF DIVING

Following surgery, illness, injury or a diving incident there is a need for a thorough review of diving fitness before a return to work. Fitness to resume diving cannot easily be judged against pre-determined guidance but usually requires an individual assessment. A number of these reviews, such as after a hernia repair, will be simple and can be conducted by a medical examiner of divers. Others, such as after "undeserved"pulmonary barotrauma, could be complex and require opinions from clinical consultants who are knowledgeable about diving, and diving medical specialists.

EPIDEMIOLOGY

At the same time as the periodic detailed assessments, the possible presence of the long term effects of diving upon health should be investigated as an epidemiological research project. This could include pulmonary diffusion capacity, somato-sensory evoked potentials and neuropsychometrics. It is felt that this should be conducted as a longitudinal research programme until the clinical significance of any changes are known, after which such surveillance may become routine.

CENTRAL MEDICAL DATA BANK

An optimum solution would be national medical data banks from which conclusions could be made on the validity of current assumptions on fitness standards and on the criteria for medical disqualification. The medical registry should be linked to a dive data bank which stores dive exposure records. Causative factors associated with specific occupational health effects could then be examined epidemiologically and the results used to enhance the safety of decompression tables and minimise the possible long term medical consequences.

The same recommendations emerged 10 years previously at a similar but unpublished HSE-sponsored conference held in Aberdeen in March 1984. One of the areas of concern noted that we should reaffirm the long-term role of a Registry to answer the uncertainties about the consequences of decisions on fitness and to assess the impact of occupational disorders such as bone necrosis. It is a reflection upon governments and industry that this recommendation is still unfunded.

THE TRAINING OF DOCTORS

In order to ensure competency in the assessment of diver fitness, it is recommended that all doctors must have attended a suitable instructional course to meet specified training objectives. These competencies need to be defined.

It is recommended that detailed training objectives and accredited experience could be defined along the following lines:

> **Medical Examiner of Divers:** A minimum course of some 30 hours plus 8 hours revision training per year (averaged over a rolling 3-year period). It is an advantage if the doctor has some personal diving experience but this is not essential. There is no requirement for such a doctor to be fit to go under pressure in a compression chamber. Regular revision training needs to be specified.

> **Diving Medical Specialist:** There is a limited but essential need for diving doctors of

consultant status. Such doctors should have received some practical diving training in order to enable them to fully understand and appreciate the hazards and demands of the working environment. They should have some experience of working with each of the different categories of diving. Competencies need to include familiarity with the practical aspects of all types of diving, knowledge and experience of treating difficult diving incidents and the ability to use applied physiology in the assessment of the divers' working environment and the associated equipment. A postgraduate qualification in occupational medicine would be an appropriate foundation but, in practice, any clinical specialist training can provide a suitable basis. A two to four week course would be a minimum introduction to this subject and must be supplemented by appropriate experience. It follows that such doctors must initially be fit to dive in order to complete their training. They would need to maintain fitness for compression chamber work for as long as they have direct responsibilities for the treatment of diving casualties, but there is no requirement to maintain fitness in order to conduct fitness examinations or to provide advice in emergencies. Regular refresher training also needs to be defined.

Clinical Consultants: Hospital specialists who accept consultations on aspects of diver fitness should have had the same introductory course as the examining doctors. Clinical consultants in the vicinity of a busy specialist centre should be able to build up adequate knowledge. Past experience suggests that only a very few such consultants in each speciality are needed nationally.

The scope of the 4-day meeting "Medical Assessment of Fitness to Dive" was comprehensive and these proceedings offer a clearer understanding of the difficulties of making a wise decision upon fitness for recreational divers and for many of those who work in a particularly unforgiving environment.

****

LIST OF PARTICIPANTS

Dr. L. Aanderud, Norway
Dr. M.D. Ahern, U.K.
Dr. M. Anderson-Upcott, U.K.
Dr. J.F. Andressen, Norway
Dr. J.A. Ask, Norway
Dr. T.M. Aune, Norway
Mrs. R. Banner, U.K.
Dr. G.M. Barker, U.K.
Mr. A.C. Barnes, U.K.
Prof. P.B. Bennett, U.S.A.
Dr. J.R. Bergin, U.K.
Dr. W. Bergöö, Sweden
Dr. B. Bertelsen, Denmark
Mrs. V.K. Bertelsen, Denmark
Dr. D.J. Bickle, U.K.
Dr. M.J. Blyth, U.K.
Surg. Lt. O. Boonstra, The Netherlands
Dr. A. Boycott, U.K.
Dr. A.J. Bray, U.K.
Dr. D. Brekke, Norway
Dr. M.D. Brooke, U.K.
Mr. S. Brooke, U.K.
Surg. Cdr. J.R. Broome, U.K.
Dr. R.M. Brown, U.K.
Dr. R. Bunting, U.K.
Dr. D.C.L. Burges, U.K.
Dr. M.W. Calder, U.K.
Dr. D. Caughey, U.K.
Dr. J. Challenor, U.K.
Dr. D.H.K. Chalmers, U.K.
Dr. J.W. Charters, U.K.
Dr. G. Clark, U.K.
Dr. A.K. Coates, U.K.
Dr. D. Connan, U.K.
Dr. D. Courtney, U.K.
Dr. D.G. Craig, U.K.
Dr. A. Crookston, U.K.
Dr. R.A. Davenport, U.K.
Dr. A.J.G. Davis, U.K.
Surg. Cdr. M.R. Dean, U.K.
Dr. F. Dick, U.K.

Dr. S. Docherty, U.K.
Dr. M. Doig, U.K.
Dr. R. Vanden Eede, Belgium
Dr. P.J.S. Farrell, U.K.
Dr. P.J. Fell, U.K.
Dr. S.R. Foster, U.K.
Dr. W.A. Freeland, U.K.
Dr. John E. Galway, U.K.
Dr. A.P. Glanvill, U.K.
Ms. C. Grainger, U.K.
Lt. Cdr. A.P. Griffin, Canada
Mrs. C. Grönkvist, Sweden
Dr. H. Grönkvist, Sweden
Dr. C. Harris, U.K.
Dr. J.P. Hawson, U.K.
Mr. A.C. Head, U.K.
Dr. H. Hepburn, U.K.
Dr. A.E. Hickish, U.K.
Dr. G. Hickish, U.K.
Mr. Jeffrey D. Hodson, U.S.A.
Dr. A.P. Hothersall, U.K.
Dr. Ø. Irtun, Norway
Dr. R.G. Jackson, U.K.
Dr. E. Jones, U.K.
Dr. Reno M. Karlson, Norway
Dr. R.B. Keston, U.K.
Dr. P. Knessl, Switzerland
Dr. J. Kuokkanen, Finland
Dr. B. Lagercrantz, Sweden
Mr. M.A. Lang, U.S.A.
Dr. K. LeDez, Canada
Dr. R.M. Lees, Canada
Dr. M. Lepawsky, Canada
Dr. N. Lewkowicz, U.K.
Dr. V.R.F. de Lima, U.K.
Dr. L. Lindholm, Norway
Dr. W.J. Lockett, U.K.
Dr. P. Longobardi, Italy
Dr. D.G.R. Lowden, U.K.
Dr. J.C.S. Lowsley-Williams, Gibraltar
Mr. P. Lowsley-Williams, Gibraltar

Dr. N. Macleod, U.K.
Dr. C.A. MacDonald, U.K.
Dr. N. MacKay, U.K.
Dr. J. Madsen, Denmark
Dr. T.W. Manson, U.K.
Dr. I. Masarik, Dubai
Dr. A. Maw, U.K.
Dr. J. Mawdsley, U.K.
Dr. C.J. May, U.K.
Dr. W.D.S. McLay, U.K.
Dr. G.J. McCleane, U.K.
Dr. G. Yancey Mebane, U.S.A.
Dr. F. Micalella, Italy
Dr. A.H. Milne, U.K.
Dr. S.I. Modahl, Norway
Dr. S.D. Mohideen, Malaysia
Dr. T. Moore, U.K.
Dr. A.G.L. Morgan, U.K.
Dr. J. Morrison, U.K.
Dr. M.S. Musgrave, U.K.
Dr. J.C. Nainby-Luxmoore,
Dr. J. Netland, Norway
Dr. M.J. O'Kane, U.K.
Dr. A. O'Malley
Dr. D. Orr, U.K.
Dr. J.J. O'Sullivan, U.K.
Dr. D.P. O'Toole, Eire
Prof. G. Page, U.K.
Dr. A. Holmes Pickering, U.K.
Dr. B. Pingree, U.K.
Dr. A. Prentiss, U.K.
Dr. N. Puttick, U.K.
Dr. C. Rae, U.K.
Dr. N. Ramanathan, U.K.
Mr. D. Rankin, U.K.
Mr. D.H. Robertson, U.K.
Dr. C. Robinson, U.K.
Dr. I. Robinson, U.K.
Dr. R. Rogerson, U.K.
Dr. L. Rudy, Switzerland
Dr. H.D. Rycroft, U.K.
Dr. G.T. Russell, U.K.
Dr. M. Saliba, Malta
Dr. I. Sibley-Calder, U.K.
Dr. R.S. Sidra, U.K.
Mrs. M. Simpson, U.K.
Dr. D. Skan, U.K.
Dr. R.A. Skeide, Norway
Dr. P.D. Slater, U.K.
Lt. Cdr. J. Sommerfelt-Pettersen, Norway
Mrs. C. Spence, U.K.

Dr. P. Staples, U.K.
Dr. R.N. Stephenson, U.K.
Dr. M.W. Stubley, U.K.
Dr. P. Suprani, Italy
Mr. Woody C. Sutherland, U.S.A.
Dr. T. Ternent, U.K.
Dr. B. Thio, Singapore
Dr. I. Thomas, U.K.
Dr. J.C.D. Turner, U.K.
Mr. M. Welham, U.K.
Dr. W. Wellens, Belgium
Cdr. W. Welslau, Germany
Dr. J. Wendling, Switzerland
Dr. J.R.E. Whitehead, U.K.
Mr. L. Willen, Norway
Dr. D.I. Wintour, U.K.
Miss R. Withnall, U.K.
Dr. J.F. Wollaston, U.K.
Dr. R. Wood, U.K.
Dr. P. Wysocki, Norway
Dr. P.L. Zacharias, U.K.

See also: List of Contributors